SUPERVISORY MANAGEMENT
For Health Care Organizations

Third Edition, Revised and Expanded

Theo Haimann, PhD
**The Mary Louise Murray Professor
of Management Sciences
St. Louis University**

**The Catholic Health Association of the United States
St. Louis, MO 63134**

First Edition published in 1965.
Second Edition published in 1973.

Library of Congress Cataloging in Publication Data

Haimann, Theo.
Supervisory management for health care organizations.

Includes index.
1. Health facilities—Administration. I. Catholic Health Association of the United States. II. Title. [DNLM: 1. Health facilities—Organization and administration. WX 150 H151s]

RA971.H22 1983	362.1'1'068	82-23570
ISBN 0-87125-081-0		

SUPERVISORY MANAGEMENT
For Health Care Organizations

To
Ruthe

CONTENTS

PREFACE

The health care field is confronted with a steady influx of more sophisticated and exotic practices and equipment as medical knowledge and technology advance. Medical doctors are able and expected to provide their patients with the most advanced tests and treatment programs. And this is happening against the background of already high costs of medical care. Nearly 10 percent of the U.S. gross national product is now spent on medical care; 20 years ago the percentage was only half that. Continuously rising medical bills is a major pressing concern to government, American industry, the health care system, and the consumer.

One of the concurrent changes of concern to us is the fact that most health care now takes place in an organizational setting. Business and industrial activities have long been the exponents of the corporate world. But now much of the delivery of health care takes place within the context of an organization, not-for-profit health care centers, health maintenance organizations, proprietary hospitals, incorporated group practices of physicians or surgeons, and many others. Without going into the multitude of reasons for this development we must recognize the fact that today's health care professionals work within an organizational setting. Therefore, it is necessary that they understand the nature and complexity of organized activity and their place within it.

In order to contribute to organizational effectiveness, administrators and managers must understand and know the practice of management. Most executive level positions are filled by individuals who have been exposed to formal health administration education. But thousands of middle and lower level administrative positions, such as department heads and supervisors, are filled by health professionals and others who have not had any formal education or training in administration, management, and supervision per se.

This book is intended for these department heads and supervisors in all types of health care facilities, hospitals, health maintenance organizations, physician's group practices, extended care facilities, nursing homes, homes for the aged, rehabilitation centers, long term care facilities, or other institutions of this type. They were placed into their supervisory positions primarily because they did an outstanding job in their chosen health care fields. Their previous experience and education, however, rarely included the area of supervision. Thus, these supervisors who rise from the ranks often find themselves in increasingly demanding positions yet have little or no familiarity with the administrative and managerial aspects of their newly attained rank. Suddenly they are confronted with the need to be an effective manager, to stay on top of a more sophisticated job, to gain new perspectives and insights into human relationships. Their position may have changed from being a good nurse, for example, to becoming an efficient head nurse, supervisor of nursing, or whatever the title may be. The primary function changes from doing things oneself to getting things done through and with employees by motivating them so that they enthusiastically go about achieving departmental and institutional objectives.

This book is written for an introductory course in management principles to acquaint students with their future roles in an organized activity. It is intended to be used as a textbook in the education of nurses, medical technologists, dietitians, therapists, medical records administrators, and all the many other health care professonals. It can be used in any of the courses where managerial, supervisory, and leadership concepts are studied.

In addition to this, this text is intended to aid people in the health care field who are already faced with such a supervisory task. Its purpose is to demonstrate to the supervisors that proficiency in supervision will better equip them to cope with the ever-increasing demands of getting the job done, will contribute more effectively to the over-all goals of the institution, and at the same time will make them more valuable to the facility's chief executive.

This book is introductory in the sense that it assumes no previous knowledge of the concepts of supervision. Although the book does include material of a sophisticated nature, this material is explained in terms that can easily be understood by the inexperienced supervisor. The book will also help newly appointed supervisors become acquainted with the many problems which they will confront and offers practical advice for their solution. For experienced supervisors, this book is intended to refresh thinking and widen horizons by taking a different and challenging look at both their own position and that of their employees.

Even though the text is written for supervisors, not for administrators, most of its content would be of great interest to the latter also. The common denominator of all levels of supervisors is the part they play as managers within the administrative hierarchy of the institution. Without going into the technical details of specific supervisory positions, the book discusses the managerial aspects common to every supervisory job whether it is in nursing, medical records, medical social work, housekeeping, dietary, pharmacy, laboratory, x-rays, respiratory therapy, security, laundry, maintenance, engineering, or any of the numerous other specialties found within the health care field.

It is important to realize that the supervisory position in any field is the most critical point in the entire organizational structure. It involves the management of people in the day-to-day running of a department within an organization. In hospitals and other health care facilities, the supervisor's position is exceptionally strategic since in most cases the recipient does not elect to receive the services provided, nor does this person understand them. The supervisor in a hospital or related health facility must contend with emotional factors involved in the care of the patients and their loved ones under conditions which make effective supervision unusually difficult. In addition to this, the supervisor is often torn between considerations of a professional nature and those of an administrative nature. But above everything else, the supervisor's activities must ultimately reflect the welfare of the patient. All of these internal factors make it more imperative for the supervisor to be a capable manager of the department.

Moreover, external factors also affect the supervisor's role. It is an established fact that hospitals and related enterprises comprise one of the largest activities in the United States today. Provisions for health care services will become more complex due to rapidly expanding areas of concern, growing government support, increasing population, and advances of medical science and technology. In addition, it is essential for all health care facilities to keep pace with the social and environmental progress of civilization. This means an ever increasing challenge for efficient management capable of coping with more sophisticated problems, whether they are of an economic, professional, scientific, or educational nature.

Thus, the focus of this book is on the managerial process, more specifically on the managerial functions of planning, organizing, staffing, influencing, and controlling and their relation to the daily job of the supervisor. Connecting these functions together are the decision-making process and communication. In reality, all of the managerial functions are closely related and such a distinct classification is not always discernible in practice. But this type of academic separation does make possible a methodological, clear, and complete analysis of the managerial functions of a supervisor.

The supervisor's job of getting things done with and through people has its foundation in the relationship between the supervisors and the people with whom they work. For this reason the supervisor must have considerable knowledge of the human aspects of supervision, of the behavioral factors that motivate the employees. This book attempts to integrate such behavioral factors into the conceptual framework of managing. Although it is obviously not an all-comprising text on management, the book does try to present a balanced picture. Thus, human relations and behavioral aspects are kept in proper perspective in relation to the other aspects of the supervisory job.

In writing this third edition, I have retained the basic concepts and the emphasis on the five basic managerial functions. All of the chapters of the previous editions have been revised and updated and some of the subject matter has been re-arranged in order to facilitate the reader's understanding of the concepts and their application. These concepts, however, are expanded and integrated with current practices, new knowledge, and recent developments to show the contemporary emphasis of this edition. Completely new materials have been added in many areas in order to make this book more usable for today's department heads and supervisors. More attention is given to the behavioral sciences, psychology, and sociology as they impact on managing human resources. New material has been added on organization design, performance appraisal, quality circles, MBO, individual and small group behavior, motivation, equal and fair employment practices, and many other aspects of managing.

A new chapter has been added, focusing on some of the legal aspects of the supervisory job. Everyone working in the health care field is aware of the importance of legal problems and their implications. Therefore, this chapter, written in layman's language, will familiarize supervisors with some of the legal aspects of health care activities. It is not intended to advise supervisors what to do or not to do and is certainly not a substitute for consultation with and legal advice by lawyers. Special thanks go to Carolyn Haimann, JD, in-house legal counsel for the Jewish Hospital of St. Louis, who has written this chapter.

Material for this text has come from the writings and research of scholars in the areas of management, behavioral and social sciences, as well as from the practical experience of many supervisors, managers, and administrators in the field. In addition, this text also reflects my own experiences in teaching management, in consulting, in conducting many supervisory development programs, and in giving lectures to administrators and supervisors at different levels in the managerial hierarchy of hospitals and related health care facilities.

In writing the book, I fully realize that most people working in health care facilities are women, and was seriously tempted to refer to supervisors as "she" and to use the female gender throughout the book. Since there are a number of men also actively engaged in the delivery of health care, however, I thought it best to give men and women "equal time" by referring to them as supervisors, department heads, or similar terms. This was accomplished by using nouns or plural pronouns or by using the expression he or she. On rare occasions when it was necessary to refer to an individual, I used the old fashioned common gender he, meaning a person of either sex. I hope that those readers who are sensitive to such terminology will forgive me and not interpret this stylist device as prejudicial to the vital managerial role of women in the health care field. Another language problem faced in this as well as in previous editions is the use of the term subordinate; it is meant to describe a person who is below a supervisor or manager in the organization's hierarchy. The term denotes position only and is not intended disparagingly.

Finally, in writing a book such as this an author is indebted to so many persons that it is impossible to give them all due credit. I owe a great obligation to so many members of Barnes Hospital, St. Louis, that it would be impossible to mention all of them by name. Invariably this health care center was a source of much information and insight. Among the many who were so helpful, special thanks to Rose Dunn, vice president of Barnes Hospital, for her helpful review of the last edition and many suggestions for this edition.

I also wish to acknowledge with thanks the help and encouragement given by The Catholic Health Association. Thanks also goes to Lynda Palazzolo who skillfully transcribed many challenging notes into readable manuscript. Last, but by no means least, special thanks go to my wife Ruthe for her patience and general assistance throughout the years. To all these I extend my grateful appreciation while bearing full responsibility for any sins of omission or commission.

Theo Haimann

Part One

Stepping Into Management

1

The Supervisor's Job

A Health Care Perspective

Today's health services are increasingly being delivered in an organizational setting, such as a hospital, nursing home, clinic, surgical center, health maintenance organization, physicians' offices, home care programs, or any other kind of health care institution. Only an organizational setting can bring together the physical facilities, professional expertise, skills, technology, and the myriad of other supports that today's health services delivery requires, whether these services are curative, rehabilitative, or preventative. Therefore, it is absolutely necessary that those who deliver or help deliver health care services understand the complexities of organizational life and administration, in addition to their professional areas of expertise.

Traditionally, health care professionals were primarily concerned with the technical and clinical aspects of their work; being a good nurse meant mastering the field of nursing. This was true even of the director of nursing who was a nurse first and a manager second. Now because of the increased pressures for better health care delivery, the health professional must be equally concerned with both aspects of the job, the administration, and the profession.

External forces are likely to continue to impose constraints on health care services and set higher expectations. This will require even increasingly better management and control over internal affairs.

Delivery of health care is a term that is becoming increasingly common in the daily press, magazine articles, and conversations in the United States. What is generally meant by this term is the problem of providing adequate health care services of all types, intended to maintain and improve the health of all people regardless of age, color, locale, or ability to pay. The reason health care delivery systems are receiving such attention in the United States is that the cost of health care has risen more steeply than any other item in our national economy. Not only have the total expenditures in the field of health services risen by leaps and bounds, but these expenditures have also become an ever-increasing percentage of the overall economy, as expressed in our gross national product. It is understandable that the delivery of health care has become a major national issue and that the institutions engaged in this service, such as hospitals and related health care facilities, are receiving continuous and increasing scrutinization.

Moreover, since the delivery of health care largely means providing a service, it is understandable that from 60 percent to 70 percent of the total expenditures within the field are for wages and salaries. Therefore, many criticisms have naturally centered around employee productivity to justify such large wage and salary expenditures. What is needed is better and more effective administration of health care centers, that is, better supervision throughout. In the final analysis it is the supervisor of the department, regardless of the title, who is responsible for the department functioning smoothly and efficiently. It is essential, therefore, that due emphasis be paid to the need for the managerial development of effective supervisors within all phases of the health care field.

The Demands of a Supervisory Position

The supervisory position within the administrative structure of a health care institution, such as a hospital, surgical center, health maintenance organization, clinic, or any other medical facility, has long been acknowledged as a difficult and demanding one. You have probably learned this from your own experience or by observing supervisors in hospitals and related institutions as they go about their daily tasks. The supervisor, whether a head nurse or a chief technologist in the clinical laboratory, can be depicted as "the person in the middle," since he or she serves as the principal link between higher administration and the hospital employees. (See Figure 1-1.)

If we look carefully at the job of almost any supervisor, regardless of who or what he or she supervises, we can see that it involves four major dimensions. First, the supervisor must be a good boss, a good manager, and a leader of the employees who work in this unit. The supervisor must have the technical, professional, and clinical competence to run the department smoothly and to see that the employees carry out their assignments success-

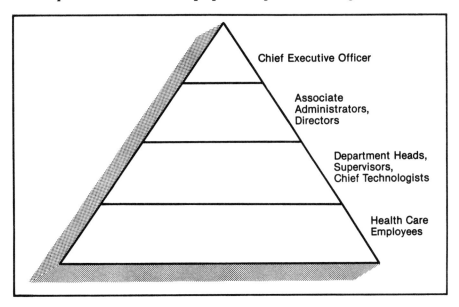

Figure 1-1. The administrative pyramid.

fully. Second, the supervisor must also be a competent subordinate to the manager above. In most instances, this person would be an administrator, associate administrator, or director of a service.

Between these two dimensions of the supervisor's role is a third area in which he or she acts as a connecting link between the employee and the administration. To the employees, such as RNs, LPNs, aides, or unit secretaries, the head nurse can be viewed as being *the* administration of the hospital, since in this example the head nurse is the primary contact that employees have with the administration. The supervisor is that member of the administration who must make certain that the work gets done.

The fourth and final part of the supervisor's role is to maintain satisfactory working relationships with the heads of all other departments and services in the medical center. The relationship to these other department heads must be that of a good colleague who is willing and eager to coordinate the department's efforts with those of the other departments in order to reach the overall objectives and goals of the institution, namely, the best possible patient care.

The four dimensions of the supervisor's job are shown more clearly in Figure 1-2. He or she must be successful in vertical relationships downward with subordinates and upward with his or her superior. In addition, he or she must be skillful in handling horizontal relationships with other supervisors, since this will facilitate getting the job done for the benefit of the client.

Partly because of the complexity of these relationships, it is commonly acknowledged that the role of the first-line supervisor in any industrial or commercial undertaking is a most difficult one. It is even more difficult for supervisors within a health care facility because their activities directly or in-

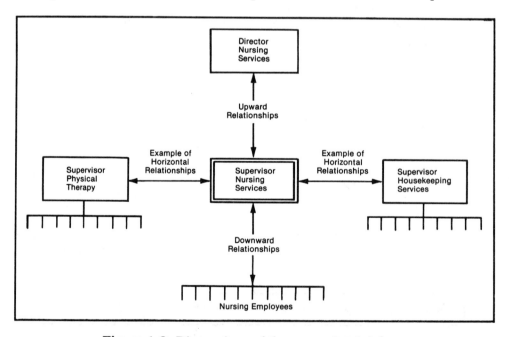

Figure 1-2. Dimensions of the supervisor's job.

directly affect the quality of patient care and the smooth overall functioning of the institution. In addition to their many professional obligations, hospital supervisors must always bear in mind the needs and desires of patients and their relatives who, at the time, are physically and emotionally upset. Thus, the supervisor should be continuously aware of the problems of human relations among medical staff members, other hospital personnel, and patients. All of these considerations make the job of the hospital supervisor a particularly demanding and challenging one.

Let us be more specific and look at the demands made on a head nurse in charge of a nursing unit. Whether the hospital practices case nursing, functional nursing, team nursing, or primary care, it still is the head nurse's duty to provide for and supervise the nursing care rendered to the patients in the unit. She does this partly by delegating a certain amount of her authority for the care of patients and the supervision of personnel to an assistant head nurse or team leaders within her area. But the head nurse must still plan, direct, and control all activities within the nursing unit. She must make the rounds of her unit with medical and nursing staff. She also is expected to make rounds for personal observation of the condition and behavior of patients and to assess the need for and quality of continued nursing care. She may even have to assume general nursing functions in the care of those patients who have complex problems.

Furthermore, the head nurse must interpret and apply the policies, procedures, rules, and regulations of the hospital in general and of the nursing services in particular. She must provide coverage of the unit for 24 hours by scheduling to have the unit properly staffed at all times. She is to communicate and report to her nursing supervisor (assuming that the nursing supervisor is the immediate superior of a number of head nurses) all pertinent information regarding patients in her unit. She must orient new personnel to the unit and acquaint them with the general philosophies of the hospital. She is also concerned with continued inservice education in her unit, in other words, with teaching personnel. Likewise, she participates in the evaluation of her subordinates. In addition, it is part of the head nurse's job to coordinate the activities of her unit with unit managers if these are available. She also must coordinate her patient care with the care and therapeutic procedures of the various departments throughout the hospital. Moreover, she is involved in the design and regular reevaluation of the budget. She serves on a number of committees, in addition to attending all head nurses' meetings. She might also be expected to help in the supervision and instruction of student nurses when necessary. Many other duties are often assigned to a head nurse, depending on what the particular health care facility specifies in its description of this very demanding position.

We might also look at the work that is required of another supervisory position in a hospital, that of the supervisor of the housekeeping department, often called the executive housekeeper or director of environmental affairs. Generally, a job description will tell you that it is this supervisor's job to maintain the hospital in a clean, sanitary, and orderly condition. She must continuously study new cleaning methods and new cleaning equipment and recommend changes of layout and location of equipment, if necessary, to facilitate the cleaning of various areas of the hospital. She also plans and directs the work schedule for the housekeeping staff, taking into consideration visiting hours, traffic, and the amount of work to be done. She is expected to write instruction sheets and training manuals for housekeeping procedures and must be able to teach staff members both prevailing and new methods and demonstrate these with equipment. Furthermore, she must periodically inspect their completed work for quality of service. In addition to this, she will plan and select furnishings for the various rooms, considering serviceability, decorative appeal, and other factors.

Moreover, the housekeeping supervisor must develop and maintain effective working relationships with the professional, administrative, and maintenance personnel of the institution. She is expected to interview and make the final selection of applicants who have been referred to her by the personnel department. It is also her job to dismiss unsatisfactory employees and to take disciplinary action whenever necessary. There may be many other duties connected with the job of executive housekeeper, making this another demanding supervisory position in a medical facility.

With our growing, complex society and the increasing demands for more sophisticated and better health care, the job of any hospital supervisor is likely to become even more challenging. This is true whether the title is head nurse, medical record administrator, operating room supervisor, director of maintenance, chief respiratory therapist, laboratory supervisor, chief technologist of radiology, food service supervisor, or supervisor of any one of the many other activities necessary for the smooth functioning of a health care center.

This supervisory position is usually the first step in a long career of administrative positions that will make increasingly more demands for competent management as the individual moves up the administrative ladder. For instance, the staff nurse is made an assistant head nurse; after having served in this capacity for some time, she is promoted to head nurse, then to supervisor of nurses, then possibly to associate director of nursing, and even eventually to director of the nursing service. Most of the tens of thousands of managerial positions in health care organizations are filled by health professionals who have not had any formal administrative training or study in management or administration *per se*. It is therefore essential that the supervisor, department head, chief technologist, or whatever the title may be, learn as much as possible of the meaning of being a competent first-line manager because this is his or her first entry into the managerial and administrative ranks.

The Managerial Aspects of a Supervisory Position

The job of a supervisor can be somewhat simplified, however, if we think of it in terms of two main requirements. First the supervisor is required to have a thorough knowledge of the job to be performed and must be clinically and technically competent to do the job in question. The second aspect of the supervisor's job is that he or she must also be a manager of the department. It is this managerial aspect and managerial competence that will significantly determine the effectiveness of a supervisor's performance.

You may have observed various supervisors on different occasions and noticed that some of them are usually harassed, disorganized, and overly involved in doing the job at hand. They are muddling through and are knee-deep in work. Such supervisors put in long hours and are never afraid of doing anything themselves. They are working exceedingly hard, but never seem to have enough time left to actually supervise. On the other hand, you may have observed supervisors who seem to be on top of the job and whose departments function smoothly and orderly. They have found time to sit at their desks at least part of the day and keep their desk work up to date. Why is there such a difference?

Of course, some supervisors are basically more capable than others, just as there are poor and good medical technologists. But if you compare two chief technologists in two hospitals to discover why one is on top of the job and the other is continuously fixing things herself, you will probably find that one understands her job better than the other. Let us assume that both are equally good professionals, both work in the same subspecialty and have similar equipment, and the conditions under which they perform are similar. Still, the results of one chief technologist are significantly better than those of the other. Why is this? The answer is that the one is simply a better manager. She is able to supervise the functions of her department in a manner that allows her to get the job done with and through the people of her department. The difference between a good supervisor and a poor supervisor, assuming that their professional skills are alike, is the difference in their managerial abilities.

Surprisingly enough, however, the managerial aspect of the supervisor's position has long been neglected. Rather, the emphasis has always been put on the clinical and technical competence for doing a particular job. Consider your own job, for example. It is very likely that you were appointed to this job from the ranks of one of the various professional services or crafts. As a result of your ingenuity, effort, and willingness to work hard, you were promoted to the supervisory level and were expected to assume the responsibilities of managing your unit. But precious little was done to acquaint you with these responsibilities or to help you cope with the managerial aspects of your new job. More or less overnight you were made a part of administration without having been prepared to be a manager. Ever since, you have done the best you could by imitating and learning from your predecessors, and your department is probably functioning reasonably well. But there are likely to be some problems, and these may be eased by a better understanding of the supervisory aspects of your job, so that you will be the manager running the department instead of the department running you.

It is the aim of this text to show the supervisor how to become a better manager. Of course, this does not mean that one can neglect or underestimate the actual work involved in getting the job done. As you know, one of the requirements of a good supervisor is a thorough understanding of the clinical, professional, and technical operations. Often the supervisor is actually the most skilled individual of the department and can do a more efficient and quicker job. But he or she must not be tempted to step in and take over the job, except for purposes of instruction or in case of an emergency. Rather, the supervisor's responsibility is to see to it that the employees can do the job and do it properly. As a manager, the supervisor must plan, guide, and manage. Let us concentrate further on these managerial requirements of the supervisory position.

The Meaning of Management

First, let us consider what is meant by management. The term management has been defined in many ways, generally as a process of coordinating and integrating human, technical, and other resources to accomplish specific results. The following is a more meaningful definition for our purposes: *management is the process of getting things done through and with people, by directing and motivating the efforts of individuals toward common objectives.* You have undoubtedly learned from your own experience that in most endeavors one person can accomplish relatively little alone. For this reason, people have found it expedient and even necessary to join with others to attain the goals of an enterprise. In every organized activity, it is the manager's function to achieve the goals of the enterprise with the help of subordinates and fellow employees.

But achieving goals through and with people is only one aspect of the manager's job. He or she must also create a working atmosphere within which subordinates can find as much satisfaction of their needs as possible. In other words, a supervisor must provide a climate conducive for the employees to fulfill such needs as recognition, achievement, and companionship. If these needs can be met right on the job, employees are more likely to strive willingly and enthusiastically toward the achievement of departmental objectives, as well as the overall objectives of the institution. Thus, we must add to our earlier definition of management by saying that the manager's job is *getting things done through and with people by enabling them to find as much satisfaction of their needs as possible, while at the same time motivating them to achieve both their own objectives and the objectives of the institution.* The better the supervisor performs these duties, the better the departmental results will be.

You may have noticed by this time that we have been using the terms supervisor, manager, and administrator interchangeably. Although the exact meaning of these titles varies with different institutions, the term *administrator,* or *executive,* is generally used for top-level management positions, whereas *manager* and *supervisor* usually connote positions within the middle or lower levels of the institutional hierarchy. There are some theoretical differences to consider, but for our purposes these terms will be used interchangeably.

Our reason for doing this will become clearer when you understand the somewhat surprising fact that the managerial aspects of all supervisory jobs are the same. This is true regardless of the supervisor's department or section or level within the administrative hierarchy. Thus, the managerial content of a supervisory position is the same whether the position is director of nursing services, head of the housekeeping division, chief engineer in the maintenance department, or chief therapeutic dietitian. By the same token, the managerial functions are the same for the supervisor on the firing line (lowest level or first-line supervisor), middle level of management, or top administrative group. In addition, it does not matter in which kind of organization you are working. Managerial functions are the same for an industrial enterprise, commercial enterprise, not-for-profit organization, fraternal organization, government, or hospital or other health care facility. Regardless of the organization, department, or level, the managerial aspects and skills are the same.

Managerial Skills and Technical Skills

Managerial skills must be distinguished from the professional, clinical, and technical skills required of a supervisor. As stated above, all supervisors must also possess special technical skills and professional know-how in their field. Naturally, technical skills vary between departments, but any supervisory position requires both professional technical skills and standard managerial skills. Mere technical and professional knowledge would not be sufficient.

It is important to note that as a supervisor advances up the administrative ladder, he or she will rely less on professional and technical skills and more on managerial skills. If you will observe your own institution, you will find that the higher you go within the administrative hierarchy, the more administrative skills are required and the less technical know-how. Therefore, the top administrator generally uses far fewer technical skills than those who are employed under him or her. But in the rise to the top, the administrator has had to acquire all the administrative skills necessary for the management of the entire enterprise. For example, the chief executive officer of a hospital is concerned primarily with the overall management of hospital activities; his or her functions are almost purely administrative. In this endeavor, of course, the chief executive depends on the technical skills of the various subordinate administrators and managers, including all the first-line supervisors, to get the job done. The chief administrator, in turn, uses managerial skills in directing the efforts of all these subordinate managers toward the common objectives of the hospital. Therefore, throughout the organization the purpose of the managerial skills is the same.

Managerial Skills Can Be Learned

At this point, you may be wondering how a supervisor acquires these very important managerial skills. First of all, let us emphatically state that the standard managerial skills can be *learned*. They are not something with which you are necessarily born. Although it is often suggested that good managers, like good athletes, are born, not made, this belief is patently false. It cannot be denied that people are born with different physiological and biological potentials and that they are endowed with an unequal amount of intelligence and many other characteristics. It is also true that a person who is not a natural athlete is not likely to run 100 yards in record time. But many individuals who are natural athletes have not come close to that goal either.

A good athlete is made when a person with some natural endowment, by practice, learning, effort, sacrifice, and experience develops this natural endowment into a mature skill. The same holds true for a good manager; by practice, learning, and experience he or she develops this natural endowment of intelligence and leadership into mature management skills. The skills involved in managing are as learnable and trainable as the skills involved in playing tennis. If you currently hold a supervisory position, it is likely that you have the necessary prerequisites of intelligence and leadership and that you are now ready to acquire the skills of a manager. Of course, it takes time and effort to develop these skills; they are not acquired overnight. The supervisor has ample opportunity to apply the principles and guidelines discussed in this text to the daily work. By applying the content of this text, the supervisor will certainly prevent many difficulties from occurring, and before too long the supervisor will reap the many benefits from practicing good supervision.

Benefits From Better Management

The benefits that you as a supervisor will derive from learning to be a better manager are obvious. First, you will have lots of opportunity to apply managerial principles and knowledge to your present job. Good management as a supervisor will make a great deal of difference in the performance of your department. It will function more smoothly, work will get done on time, you will probably find it easier to stay within your budget, and your workers will more willingly and enthusiastically contribute toward the ultimate objectives. The application of management principles will put you as a supervisor on top of your job, instead of being completely "swallowed up" by it. You will also have more time to be concerned with the overall aspects of your department, and, in so doing, you will become more valuable to those to whom you are responsible. For example, you will be more likely to contribute significant suggestions and advice to your superiors, perhaps in areas about which you have never before been consulted but that ultimately affect your department. You will also find it easier to see the complex interrelationships of the various departments throughout the health care center, and this in turn will help you to work in closer harmony with your colleagues who are supervising other departments. Briefly, you will be able to do a more effective supervisory job with much less effort.

In addition to the direct benefits of doing a better supervisory job for the hospital, there are other benefits for you personally. As a supervisor applying sound management principles, you will grow in stature. As time goes on you will be capable of handling more important and more complicated assignments. You will be able to fill better and higher paying jobs. You will move up within the managerial hierarchy and will naturally want to improve your managerial skills as you advance.

As noted above, an additional satisfying thought is that the functions of management are equally applicable in any organization and in any managerial or supervisory position. That is, the principles of management required to produce microwave ovens, manage a retail department, supervise office work, or run a garage are all the same. Moreover, these principles are applicable not only in the United States, but in other parts of the world. Aside from local peculiarities and questions of personality, it would not matter whether you are a supervisor in a textile mill in India, a supervisor in a chemical plant in Italy, the foreman of a department in a steel mill in Gary, Indiana, or the supervisor of the medical records section in a hospital in St. Louis. By becoming a manager, you will become more mobile in every direction and in every respect.

Obviously, then, there are great inducements for you to learn the principles of good management. However, you cannot expect to learn them overnight. You can only become a good manager by actually managing, that is, by applying the principles of management to your own work situation. You will undoubtedly make mistakes here and there but will, in turn, learn from those mistakes. The principles and guidelines of management discussed in this book can be applied to most situations. They will help you avoid errors that often take a long time to correct. Your efforts to become an outstanding manager will pay handsome dividends. As your managerial competence increases, you will be able to prevent many of the difficulties that make a supervisory job a burden instead of a challenging and satisfying task.

Summary

The role of the supervisor is a most demanding one. To the employees in the department, the supervisor represents management. To a superior, he or she is a subordinate. To the supervisors in other departments, he or she must be a good colleague, coordinating efforts with theirs to achieve the institution's objectives. The supervisor must possess clinical and technical competence for the functions to be performed in the department and at the same time be the manager of that department. Management is the function of getting things done through and with people. The way a supervisor handles the managerial aspects of the job will make the difference between running the department and being run by the department. The managerial aspects of any supervisory job are the same, regardless of the particular kind of work involved or the position on the administrative ladder. As a supervisor climbs up this ladder, the managerial skills will increase in importance, and the technical and professional skills will gradually become less important. These managerial skills can be learned; a manager is not "born," he or she is made. A supervisor will benefit greatly both in a professional sense and in a personal sense if he or she takes the time to acquire the managerial skills.

2

Managerial Functions and Authority

Chapter 1 discussed the importance of managerial skills to a supervisor, the fact that they can be learned, and the benefits of acquiring them. But we have not yet stated exactly what these all-important managerial skills are. Managerial skills are the functions a manager *must* perform to be considered a true manager. They are the functions necessary to carry out the managerial job.

The Managerial Functions

In this text, the five managerial functions are classified in the major categories of *planning, organizing, staffing, influencing,* and *controlling*. The labels used to describe these functions vary to some minor degree in management literature; some textbooks list one more or one less managerial function. Regardless of the terms or number used, the managerial functions collectively constitute one of the two major responsibilities of a manager. The other major characteristic of the managerial position is the concept of authority, which will be discussed later in this chapter.

A person who does not perform all of these functions is not a manager in the true sense of the word, regardless of title. Of course, we must specify more precisely the managerial functions of planning, organizing, staffing, influencing, and controlling. The following explanation is general and brief, since most of the book is devoted to the discussion and ramifications of each of these functions.

Planning

Planning is the function that determines in advance what should be done in the future. It consists of determining the goals, objectives, policies, procedures, methods, and other plans needed to achieve the purpose of the organization. In planning, the manager must think of, contemplate, and decide among various available alternatives. Thus, planning is mental work. It involves thinking before acting, looking ahead, and preparing for the future. It is laying out in advance the road to be followed and the way the job should be done.

You may have observed supervisors who are constantly fighting one crisis after another. The probable reason is that they did not plan. They did not look ahead. It is every manager's duty to plan; this function cannot be delegated to someone else. Certain specialists may be called on to give some assistance in laying out various plans, but it is up to the supervisor as the manager of the department to make departmental plans. Of course, these plans must coincide with the general overall objectives of the hospital as laid down by the chief administrator. But within the overall directives and general boundaries, the manager has considerable leeway in mapping the departmental course.

Planning must come before any of the other managerial functions. Even after the initial plans are laid out and the manager proceeds with the other managerial functions, the function of planning continues in revising the course of action and choosing different alternatives as the need arises. Therefore, although planning is the first function a manager must tackle, it does not end at the initiation of other functions. The manager continues to plan while performing the organizing, staffing, influencing, and controlling functions.

Organizing

The organizing process determines how the work in a particular department will be divided and accomplished. It requires the manager to define, group, and assign job duties. More specifically, with organizing the manager determines and enumerates the various activities to be accomplished, combines these activities into distinct groups (departments, divisions, sections, teams, or any other unit), and then further divides the group work into individual jobs, assigns these activities, and, at the same time, provides subordinates with the authority needed to carry out these activities.

In other words, to organize means to design a structural framework that sets up all the positions needed to perform the work of the department and to assign particular duties to these positions. Of course, the structural framework of any department must fit into the overall structure of the institution. When the manager organizes the structural framework, it is also imperative that the authority relationships between the various subordinates are appropriately aligned. While organizing, the manager will of necessity delegate a certain amount of authority to the subordinate managers, so that they can carry out the duties for which they are responsible. It is through this organizing function that the manager clarifies problems of authority and responsibility within the department. The result of the organizing function is the creation of an activity-authority network for the department, which is a subsystem of the total hospital network.

Staffing

Staffing is the manager's responsibility to recruit new employees to ensure that there are enough qualified employees to fill the various positions needed and budgeted for in the department. Staffing involves not only the selection but also the training of these employees. It involves the problem of promoting them, appraising their performance, and giving them opportunities for further development. In addition, staffing includes a wise and appropriate system of compensation. In most health care institutions the personnel department helps with and facilitates the technical aspects of staffing. But the authority and responsibility for staffing remain with the supervisor.

Influencing

Influencing is the managerial function of issuing directives and orders to get the job done. This function is also known as directing, leading, or motivating. The influencing function of a manager includes directing, guiding, teaching, coaching, and supervising subordinates. It is not sufficient for a manager to plan, organize, and staff. The supervisor must also stimulate action by giving directives and orders to the subordinates and by supervising and guiding them as they go about their work. Moreover, it is the manager's job to develop the abilities of the subordinates by leading, teaching, and coaching them effectively. Influencing is concerned with motivating people at work to achieve their maximum potential and to stimulate them to act in ways they may not on their own.

Thus, influencing is the process around which all performance revolves; it is the essence of all operations. This process has many dimensions, such as employee morale, job satisfaction, productivity, leadership, and communication. It is through the influencing function that the supervisor seeks to create a climate conducive to employee satisfaction and, at the same time, achieves the objectives of the institution. As you know from personal experience, much time is spent in influencing subordinates. In fact, most of your time is probably spent this way.

Controlling

The managerial function of controlling involves those activities which are necessary for events to proceed and objectives to be achieved as planned. In other words, to control means to determine whether or not the plans are being carried out, whether or not progress is being made toward objectives, and what actions to take to correct any deviations and shortcomings. Again this brings up the importance of planning as the primary function of the manager. It would not be possible for a supervisor to check on whether work was proceeding properly if there were no plans against which to check. Controlling therefore includes taking corrective action if objectives are not being met and revising the plans and objectives if circumstances require it.

The Interrelationships of Managerial Functions

It is helpful to think of the five managerial functions as a continuous circular movement, a management cycle. A cycle is a system of interdependent processes and activities. Each activity blends into another and each affects the performance of the others. In daily supervisory activities you may have often felt that your job is a vicious cycle, without a beginning or an end. However, if you think of the managerial process as a cycle consisting of the five different functions, it will greatly simplify your job of supervising. As shown in Figure 2-1, the five functions flow into each other, and at times there is no clear line indicating where one function ends and the other begins. Because of this interrelationship, it is not possible for any manager to set aside a specific amount of time each day for one or another function. The effort spent on each function will vary as conditions and circumstances change. But there is little doubt that the planning function must come first. Without plans the manager cannot organize, staff, influence, or control. Therefore, throughout this text, we shall follow this sequence of planning first, then organizing, staffing, influencing, and controlling.

It should be emphasized that although the five managerial functions can be separated theoretically, in the daily job of the manager these activities are inseparable. Each function blends into the other, and each affects the performance of the others. The output of one provides the input for another. That is why these functions are viewed as elements of a system. (See Figure 2-2.)

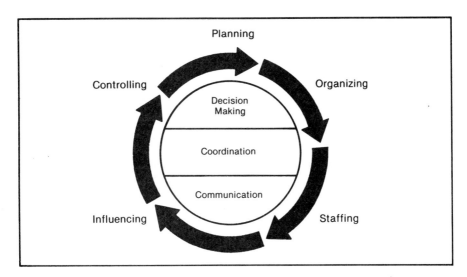

Figure 2-1

The Universality of the Managerial Functions and their Relation to Position and Time

As stated earlier, the managerial functions are universal. They are the responsibility of all managers, regardless of whether they are the chairman of the board, the president of the health care center, the vice president for patient care, or the supervisor on the firing line. All of them perform all five functions. The time and effort that each manager devotes to a particular function will vary, however, depending on the individual's level within the administrative hierarchy. For example, a chief administrator will spend more time in the planning, organizing, and controlling functions and less time staff-

Figure 2-2

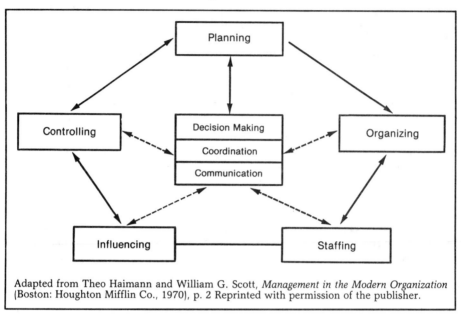

Adapted from Theo Haimann and William G. Scott, *Management in the Modern Organization* (Boston: Houghton Mifflin Co., 1970), p. 2 Reprinted with permission of the publisher.

ing and influencing. A supervisor of a department, on the other hand, will probably spend less time in planning and organizing and more time in staffing and, particularly, influencing and controlling. But the supervisor must still do some planning. The chief executive officer is bound to plan, let us say, for 1 year ahead, 5 years ahead, or even 10 or 20 years ahead. A supervisor will make plans of much shorter duration. There are times when a supervisor will have to make plans for 6 or 12 months, but more frequently will just make plans for the next month, week, or even for the same day or shift. In other words, the span and magnitude of plans will be smaller. Nevertheless, a supervisor plans, just as the administrator plans.

The same is true of the influencing function. The chief executive officer, if he or she is a capable administrator, will assign tasks to subordinate managers, delegate authority, depend on their getting the job done, and spend a minimum of time in direct supervision. As a supervisor, however, you are concerned with getting the job done each and every day and all day long, and you will have to spend a large part of your time in this influencing or directing function. Therefore, all managers perform the same managerial functions, regardless of their level in the hierarchy, but the time and effort involved in each function will depend on your rung on the administrative ladder and managerial skills. (See Figure 2-3.) Unless a manager performs all five functions, however, the managerial duties are not being fulfilled.

Authority

The second factor that characterizes a manager is authority. As with managerial functions, a person without authority is not a true manager. What

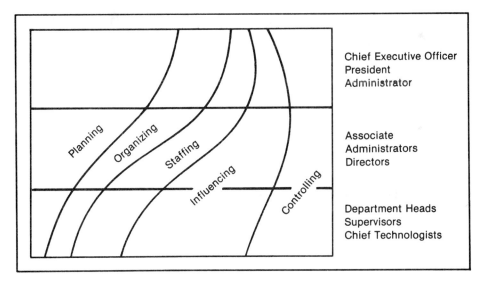

Figure 2-3. Amount of time spent on each function.

is this authority that makes a supervisor a manager? Why is authority a characteristic which makes the managerial position? Briefly, authority can be defined as legal or rightful power, the right to act. It is the power by which a manager can ask subordinates to do or not do a certain thing that the manager, as the possessor of authority, deems appropriate and necessary to realize the objectives of the department. Authority is not actually delegated to people but to positions within the enterprise. It belongs to the formal position the supervisor holds and not to the supervisor as an individual. Unless these positions are held by people, however, the delegation of authority would be meaningless. That is why one commonly speaks of the manager's authority, rather than the authority of the managerial position. This kind of managerial authority ceases when the supervisor resigns from the job or is discharged. Whoever succeeds will then have this authority.

This formal, organizational authority gives the supervisor the power and right to give directives to the members of the department to achieve the objectives and tasks assigned to it. Our concept of authority must also include the possession of power to impose sanctions and coerce. Without such power to enforce an order, the enterprise could become disorganized, and chaos could result. If a subordinate refuses to carry out the manager's directive, this authority must include the right to take disciplinary action and, in the last instance, to discharge the employee.

Of course, this aspect of authority has many restrictions. These may be in the form of legal restrictions, union contracts, or considerations of morals, ethics, and human behavior. Every successful manager knows that to influence subordinates to perform required duties it is best not to depend on this formal managerial authority, but to utilize other ways and means to get the job done. In other words, it is far better not to depend on the negative aspects of power and authority. In fact, most managers do not speak of authority at all. They prefer to speak of the "responsibility" or "tasks" or "duties" they have. Such managers rightfully consider it better human relations to say that they have the responsibility for certain activities instead of saying that they possess the authority within that area. Using the words responsibility, tasks, and duties in a loose sense allows the manager to avoid the big stick.

But as a supervisor you should not be misled by the loose use of these terms. Having authority means having the power and right to issue directives. You should know that tasks and duties have been asssigned to you and that you have accepted the responsibility for getting them done. This responsibility has been exacted from you by your superior. It is important to understand that the concept of responsibility is always connected with authority. They go hand in hand, and one cannot exist without the other. Regardless of how the supervisor applies authority, it must be stated again that the supervisory position must have it. Otherwise chaos would follow.

In Chapter 11 the concepts of authority and responsibility will be discussed in greater detail. At that time, how subordinates and workers react to authority and how authority is delegated will be examined. This latter means the process by which a supervisor receives authority from the superior manager, as well as the process by which some of the authority delegated to this position is delegated to subordinates. Just as authority is the lifeblood of any managerial position, delegating authority to the lower ranks within the managerial hierarchy makes it possible to build an organizational structure with effective managers on every level. These points will become clearer in our later discussions. Throughout this text the concept of authority will be discussed frequently and play an important role in supervisory management. This concept of formal positional authority will merge into an entire spectrum of influence, power, and authority.

At this time, it will suffice to remember that authority is one of the basic characteristics of the managerial job. Without authority, managerial functions would be meaningless, and management itself would cease to exist.

Summary

The five managerial functions of planning, organizing, staffing, influencing, and controlling are one of the two earmarks of the manager's job. Each blends into another, and each affects the performance of the others. The output of one provides the input for another. These five functions are universal for all managers, regardless of position in the managerial hierarchy. The time and effort involved in each function will vary depending on the rung of the administrative ladder the manager occupies.

The second benchmark of the managerial job is authority; it makes the managerial position real. This organizational authority is delegated to positions within the organization. Since these positions are staffed by people, one commonly speaks of the manager's authority, rather than of the authority of the managerial position.

Part Two

Connective Processes

3

Deciding

The responsibilities of a manager are the possession of authority and the performance of the five managerial functions. These five functions are interrelated and interconnected. Binding the five managerial functions together are three connecting processes, decision making, coordination, and communication. These connecting processes are not functions in and of themselves; rather, they link the five functions together into a continuous management system and make it possible for the manager to run the department as a smoothly working unit that is a subsystem within the larger system of the health care institution.

Decision making, coordination, and communication are essential to the performance of each of the managerial functions. For example, when the manager plans, decisions most certainly must be made. These decisions must also be coordinated to not contradict one another or result in duplication of effort. Finally, these decisions must be communicated to those who are to carry them out. Similarly, when the manager performs the organizing function, decisions as to the kind of organizational structure to be set up are needed, this structure must be coordinated with that of the rest of the institution, and communications and explanations to the subordinates are essential, so that they will understand their place and their duties in relation to each other and to the whole. The same pattern of deciding, coordinating, and communicating holds true for the other functions of staffing, influencing, and controlling.

Thus, the three connecting processes are a vital force for all the managerial functions and must be developed to hold the managerial system together. Since they overlay the functions, these three processes will be discussed in separate chapters before analyzing each of the managerial functions.

Decision Making

If practicing managers were asked to define in one or two words the essence of their jobs, they would very likely reply that what permeates their jobs more than anything else is "making decisions." This process of decision making is the heart of all five managerial functions. To make decisions is a substantial part of everybody's activities. All of us have to solve problems in many areas of endeavor. Therefore, decision making or problem solving should not be foreign to us. Decision making is a basic human activity that begins in early childhood and continues throughout a person's life.

Programmed and Nonprogrammed Decisions

For many of the problems with which we are confronted in our daily lives we have a pat answer. Solving these problems does not usually cause us much difficulty because we are quite familiar with them. These decisions are commonly called *programmed decisions*, because they refer to repetitive routine problems for which there are fixed answers, methods, rules, and standardized operating procedures. For instance, the staff nurse finds that a patient has an elevation of temperature. To verify the finding she measures it again with a different thermometer and finds out whether the patient just had a cup of hot coffee or a cigarette. The elevation registers the same degree. Reinforced with these facts, the nurse has a solution for the problem, namely, to check again after an hour or so. Again the results are the same. Her next decision is to see whether the attending physician left orders to cover this problem, and, if not, the nurse automatically decides to consult the physician for further action. The staff nurse had to make a number of decisions up to this point. All of them were programmed; a standard procedure had anticipated these kinds of problems. For other departments the use of computers and operations research are a great aid in making programmed decisions, e.g., the reorder point and the quantity to be ordered by the purchasing agent. A program has been designed for this particular problem, and it is being called on to come up with the answer.

For new problems, problems that are of considerable significance, and those which cover unfamiliar situations, it is increasingly difficult to make decisions. These are the *nonprogrammed decisions.* In this situation the manager should utilize a logical decision-making process; and all of the following is directed to these kinds of nonprogrammed situations.

The Importance of Decision-Making Skills

As a supervisor you are constantly called on to find practical solutions to problems that are caused by changing situations or unusual circumstances. Normally, you are able to arrive at a satisfactory decision. As a matter of fact, one reason why you are in a supervisory position is that you have made many more correct decisions than wrong decisions as problems presented themselves. Many of the decisions you have made cover problems that arise out of the daily working situation; nevertheless, they are real problems that required a solution.

All managers, at all levels of the organization in all functions, make decisions. Decisions are not made in a vacuum, since each has some effect on the entire system. All managers go through, or should go through, the same process of problem solving or decision making that you go through as a supervisor. The only difference is that the decisions made at the top of the administrative hierarchy are usually more far reaching and affect more people and areas than those which are made by a supervisor. Thus, decision making, like the five managerial functions, is an essential process that permeates the entire administrative hierarchy.

Of course, once a decision has been made, effective action is necessary. Every decision made should be put into practice and carried out. Obviously, a good decision is useless if nobody does anything about it. But getting effective action is not the problem with which we are concerned in this chapter. Other chapters will deal mainly with ways in which the manager can achieve effective action. This discussion will explain the process that should come *before* the action, the process that you as a manager should go through to decide what action to take.

Let us be more specific about the timing of this decision-making process. When viewing a person as a decision maker, a picture often comes to mind of an executive with horn-rimmed glasses bent over some papers, pen in hand, ready to sign on the dotted line. Or we picture a person in a board of directors meeting, raising an arm to vote a certain way. Such images have one point in common; they portray the decision makers at the very moment of choice, ready to select one alternative that leads from the crossroads down a particular path of action. This moment of decision making should not be emphasized here, because it does not describe the long difficult process that must come before the final moment of selecting one alternative over the others.

Although it is long and difficult, the decision-making process is worthwhile knowing. Like the managerial skills, the skills involved in decision making can be learned, and once learned they provide great benefits for the manager. These benefits will, of course, accrue to the manager, no matter what position he or she holds, because the decision-making process is used throughout the entire administrative organization.

Moreover, it is important to note that your managerial job involves not only making decisions yourself, but also seeing that those who work under you make decisions effectively. Obviously, a supervisor cannot make all the decisions necessary for running the department. Many of the daily decision-making activities for which you as a supervisor are responsible will be delegated to your subordinates. It is therefore necessary that you develop better decision-making skills, as well as train your subordinates in this process of making decisions.

The Decision-Making Process

A decision is something that takes place prior to the actual performance of the action that has been decided on. It is a conclusion that the manager has reached as to what should be done at some later time. Thus, to make a decision means to cut off deliberation and come to a conclusion. It is this deliberation, however, that is the essence of the decision-making *process*. That process requires the manager to proceed with certain steps, arranged in the following sequence:
  (1) Define the problem.
  (2) Analyze the problem.
  (3) Develop alternative solutions.
  (4) Decide on the best solution.
  (5) Action and follow-up.

Definition of the Problem

Supervisors have often been heard to say, "I wish I had the answer," or "I wish I had the solution to this," or "I wish I knew what to do about this." All of these "wishes" indicate that the supervisor is overly concerned with having an *answer*. Instead of seeking an answer, however, the supervisor should be looking for the real problem. The first task is always to find out what the problem is in the particular situation; only then can one work toward the solution, the answer. As someone has put it, "There really is nothing as useless as having the right answer to the wrong question."

To define the problem, in most cases, is not an easy task. What often appears to be the problem might be merely a symptom of it that shows up on the surface. It is necessary to dig deeper to locate the real problem and define it. For example, it might appear that a supervisor is confronted with a problem of conflicting personalities within the department. Two of the employees are continually quarreling and cannot get along together. On checking into this situation, however, the supervisor may find that the problem is not one of personalities, but that the functions and duties of each employee have never really been defined.

Thus, what appeared on the surface to be a problem of personal conflict was actually a problem of organization and structure. Only after the true nature of the problem has been realized can the supervisor do something about it, and the chances are good that once the activities and duties of the two employees are delineated, the friction will stop. There is little doubt that defining a problem like this may be a time-consuming chore, but it is time well spent. The process of decision making cannot proceed until the problem is clearly defined.

Analysis of the Problem

After the problem, and not just the symptoms, has been defined, the manager can set out to analyze it. The first step in the analysis is to assemble the facts, to gather all pertinent information. Only after a clear definition of the problem can the supervisor decide how important certain data are and what additional information may be needed. The supervisor will then gather as many facts as possible.

Many supervisors complain, however, that they never have enough facts. Although it is normal for a supervisor to feel that he or she does not have all the facts, this complaint is often just an excuse to delay a decision. A manager will never have *all* the facts available. Therefore, it is necessary to make decisions on those facts which are available and also on those additional facts which can be gathered without undue delay in time or undue cost.

At the same time, it is wise to remember that what is considered a fact is to a certain extent colored by subjectivity. One cannot be completely freed of the subjective elements involved. As much as we may want to exclude prejudice and bias, we are only human, and subjectivity will creep in somehow. Of course, we should make an effort to be as objective and impersonal as possible in gathering and examining the facts. This process of analysis, however, requires the supervisor to think not only of objective considerations but also of intangible factors that may be involved. These are difficult to assess and analyze, but they do play a significant role, especially in health care institutions. These intangibles may be factors of reputation, quality of patient care, morale, discipline, etc. It is hard to be specific about such factors, but they should nevertheless be considered in analyzing the problem.

Development of Alternative Courses of Action

After having defined and analyzed the problem, the manager's next step is to search for and develop various alternative solutions. An absolute rule is that all possible alternatives will be taken into consideration. Always bear in mind that the final decision can only be as good as the best of the alternatives considered. It can never be better than the best alternative you thought of. Each reasonable alternative should be considered as a possible way for reaching the objective. Therefore, the more alternatives you have, the greater the likelihood that the best is among them.

It is almost unthinkable that a situation should not offer at least several alternatives. These choices, however, might not always be obvious, yet it is the duty of the manager to search for them. Also, some of the alternatives may not be desirable, but the manager should not decide this until all of them have been carefully considered. If this is not done, one is likely to fall into the "either-or" kind of thinking. You have often heard it said after one minute's deliberation: "There is only one of two things that we can do, ... or ... ." The type of manager who says this is too easily inclined to see only one of these two alternatives as the right one to follow.

Nor is it enough for you as a supervisor to decide between the various alternatives that have been presented by subordinates. The routine alternatives normally suggested by them may not include all the possible choices. It is your job as a manager to conceive of more, and possibly better, alternatives. Even in the most discouraging situations there are several choices, and, although none of them may be desirable, the manager still has a choice to make.

Consider the following situation. Hospital regulations state that patients leaving their rooms after 10 AM will be charged a late-stay charge. This time limit is necessary to have the room vacated and cleaned in time for the new admission influx at 1 to 2 PM. The patient was admitted on July 1 at 2 PM to the room and leaves at 11 AM on July 2. The bill arrives with an additional day's charge as the late-stay charge, but the patient stayed less than 24 hours and refuses to pay for 48 hours. Even in this unpleasant dilemma, there are several alternatives, although none of them is completely desirable. The hospital could insist on having the patient pay the bill, although this would cause ill will. Or one could ask the attending physician to justify why the patient could not be discharged earlier if medically related. This may be sufficient to get insurance to pay the charge if an insurer is involved. Or the hospital could write off the charge.

Evaluation and Selection From Among Alternatives

As stated above, the purpose of decision making is to select or choose from among the various alternatives that course of action which will provide the greatest number of wanted consequences and the smallest number of unwanted consequences. After developing the alternatives, the manager should test each of them by imagining that each has already been put into effect. The supervisor should try to foresee the probable desirable and undesirable consequences of each. Once they have been thought through and their consequences appraised, the decision maker will be in a position to compare the desirability of the various alternatives.

In making this comparison, the supervisor should bear in mind the degree of *risk* that is involved in each course of action. One must remain aware that there is no such thing as a riskless decision; one alternative will simply have more or less risk than another. It is also possible that the question of *time* will make one alternative preferable to another. There is usually a difference in the amount of time required to carry out each alternative, and this should be considered by the supervisor. Moreover, in this process of evaluating the different alternatives, the supervisor should also bear in mind the resources, facilities, know how, equipment, and records that are available. Finally, the manager should not forget to judge the different alternatives along the lines of *economy of effort;* in other words, which action will give the greatest result for the least amount of effort and expenditure.

It is important that the decision be of high quality, but it must also be *acceptable* to the group affected by it. If the highest quality decision is not acceptable to the group, it is likely that its effectiveness is diminished, since it will be carried out at best grudgingly, or it might even be quietly sabotaged. In such a situation, it might be advisable for the supervisor to choose a more acceptable decision that is not of the highest quality. Acceptability is one more consideration in this process of choice.

Using the above criteria of risk, timing, acceptability, resources, and economy, it is often possible for the manager to see that one alternative clearly provides a greater number of desirable consequences and fewer unwanted consequences than any other alternative. In such cases, the decision is a relatively easy one. The best alternative, however, is not always so obvious. It is conceivable that at certain times two or more alternatives may seem equally desirable. In such a case, the choice is simply a matter of the manager's personal preference. On the other hand, it is also possible for the manager to feel that no single alternative far outweighs any of the others or is sufficiently stronger. In this case, it might be advisable to combine two of the better alternatives and come up with a compromise solution.

But what about a situation where the manager finds that none of the alternatives is satisfactory and that all of them have too many undesirable effects? As a supervisor, you might have been in a situation where the undesirable consequences of all the alternatives were so overwhelmingly bad that they paralyzed any action. You might have thought that there was only one available solution to the problem, namely, to take no action at all. Such a solution, however, is deceptive. A supervisor is wrong to believe that taking no action will get him or her "off the hook." In practice, taking no action is as much a decision as deciding to take a specific action, although few people are aware of this. Most people feel that taking no action relieves them of making an unpleasant decision. The only way for the manager to avoid this pitfall is to try to visualize the consequences of inaction. The manager need only think through what would happen if no action were taken and will probably see that, in so doing, an undesirable alternative is chosen.

Having ruled out inaction in most cases, you may still be in a position where all alternatives seem undesirable. In such a case, you would do well to search for new and different alternatives. Be a bit creative and try to develop at least a couple of new solutions. Also check to see that all the steps of the decision-making process have been followed. Has the problem been clearly defined? Have all the pertinent facts been gathered and analyzed? Have all possible alternatives been considered? Chances are that some new solutions will be thought of, and a good decision can then be made. In making this decision, however, you might have to employ some additional factors, such as experience, intuition, actual testing, and scientific decision making.

Experience

The manager's final selection from among the various alternatives is frequently influenced and guided by past experience. History often repeats itself, and the old saying that "experience is the best teacher" still holds true. There is no denying that managers can often decide wisely on the basis of their own experience or that of other managers. Knowledge gained by past experience can frequently be applied to new situations, and no manager should ever underestimate the importance of such knowledge. On the other hand, it is dangerous to follow past experience blindly.

Therefore, whenever the manager calls on experience as a basis for choice among alternatives, the supervisor should examine the situation and conditions that prevailed at the time of the past decision. It may be that current conditions are still very much the same, and thus the present decision should be the same as the one made on that previous occasion. More often than not, however, conditions have changed considerably, and the underlying circumstances and assumptions are no longer valid. In these cases, of course, the decision should not be the same.

Previous experience can also be helpful if the manager is called on to substantiate the reasons for making a particular decision. Experience is a good defense tactic, and many superiors use it as valid evidence. But there is still no excuse for following experience blindly. Past experience must always be viewed with the future in mind. The underlying circumstances of the past, present, and future must be considered. Only within this framework is experience a helpful approach to the selection from alternatives.

Hunch and Intuition

Managers will at times admit that they have based their decisions on hunch and intuition. At first glance, it might seem that certain managers have an unusual ability for solving problems satisfactorily by intuitive means. A deeper search, however, will disclose that the "intuition" on which the manager thought a decision was based was actually past experience or knowledge. In reality, the manager is recalling similar situations from the past that are now stored in the memory; this type of recall is labeled "having a hunch." No superior would look favorably on a subordinate who continually justifies decisions on the basis of intuition or hunch alone. These factors might come into play once in a while, but they must always be supplemented by more concrete considerations.

Experimentation

The avenue of experimentation, or testing, is a valid approach to decision making in the scientific world; conclusions reached through laboratory tests and experimentation are essential. But in management, to experiment and see what happens is inappropriate and often too costly and time consuming. Moreover, it is difficult to maintain controlled conditions and test various alternatives fairly in a normal workday environment. There may be certain instances, however, when a limited amount of testing and experimenting is admissible, as long as the consequences are not too disruptive. For example, a supervisor might decide to test out different work schedules or different assignments of duties. In this small restricted sense, experimentation may at times be valid. But, normally, in a supervisory situation experimentation is at best a most expensive way of reaching a decision.

Scientific Decision Making

During the last 25 to 40 years a new group of highly sophisticated tools has become available to aid the manager in decision making. These tools are quantitative, involving linear programming, operations research, probability, and simulation; they are sophisticated mathematical techniques applied by mathematicians, statisticians, programmers, systems analysts, or other types of scientists working with computers. The overall process is known as scientific decision making, or operations research.

Of course, only certain kinds of management problems lend themselves to this type of quantitative analysis and solution. In a hospital situation, for example, it could be applicable to problems involving scheduling, inventory, arranging for the best possible use of facilities and employees during various shifts, planning for the most effective utilization of existing facilities, etc. Such scientific problem solving is a complicated and costly way of reaching decisions, however, and it should be used only with the permission and knowledge of top administration when the magnitude of a problem warrants considerable effort and expenditure. Normally, the problems with which a single supervisor is confronted are not of this magnitude. But if there is a major problem affecting the entire hospital, or if similar problems are found in several departments, it may be advisable for top management to employ the quantitative approach. Since many health care centers today have easy access to a computer, it should not be difficult to contact someone within the computer center to see if they could lend some quantitative assistance in solving the problem. The programmers and systems analysts may produce not only an optimum solution, but their research may also lead to other findings that are welcome by-products. Management, however, should not forget that it could be a long and tedious, as well as an expensive, process. If the problem is of sufficient magnitude, such effort and expense are certainly worthwhile.

Action and Follow-Up

No matter what method has been used to arrive at the solution, effective action is necessary once the decision has been made. There is no use going through the lengthy and tedious decision-making process, unless the manager goes all the way and sees the decision carried out effectively. As stated before, there is nothing so useless as a good decision that is not carried out. In other words, decision making is only one aspect of the manager's job; achieving effective execution of the decision is at least as important. Even after action has been taken, decision making is not complete without follow-up and appraisal of the outcome. If all is well and the results are as expected and satisfactory, we can stop here. But if the results are not as expected, or if something did not work out as decided, then the supervisor should look at the situation as a new problem and go through all the steps of the decision-making process again from a new point of view.

Action and follow-up are impossible without two other essential processes, communication and coordination. Unless a decision is clearly communicated to the people who must carry it out and unless it is coordinated with other decisions and other departments, it will be quite meaningless. Thus, the two additional connecting processes that are vital to management's overall task of "getting things done through and with people" must be examined.

Summary

To select the best alternative by facts, study, and analysis of various proposals is still the most generally approved avenue of making a managerial decision. If an objective, rational, systematic method is used in the selection, the manager is likely to make better decisions. The first step in such a method is to define the problem. After a problem is defined, you must analyze it. Then you must develop all the alternatives you possibly can, think them through as if you had already put them into action, and consider the consequences of each and every one of them. Each alternative must be evaluated on the basis of past experience. By following this method, you will most likely be able to select the best alternative, the one with the greatest number of wanted and the least number of unwanted consequences.

Not only can you learn this sound method of decision making, but as a supervisor you can teach the same systematic step approach to your subordinates. In so doing, you have the assurance that whenever they are confronted with a situation where they have to make a decision, they will do it in a systematic manner also. Although this is not always a guarantee for arriving at the best decisions, it is likely to produce more good decisions than would otherwise be the case.

Scientific decision making, or operations research, is an approach to problem solving that involves quantitative analysis, models, and computers. If the problem is of sufficient magnitude to warrant such an effort, sophisticated scientific decision-making techniques involving mathematicians, statisticians, systems analysts, and other specialists are available.

4

Coordinating

The Meaning of Coordination

Supervisory management was defined as the process of getting things done through and with people by directing their efforts toward common objectives. This means that management involves the coordination of the efforts of all members of an organization. As a matter of fact, some writers have even defined management as the task of achieving coordination, or more specifically, of achieving the orderly synchronization of the efforts of employees to provide the proper amount, timing, and quality of execution so that their unified efforts lead to the stated objectives of the enterprise. Other writers have preferred to look at coordination as a separate managerial function.

We prefer to view coordination, however, not as a separate activity of the manager and not as *the* defining characteristic of management, but as a *process* by which the manager achieves orderly group effort and unity of action in pursuit of the common purpose. The manager engages in this process *while* performing the five basic managerial functions of planning, organizing, staffing, influencing, and controlling. The resulting coordination, the resulting synchronization of efforts, should be one of the goals that the manager keeps in mind when each of the five managerial functions is being performed. Coordination, therefore, is a byproduct the manager brings about while performing the five managerial functions appropriately.

It is evident that the task of achieving coordination is a much more difficult one on the top administrative level than on your supervisory level. The administrator has to achieve the synchronization of efforts throughout the entire organization. As a supervisor of only one department, you have to carry out this task primarily within your own division. Nevertheless, the achievement of coordination is necessary, regardless of the scope of your division. We have suggested that you look at coordination as something which comes about as you perform your five managerial functions appropriately. Coordination should result as a byproduct and should not be looked upon as a separate managerial function. As a supervisor, you should bear coordination in mind in everything you do. Thus, synchronizing the efforts of subordinates should be a prominent consideration whenever you plan, organize, staff, influence, and control.

Coordination and Cooperation

The term *coordination*, however, must not be confused with *coopera-tion*, since there is a considerable difference between them. Cooperation merely indicates the willingness of individuals to help each other. It is the result of a voluntary attitude of a group of people. Coordination is much more inclusive, requiring more than the mere desire and willingness of the par-ticipants. For example, consider a group of people attempting to move a heavy object. They are sufficient in number, willing and eager to cooperate with each other, and trying to do their best to move the object. They are also fully aware of their common purpose. In all likelihood, however, their efforts will be of little avail until one of them, the manager, gives the proper orders to app-ly the right amount of force at the right place and time. Only then will their ef-forts be sufficiently coordinated to actually move the object. It is possible that by coincidence mere cooperation could have brought about the desired result. But no manager can afford to rely upon such coincidental occurrence. Although cooperation is always helpful and its absence could prevent all possibility of coordination, its mere presence will not necessarily assure that process. Coordination is therefore superior to cooperation in order of impor-tance.

Attaining Coordination

Coordination is not easily attained, and the task of coordination is becoming increasingly complex the more difficult the various duties become. With the growth of an organization, the task of synchronizing the daily ac-tivities becomes more and more complicated. As the number of positions in your department increases, the need for coordination and synchronization to secure the unified result increases. Specialization is another source from which problems of coordination stem. And human nature in itself presents problems of coordination, since each of your employees is preoccupied with his or her own work and hesitates to become involved in other areas.

Coordination and the Five Managerial Functions

We have already stated that as a manager performs the managerial functions, one must remember that coordination is one of the desired by-products. Let us look more carefully at how this important byproduct is related to each of the five functions, as well as to the other connecting processes.

When the manager plans, efforts of striving for coordination must be made immediately. As a matter of fact, the planning stage is the ideal time to bring about coordination. As a supervisor, you must see to it that the various plans within your department are properly interrelated. You should discuss these plans and alternatives with the employees who are to carry them out, so that they have an opportunity to express any doubts or objections about synchronization. If employees are involved in departmental planning at the initial stages, then the supervisor's chances for coordination are much improved. The employees will get a clear picture of the purpose and direction of their department and will be better able to help achieve departmental and institutional goals.

The same concern for coordination should exist when the manager organizes. Indeed, the prime purpose for setting up a structural framework outlining who is to do what, when, where, and how is to assure coordination. This is the only way to obtain stated objectives in a synchronized fashion. Thus, whenever a manager groups activities and assigns them to various subordinates, the task of coordination should be in the supervisor's mind. By placing related activities that need to be closely synchronized within the same administrative area, coordination will, of course, be facilitated.

Moreover, in the process of organizing, management defines authority relationships among departments and employees. It should define them in such a way that coordination will result. Often poor coordination is caused by a lack of understanding of who is to perform what or by the failure of a manager to delegate authority and exact responsibility clearly. Such fuzziness can easily lead to duplication of efforts instead of synchronization. This is most likely to happen when two subordinates or two departments both feel they are responsible for the same activity.

Coordination should also be of great concern when the supervisor performs the staffing function. It is important that the right number of employees are in the various positions to assure the proper performance of their functions. The manager should see to it that they have the proper qualifications and training to coordinate their efforts willingly.

When a manager influences and directs, he or she is also involved in coordination. The very essence of giving instructions, coaching, teaching, and generally supervising subordinates is to coordinate their activities so that the overall objectives of the institution will be reached in the most efficient way. Or, as some writers have stated, coordination is that phase of supervision which is devoted to obtaining the harmonious and reciprocal performance of responsibilities of two or more subordinates. As a supervisor, you must continuously watch the performance of the different jobs under your direction to be sure that they are proceeding harmoniously.

Last, but not least, when the manager performs the controlling function the concern for coordination is present. By checking to see whether or not the activities of the department conform with the preestablished goals and standards, any discrepancy will be discovered and immediate remedial action should follow, so that the goals will be achieved and coordination will be assured at least from then on. Frequent evaluation and correction of departmental operations help to synchronize not only the efforts of employees, but also the activities of the entire organization. Thus, by its very nature, the controlling process is the last one to bring about the overall coordination necessary to lead the organization to its desired objectives.

Coordination and Decision Making

Since the process of decision making is at the heart of all managerial functions, achieving coordination must be an overriding thought in every manager's mind whenever decisions are made. When choosing from the various alternatives, the manager must never forget the importance of achieving synchronization of all efforts. Thus, that alternative will be selected which is most likely to bring about the best coordination within the department. There may be times when a certain alternative *taken by itself* would seem to constitute the best choice. A second choice, however, might result in better coordination throughout the department. This is why the previous chapter stresses the importance of the acceptability of the solution as one of the supervisor's considerations in choosing from alternatives. The supervisor would be far better off to follow the second solution, since achieving coordination is an important objective. In other words, each decision a manager makes is an exercise in the synchronization and integration of the department's activities.

Coordination and Communication

In all coordination efforts, good communication will be of immeasurable help. It is not enough for a manager to make decisions that are likely to bring about coordination. It is at least as important to have them carried out effectively. To achieve successful execution, the supervisor must first be able to communicate the decisions to the subordinates so that they understand them correctly. Therefore, good communication is actually essential for achieving coordination. Personal, oral face-to-face contact is probably the most effective means of communicating to obtain coordination. Other means, however, such as written communications, reports, procedures, rules, bulletins, as well as numerous modern mechanical devices, ensure the speedy dissemination of information to employees. Recent developments in electronic data processing can also be of considerable help in communicating and coordinating. The importance of good communication for achieving coordination will become even more obvious as we discuss this final connecting process in Chapter 5.

Internal Coordination in Health Care Centers

Because of the proliferation and specialization of medical sciences and technologies, health care centers have become large and complex organizational structures. More and more positions have had to be created, and this increasing specialization and division of work has generated a need for more and better coordination. Of course, the division of labor arises from the recognition that work divided into smaller specialized tasks permits a group of people, performing together, to accomplish more than one individual attempting the whole task alone. As a result of such specialization, however, the synchronization of daily activities has become extremely complicated, and coordination has become increasingly difficult to attain. This is especially true in the health care field. You know that as the number of positions in your department and in the hospital increases and as more specialized tasks are to be performed, the greater is your need and effort for coordination and synchronization to secure the unified result, namely, the best possible patient care.

Coordination With Other Departments

As a supervisor in a health care center, you also know that you must be concerned with more than just coordination inside your department. You also have to coordinate the efforts of your department with those of the many other departments involved in the care of the client. Of course, the process of bringing about the total coordination of *all* divisions and levels within a health care facility is primarily the concern of the chief administrator. It is the chief executive officer who must deal with the fact that each special departmental interest in the health care center is likely to stress its own opinion of how the best possible patient care should be accomplished, and each is likely to favor one route or another, depending on its particular functions and experience. This problem of different viewpoints also holds true among the numerous levels of the administrative hierarchy. It takes considerable thoughtfulness and understanding on the part of the chief administrator and all the other managerial and supervisory personnel to coordinate the working relationships of the groups above, below, and alongside each department. Even with cooperative attitudes, self-coordination, and self-adjustment by most members of the health care center, there can still be duplication of actions and conflicts of efforts unless good administration very carefully synchronizes all activities. Only through such coordination can management bring about a total accomplishment that exceeds the sum of the individual parts. Although each part is significant, the result can be of greater significance if management achieves success in coordination.

Dimensions of Coordination

One can see the need for coordination in three directions: vertical, horizontal, and diagonal coordination.

Vertical Coordination

Coordination between the different levels of an organization can be considered as *vertical* coordination, for instance, between the administrator and the director of nursing and between the director of nursing and a supervisor of nursing. Vertical coordination is achieved by delegating authority, assigning duties, and supervising and controlling. Although authority carries great power with it, vertical coordination is better achieved by the various managers performing their managerial functions expertly, instead of relying on the sheer threat of formal authority. (See Figure 4-1.)

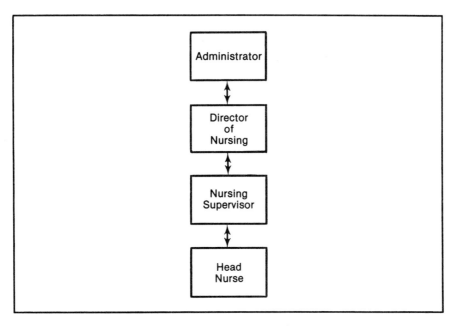

Figure 4-1. Vertical coordination

Horizontal Coordination

Horizontal coordination exists between people and departments on the same organizational level. For example, to achieve better hospital room utilization, the need for an earlier checkout hour has been targeted as the solution. To work out this problem, new arrangements have to be made between the various managers of the activities affected. Therefore, the director of admissions, together with the director of nursing, chief of the pharmacy, head of patients accounts, executive housekeeper, and director of the ancillary escort services, all involved in the discharge process, will try to coordinate their activities to achieve this goal. (See Figure 4-2.) Each of the executives involved manages his or her own department and has no authority over the other executives. It is obvious that horizontal coordination cannot be ordered by any one of them. If horizontal coordination cannot be achieved, such a problem must be referred to a level in the managerial hierarchy with authority over all of these departments. In all likelihood this is the chief executive officer, who will simply issue the necessary directives.

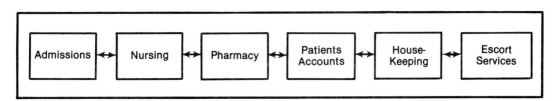

Figure 4-2. Horizontal coordination

Diagonal Coordination

Diagonal coordination exists when all departments have access to a centralized service. For example, the services of a centralized plant engineering and maintenance department have to be coordinated by negotiations between this department and the users. (See Figure 4-3.) They are responsible for working this out. Coordination cannot be accomplished simply by referring the problem to the next level in the chain of command.

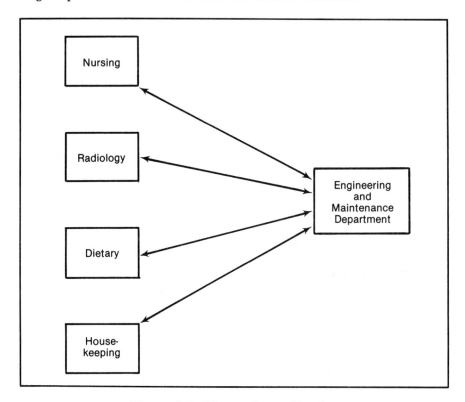

Figure 4-3. Diagonal coordination

The Coordinator

The task of securing harmonious action and internal coordination within a health care center belongs primarily to those who are in a managerial position. This task cannot be delegated to a specialist, often called a "coordinator." The managers are in a far better position than any special coordinator to view the various functions and determine how they should be coordinated to bring about the desired objective and get the job done. Although some hospitals do have positions labeled coordinator, these are often regular managerial and supervisory jobs and should be named as such. In these cases, the title coordinator is a misnomer. For instance, instead of having a group of nurses known as nursing supervisors, they might be called nursing coordinators. Their positions are likely to be managerial, regardless of the incorrect title. Some health care centers simply prefer the word coordinator to that of supervisor. On the other hand, a number of positions in many health care centers are properly known and labeled coordinator, such as inservice coordinator or education and training coordinator. These are usually staff positions providing service and assistance in their area of expertise to whomever would need and benefit from it. The important point is that *all* managers must coordinate as they perform their five managerial functions, and therefore it is questionable whether the task of securing internal coordination within the health care center can be shifted or assigned to a special department or a number of individuals.*

External Coordination

In addition to this need for internal coordination, however, there exists a need for coordination with factors *external* to the institution, such as changes in the general economy, governmental activities, medical and technological advances, and the interests of the general public in health care. A certain amount of external coordination should exist between each hospital and other health care institutions and the many aspects of the health care system at large. In those situations where a hospital is trying to coordinate some of its activities with other health care institutions or with any other external factors, such as a social work agency, a visiting nurses agency, etc., a special coordinator or liaison person may be utilized. Such a person should be thoroughly familiar with the conditions and thinking of his or her institution, be able to explain these to the others, and report the findings and intentions back to his or her institution. Normally, however, an external coordinator does not have any authority to commit the institution to action. In most instances, it is necessary to check back with the administrator or executive director as to how far the institution will go to support whatever action has been decided upon. In this situation, then, we are not dealing with a manager in the sense of the term used in this text.

Nevertheless, the importance of such external coordination should not be underestimated. Obviously, the more external coordination among medical centers and related institutions, the better will be our overall health care system. Thus, a great deal is being said today about interface relationships, that is, analyzing behavior among health care centers at the point where they are tangent to one another.

---

*Professors Lawrence and Lorsch conducted some of the best recent studies on coordination and integration. They examined various managerial coordinating efforts in different industrial environments, namely, in highly dynamic settings, in relatively dynamic settings, and in a predictable and stable environment. Their findings could be taken into consideration in certain health care settings. Paul R. Lawrence and Jay W. Lorsch. *Organization and Environment, Managing Differentiation and Integration* (Homewood, IL: Richard D. Irwin, Inc., 1969); first published in 1967 by Division of Research, Graduate School of Business Administration, Harvard University, Cambridge, MA, "New Management Job: The Integrator," *Harvard Business Review* 45 (November-December 1967): 142-151.

In the final analysis, management's ever-increasing problems of coordination, both internal and external, can only be offset by ever-increasing knowledge of how to perform the managerial job. Fortunately, this knowledge is becoming broader because of the emergence of new tools and devices and a more thorough understanding of the overall dependence and relationships among health care systems within the community, state, and country.

Summary

Coordination is the orderly synchronization of all efforts of the members of the organization to achieve the stated objectives. It is not a separate managerial function but a byproduct that comes about when the manager performs the five managerial functions. There is a significant difference, however, between cooperation and coordination. Although cooperation is always helpful in achieving coordination, the latter is superior in importance to the former.

As a supervisor plans, organizes, staffs, influences, and controls, it must be remembered that the ultimate goal is to achieve coordination or the synchronization of all efforts. The same overriding thought permeates the manager's mind whenever decisions are made and communicated to the employees. Achieving coordination is a valid consideration for all managers, regardless of their positions, level within the administrative hierarchy, or the kind of enterprise in which they work. Because of the proliferation and specialization of medical sciences and technologies, the task of obtaining coordination in a health care center has become increasingly difficult. However, coordination is clearly a part of the regular managerial positions in a hospital and should not be shifted or assigned to a special position labeled coordinator.

In addition to the need for internal coordination in a hospital, there exists a need for coordination with factors external to the institution, such as government agencies and local health councils. For this external coordination, a liaison person or special coordinator can be utilized to provide the necessary contacts between the hospital and outside factors.

5

Communicating

Like all organizations, a health care center needs valid information as one of its important resources. Communication provides the key for this. A hospital devotes a great deal of activity to gathering and processing information from the moment the client enters the facility until discharge. Serious consequences can arise when communications are minimal, become misunderstood, break down, or do not exist. A spectacular example of the impact of no communication is the following incident.

A few years ago, an incident took place in a Chicago area hospital in which a patient was "lost" for 25 hours. A patient whose condition left him unable to speak or otherwise communicate, and needing support to sit up in a wheelchair, was secured to a wheelchair with a restraint belt, pillow, and lapboard. He had been in the occupational therapy department in the lower level of the hospital and was wheeled by a volunteer escort, supposedly back to his ward. The escort wheeled him, along with another patient, to the passenger elevator(s). The volunteer escort was to complete the assignment. About 45 minutes later, a nurse, assuming the patient was back in his ward, could not locate him there. Intensive investigation began immediately, searching the hospital and adjoining buildings with the assistance of the hospital police unit, ward staff, physicians, nurses, etc. The patient could not be located. The search continued for 25 hours, when a member of the hospital personnel stepped onto an elevator in the basement to find the patient secured in a wheelchair and bent over. This person was unaware that the patient had been missing and leaned over to speak to him, offering assistance. He quickly observed that the patient was unable to respond, and after reading forms attached to the chair, returned the patient to his floor, where he was recognized by a medical student and returned to his proper ward. During the "lost patient's" absence, several hospital employees who would have recognized the patient told investigators they rode the elevator on which he was later found and did not see him. An elevator repairman also said he and an inspector took the elevator out of service for some time during the patient's absence and that no one was on the elevator. Despite a thorough month-long investigation, the hospital was unable to account for the patient's whereabouts during the 25-hour period.

Unfortunately the patient died from cerebral hemorrhage after undergoing brain surgery several weeks later. The hospital stated that his death was in no way connected with any ill effects caused by this incident.

Communication is the third process that serves to link the managerial functions in an organization. Employees look for and expect communication, since it is a means of motivating and influencing people. Communication is vital to them not only for purposes of social satisfaction but also to carry out their jobs effectively. Thus, the communication process fulfills both human needs and institutional needs.

You already know that as a supervisor your job is to plan, organize, staff, influence, and control the work of the employees of your department and to coordinate their efforts for the purpose of achieving departmental objectives. But to do this you must explain and discuss the arrangement of the work. You must give directives. You must describe to each subordinate what is expected of him or her. It is likely that you will need to speak to your employees regarding their performance. All of this is communication.

As you continue supervising employees, you probably will come to realize that your skill in communication determines your success. Communication is the most effective tool for building and keeping a well-functioning team. Just consider your own job and you will quickly see why communication is essential to successful supervision. Is there any area of responsibility within your job as a supervisor that you could fulfill without communicating? Certainly not.

You probably know some supervisors who are competent, professionally knowledgeable, and well mannered. Nevertheless, they do not seem to accomplish anything. Deep down, you probably know the reason: they cannot use words to sell themselves or to sell their plans; they cannot communicate. You may also have observed supervisors who have lost their skill in communicating or who think that communication is no longer worth the effort. Before they knew it, they lost touch with their employees because they failed to communicate. This ability to communicate is absolutely essential to leadership. It is the only means a supervisor has to take charge of and train a group of employees, to direct them, motivate them, and coordinate their activities so that the goals can be reached. The problem of communication is vital for any organization. Without effective communication the organizational structure cannot survive.

The Nature of Communication

Communication is the process of transmitting information and understanding from one person to another. Communication, fundamental and vital to all managerial functions, is a means of imparting ideas and making oneself understood by others. The exchange is successful only when mutual understanding results. It is not necessary to have agreement, as long as the sender and receiver have successfully exchanged ideas and understand each other. Since managing is getting things done through others, it is an obvious requirement that the manager communicate with the members of the group.

As a supervisor, you spend approximately 90% of your time in either sending or receiving information. Of course, it would be incorrect to assume that real communication is actually taking place all of this time. The mere fact that a supervisor is constantly engaged in sending and receiving messages is most certainly not any assurance that he or she is an expert in communicating.

In the many instances where communication has not taken place, the result has been confusion and error.

Communication was defined as the process of passing information and understanding from one person to another. The significant point here is that communication always involves two people: a sender and a receiver. It is wrong to think of communication as merely a matter of sending. There must be a receiver. One person alone cannot communicate; communication is not a one-way street. For example, a person who is stranded on a deserted island, shouting for help, does not communicate because there is no receiver. This is an obvious example, but it may not be so obvious to managers who send out a large number of memoranda. Once a memorandum has been mailed, they are inclined to believe that communication has occurred. However, communication does not occur until information and understanding have passed *between the senders and the intended receivers.*

This understanding aspect of communication is another important part of our definition. A receiver may hear a sender because he has ears but still not understand what the sender means. Understanding is a personal matter between people. If the idea received is the one intended, then communication has taken place. However, people may interpret messages differently. If the idea received is not the one intended, then communication has not taken place; the sender has merely spoken or written. "Simply telling" somebody something is not enough to guarantee successful communication. As long as there is no reception or imperfect reception of the idea intended, we cannot speak of having communicated.

As stated before, communication does not require the receiver to agree with the statement of the sender. Communication occurs whenever the receiver at least understands what the sender means to convey. Two people can fully understand each other and still not agree. Thus, as a supervisor your subordinates do not have to agree with everything you communicate to them. But they must understand it. No subordinate can be expected to comply with a directive unless there is understanding on his or her part. Similarly, supervisors must know how to receive knowledge and understanding in the messages sent to them by their subordinates, fellow supervisors, and superiors.

Only through such communication can policies, procedures, and rules be formulated and carried out. Only with such communication can misunderstandings be ironed out, long-term and short-term plans achieved, and activities within a department coordinated and controlled. The success of all managerial functions depends on effective communication.

Channels of Communication

In every organization, the communication network has two distinct but equally important channels: the formal channel of communication and the informal channel, usually called the grapevine. Each carries messages from one person or group to another in downward, upward, sideward, and diagonal directions. (See Figure 5-1.)

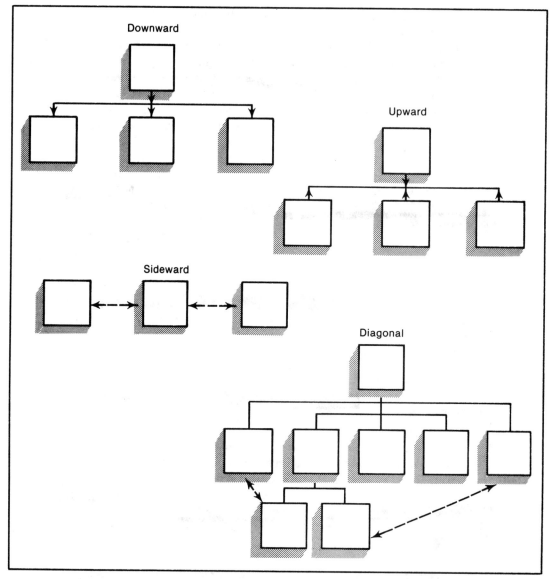

Figure 5-1. The directions of information along formal communication channels.

Formal Channels

The formal channels are established mainly by the organizational structure. They follow the lines of authority from the chief administrator all the way down. You are probably familiar with the expression that messages and information "must go through channels." This, of course, refers to the formal flow of communication through the organizational hierarchy.

Downward Communication

When it moves in a downward direction, this formal flow of communication begins with someone at the top issuing a directive, and the next person in the hierarchy passing it along to those who report to him or her, and so on down the line. The downward direction is the one management relies on the most for its communication. Generally, downward communication starts action by subordinates. Its content is mostly of a directive nature. It is used to convey not only directives, but also information, objectives, policies, procedures, and so forth to subordinates for implementation. The downward flow thus helps to tie the levels of the organizational structure together and to coordinate activities.

Upward Communication

Upward communication is a second but equally important direction in which messages flow through the official network. Any person who is charged with supervisory authority accepts an obligation to keep the superior informed. Moreover, the subordinates must feel free to convey to their superior their opinions and attitudes and to report on activities and actions regarding their work. Management should encourage a free flow of upward communication, since this is the only means by which it can determine whether its messages have been transmitted and received properly and whether appropriate action is taking place.

Upward communication is of an informative and reporting nature. It carries information about what has happened, as well as opinions of subordinates to their superiors. It reports on work-related activities and provides a lot of control information. This is how the manager will learn whether or not proper action is taking place.

As a supervisor, you should encourage and maintain upward communication channels and pay proper attention to the information transmitted through them. You must show that you want the facts and want them promptly. Unfortunately, the reaction of many managers to upward communication is still very much like that of ancient tyrants who executed the "bearer of bad news." In your supervisory capacity, you must make a deliberate effort to encourage upward communication by showing a genuine desire to obtain and use the ideas and reports of your subordinates, by being approachable, and by recognizing the importance of upward communication. Lack of an effective upward flow will throttle the natural desire of your employees to communicate, lead to frustration, and ultimately cause your employees to seek different outlets, such as the grapevine.

In addition to encouraging your employees to communicate upward to you, you must likewise communicate upward to your own superior. Persons who have been put into a supervisory position accept the obligation to keep their superiors informed. As stated at the outset, supervisors are the people in the middle. They are not only responsible for providing good communication downward *to* their employees, but they are also responsible for stimulating good communication upward *from* their workers and then for passing this and other information to the next higher level in the administrative hierarchy.

However, most supervisors will agree with the statement that it is much easier for them to "talk down" to their subordinates than to "speak up" to their
superior, especially if they have ever had to tell their boss that they did not
meet a certain schedule due to bad planning or that they forgot to carry out an
order or that something else went wrong.

Nevertheless, it is the supervisor's job to keep his or her superior advised of up-to-date facts concerning the department. The supervisor should
inform the superior of any significant developments as soon as possible after
they occur. It would be most unfortunate if the boss were to learn such news
elsewhere, because this would indicate that proper upward communication
was not allowed or that you were not providing it. It is a supervisor's duty to
keep a superior up-to-date, even if the information reveals errors that have
occured. It is your superior's right to have complete information, and it is
your duty to provide complete information about the functioning of your
department. After all, your boss is still responsible if anything goes wrong.

Your superior may have to act on what you report. Therefore, the information must get there in time and in a form that will enable your superior
to take the necessary action. As a supervisor, you must assemble all facts that
are needed and check them carefully before passing them on to your boss. Try
to be as objective as possible. This, of course, will be quite difficult at times,
since all subordinates want to appear favorably in the eyes of their boss. Thus,
there is a danger that you may want to soften the information a bit so that
things will not look quite so bad as they actually are. However, it is likely that
sooner or later the full extent of the malfunctioning will be discovered. When
difficulties arise, it is best to tell your superior the complete score, even if this
means admitting mistakes. Always keep in mind that your boss depends on
the supervisors for upward communication, just as you depend on your
employees to pass along their bits of information to you.

Sideward Communication

In addition to downward and upward communication, a third direction of communication is essential for the efficient functioning of an enterprise. This is sideward, or lateral, communication. It is concerned mainly
with communication across departments or among people on the same level
in the hierarchy but in charge of different functions. For example, lateral
communication will often take place between the operating room supervisor
and the head nurse on the surgical floor.

Diagonal Communication

Diagonal communication, on the other hand, is the flow of messages
between positions that are not on the same lateral plane of the organization
structure. Communication between line groups, such as nursing personnel,
and staff groups, such as the laundry department, is an example of diagonal
communication, or messages between the floor nurse and the radiology
department, or therapy, dietary, the laboratories, etc. (See Chapter 12.) To
achieve coordination among the various functions in any organization, especially in a health care organization, a free flow of both lateral and diagonal

commmunication is absolutely essential. Without it, good patient care would be difficult to achieve.

The Grapevine:
An Informal Channel of Communication

Although it is essential to develop sound formal channels, the dynamics of organizational life tend to create additional channels of communication. An informal network of communication commonly referred to as the grapevine emerges. Every organization has its grapevine, a network of spontaneous channels.

It is a logical and normal outgrowth of the informal groupings of people, their social interaction, and their natural desire to communicate with each other. The grapevine must be looked on as a perfectly natural activity. It fulfills the subordinate's desire to be "in the know" and to be kept posted on the latest information. The grapevine also gives the members of the organization an outlet for their imagination and an opportunity to relieve their apprehensions in the form of rumors. At the same time, it offers the supervisor excellent insight into what the subordinates think and feel. An efficient manager will acknowledge the grapevine's presence and put it to good use if possible.

Operation of the Grapevine

Sometimes the grapevine carries factual information and news, but most of the time it carries inaccurate information, half-truths, rumors, private interpretations, wishful thinking, suspicions, and other various bits of distorted information. The grapevine is active all day long, and it spreads information with amazing speed, often faster than most official channels could. The grapevine has no definite pattern or stable membership. It carries information in all directions, up, down, laterally, and diagonally. The news is carried in a flexible, meandering pattern, ignoring organization charts. Its path and behavior cannot be predicted, and the path followed yesterday is not necessarily the same as today or tomorrow.

Most of the time only a small number of employees will be active participants in the grapevine. The vast majority of employees hear information through the grapevine but do not pass it along. Any person within an organization is likely to become active in the grapevine on one occasion or another. However, some individuals tend to be active more regularly than others. They believe that their prestige is enhanced by providing the latest news, and hence they do not hesitate to spread the news or even change it, so as to augment its "completeness" and "accuracy." These active participants in the grapevine know that they cannot be held accountable, so it is understandable that they exercise a considerable degree of imagination whenever they pass information along. The resulting "rumors" give them, as well as other members of the organization, an outlet for getting rid of their apprehensions. During periods of insecurity, upheaval, and great anxiety the grapevine works overtime. In general, the grapevine serves as a safety valve for the emotions of all subordinates, providing them with the means to freely say what they please without the danger of being held accountable. Since everyone knows that it is nearly impossible to trace the origins of a rumor, employees can feel quite safe in their anonymity as they participate in the grapevine.

Uses of the Grapevine

Because the grapevine often carries a considerable amount of useful information, in addition to distortions, rumors, and half-truths, it can help to clarify and disseminate formal communication. It often spreads information that could not be disseminated through the official channels of communication. For instance, the nursing director "resigns" suddenly. Although top administration does not want to say publicly what happened, it does not want to leave the impression that she was treated unfairly or discriminated against. In such a situation, someone in administration may tell someone in the hospital, who "promises" not to tell it further, what really happened.

Managers should accept the fact that they can no more eliminate the grapevine than they can abolish the informal organization that develops among employees. It is unrealistic to expect that rumors can be stamped out; the grapevine is bound to flourish in every organization. To deal with it, the supervisors must tune in on the grapevine and learn what it is saying. They must look for the meaning of the grapevine's communication, not merely for its words. They must learn who the leaders are and who is likely to spread the information. They must also learn that by feeding the grapevine facts, they can counter rumors and half-truths. This is one way to utilize the grapevine's energy in the interest of management.

Rumors can be caused by several different factors, such as wishful thinking and anticipation, uncertainty and fear, or even malice and dislike. For example, it is quite common for employees who want something badly enough to suddenly start passing the word. If they want a raise, they may start a rumor that management will give everybody an across-the-board pay increase. No one knows for certain where or how it started, but this story spreads like wildfire. Everyone wants to believe it. Of course, it is bad for the morale of a group to build up their hopes in anticipation of something that will not happen. If a story is getting around that the supervior realizes will lead to disappointment, the manager should move quickly to debunk it by presenting the facts. A straight answer is almost always the best answer. In other words, the best prescription for curing this type of rumor is factual medicine.

The same prescription applies to rumors caused by fear or uncertainty. If, for example, the activities of the institution decline, and management is forced to lay off some employees, stories and rumors will quickly multiply. In such periods of insecurity and anxiety the grapevine will become more active than at other times. Usually the rumors are far worse than what actually happens. Here again, it is better to give the facts than to conceal them. If the supervisor does not disclose the facts, the employees will make up their own "facts," which are usually a distortion of reality. In many instances, much of the fear and anxiety can be eliminated if the facts of what will happen are disclosed. Continuing rumors and uncertainty are likely to be more demoralizing than even the most unpleasant facts. Thus, it is usually best to explain immediately why employees are being laid off, why orders are being given, and so on. When emergencies occur, when new procedures are introduced, when policies are changed, explain why. Otherwise your subordinates will make up their own explanations, and often they will be incorrect.

There may be situations, however, where you as a supervisor do not have the correct facts either. In such instances, let your superior know what is bothering your employees. Ask your superior for specific instructions as to what information you may give, how much you may tell, and when. Next, meet with your chief assistants and lead employees. Give them the story and guide their thinking. Then they can spread the facts before anyone else can spread the rumors.

Although this procedure may work with rumors caused by fear or uncertainty, it might not be appropriate for rumors that arise out of dislike, anger, or malice. Once again, the best prescription is to try to be objective and impersonal and to come out with the facts, if this is possible. Sometimes, however, a supervisor will find that the only way to stop a malicious rumor peddler is to expose him or her personally and then reveal the untruthfulness of the statement.

A superior should always bear in mind that the receptiveness of any group to rumors of this type is directly related to the strength of the supervisor's leadership and the respect the subordinates have for the manager. If employees believe in your fairness and good supervision, they will quickly debunk any malicious rumor, once you have exposed the person who started it or given your answer to it. Thus, although there is no way to eliminate the grapevine, even its most threatening rumors can be counteracted to management's advantage. Every supervisor, therefore, will do well to listen to the informal channels of communication and to develop the skill in dealing with them.

The Communication Media

The media for communication can be words, pictures, and actions. Spoken and written words are, of course, the most important symbols used. But it would be wrong to ignore or underestimate the power of pictures and actions in conveying meaning and understanding.

Pictures

Pictures, the visual aids that a manager will resort to from time to time, are particularly effective in connection with well-chosen words to complete a message. Most enterprises make extensive use of pictures in the form of blueprints, charts, drafts, three-dimensional models, posters, and so on. Motion pictures and comic strips offer clear proof of the power of pictures to communicate and bring about understanding.

Actions

Actions and behavior are other media used in communication. As managers, supervisors must not forget that what they do is interpreted as a symbol by their subordinates and that actions often speak louder than words. Because of the managerial status, all observable acts communicate something to employees, whether they intended them to or not. Purposeful silence, gestures, a handshake, a shrug of the shoulder, a smile, and a frown all have meaning. For instance, a frown on the supervisor's face may at times mean more than 10 minutes of oral discussion. These are examples of nonverbal communications known as *body language*.

By the same token, a manager's inaction is also a way of communication. An unexplained action can often communicate a meaning that was not intended. Suppose, for example, that a piece of equipment has been removed from the laboratory for overhaul without telling the employees the reason why. To the technologists apprehensive of a reduction or change in activities, such unexplained action could convey a message that the supervisor probably had no intention of sending.

Spoken and Written Words

Words are the most widely used forms of communication. This is a real challenge to the supervisor because words can be tricky, and messages that mean one thing to one employee can have a completely different meaning to someone else. Therefore, supervisors must make an effort to improve their skills in speaking, writing, listening, and reading. You may have heard the often told story about the maintenance foreman who asked the new worker to go out and paint the canopy in front of the hospital green. When the foreman checked on the job an hour later, he found that the waste can had been painted bright green. The new employee did not know what a canopy was. Perhaps he should have known, but no one had ever told him.

Written Communication

A well-balanced communication system, of course, will include both the oral and written media. Although oral communication is the most frequently used, written messages are indispensable and very much in use in the health care field. They provide a permanent record to which references can be made as often as necessary. The spoken word, in contrast, generally exists only for an instant. Often, detailed and specific instructions may be so lengthy and cumbersome that they must be put into writing so that they can be studied for a longer period of time. It is advisable to use the written medium for widespread dissemination of information that may concern a number of people. Furthermore, there is a degree of formality connected with written communications which orally delivered messages usually do not carry. Although there are many occasions in the health care field where the written form is absolutely necessary, most of the supervisor's communication will take place by word of mouth. Therefore, the following discussions primarily refer to spoken, or oral, communication.

Oral Communication

In most instances, oral communication is superior to the written medium, since it normally achieves better understanding and saves time. This is true of both oral telephone and face-to-face communication. In daily performance, face-to-face discussions between the supervisor and subordinate are the principal means of two-way communication. Such daily contacts are at the heart of an effective communication system. They provide the most frequently used channels for the exchange of information, points of view, instructions, and motivation. There is no form of written communication that can equal oral, especially the face-to-face oral, communication between a supervisor and the employees. Therefore, the effective supervisor will utilize this medium more than any other. He or she knows that subordinates like to see and hear their boss in person and that oral communication is usually well received because most people can express themselves more easily and more completely by voice than by writing.

Aside from these features, the greatest single advantage of oral communication is that it provides immediate *feedback*, even if the feedback is only an expression on the listener's face. By merely looking at the receiver, the sender can judge how the receiver is reacting to what is being said. Oral communication thus enables the sender to find out immediately what the receiver is hearing or not hearing. Oral communication also enables the receiver to ask questions right then and there if the meaning is not clear, and the sender can explain the message more thoroughly and clarify unexpected problems raised by the communication. Moreover, the manner and tone of the human voice can endow the message with meaning and shading that even long pages of written words simply could not convey. The manner and tone create the atmosphere of communication, and the response is influenced accordingly.

The good communicator must be concerned with the total impact of his or her message. The sender must be aware of the listener and of the responses, both verbal and nonverbal. These responses provide feedback that indicates whether or not the message is getting across. If not, the communicator must search for the reason why.

Roadblocks to Communication

The supervisor must be familiar with the many barriers to effective communication. The effective communicator must realize that the speaker and the listener are two separate individuals who live in different worlds and that many factors can interfere and play havoc with the messages which pass between them. Always remember that there is no communication until and unless the meaning received by the listener is the same as that which the sender intended to send. Let us now turn to those factors which may create roadblocks to the intended meaning of a communication and discuss the ways and means of successfully overcoming these blocks.

Most organizational structures today are intricate and create several layers of supervision, long lines of communications, and distance between the employees and top administration. Breakdowns of communication can occur at any level of supervision. All of you are familiar with the confusions, frictions, and inconveniences that arise when communications break down. These breakdowns are not only costly in terms of money, but they also create misunderstandings that may hurt your teamwork morale and even patient care. Indeed, many of a supervisor's problems are due to faulty communication. That is, the way you as a supervisor communicate with your subordinates is the essence of your relationship, and most problems of human relations grow out of poor or nonexistent communication. Although the number of communication barriers is large, the more important ones can be grouped into three general categories: language barriers, status and position barriers, and general resistance to change.

Language

Normally, words serve us well and we generally understand each other. But sometimes the same words suggest different meanings to different people. The words themselves create a barrier to communication. It is often said that people on different levels "speak a different language." There are many instances when a frustrating conversation ends with the admission that "we are just not speaking the same language," yet both participants have been conversing in English. To avoid such a breakdown in communication, the communicator should use the language of the receiver and not his or her own language. The sender should speak a language that the receiver is accustomed to and that the latter understands. It is not a question of whether the receiver *should* understand it; the question is simply, does he or she? The supervisor must therefore use plain simple words, direct uncomplicated language.

Of course, this is difficult at times because the English language assigns several meanings to one word. This problem is often referred to as one of semantics. For example, the word "round" has many meanings. We speak of round as a ball, he walks round and round, a round dozen of eggs, a round trip, a round of beef, a round of boxing, round as a cylinder, etc. When using words that have such different meanings, the communicator must be certain the exact meaning intended is clarified. The sender should not just assume that the receiver will interpret the word in the same way he or she does.

Many words in our language have reasonably similar meanings, yet they convey different messages, as evidenced in the following two lists:*

List A	*List B*
Firm	Unyielding
Aggressive	Ruthless
Compassionate	Weak
Concerned with detail	Nit picking
Certain	Cocky
Easygoing	Unconcerned
Selective	Arbitrary
Respects lines of authority	Bureaucratic
An independent thinker	A nonconformist
Blunt and direct	Tactless

For most people, the words in list B convey a less favorable message than those in list A. When describing someone you care for, you are likely to use the words in list A. However, the listener tends to listen and interpret the language based on *his or her own* experience and frame of reference, not yours.

Status and Position

It cannot be denied that an organizational structure and the resulting administrative hierarchy create a number of different status levels among the members of a health care center. Status refers to the regard and attitude displayed and held toward a particular position and its occupant by the members of the organization. There is certainly a difference in status between the level of the president and that of the supervisors and between the level of the supervisors and that of their employees. This difference in status and position becomes more apparent as one level communicates with the other.

For example, when employees listen to a message from the supervisor, several factors become operative. First, the employees evaluate what they hear in relation to their own position, background, and experience; they also take the sender into account. It is difficult for a receiver to separate what he or she hears from the feelings he or she has about the person who sends the message. It often happens, therefore, that the receiver adds nonexistent motives to the sender. Union members are frequently inclined to interpret a statement coming from administration in a negative manner because they are often con-

---

*From Richard M. Hodgetts and Steven Altman, *Organizational Behavior* (Philadelphia: W. B. Saunders Company, 1979), 306. Reprinted by permission of Holt, Rinehart and Winston, CBS College Publishing.

vinced that management is trying to weaken and undermine the union. Often a hospital's newspaper is considered a propaganda organ and mouthpiece of administration, and its contents are viewed with suspicion. Such mental blocks and attitudes obviously do not make for good understanding.

The supervisor who is trying to be an effective communicator must realize that these status and position differences influence feelings and prejudices of the employees and thus create barriers to efforts to communicate with them. To overcome these barriers, managers should put themselves in the employees' place and try to analyze and anticipate the employees' reaction before sending their message. Moreover, not only might the employee evaluate the boss' words differently, but undue importance might also be placed on a superior's gesture, silence, smile, or other facial expression. Simply speaking, the boss' words are not just words; they are words that come from a boss. This is how barriers due to status work in the downward flow of communication.

Similar obstacles due to status and position also arise in the upward flow of communication, since all subordinates are eager to appear favorably in their boss' eyes. Therefore, employees may conveniently and protectively screen the information that is passed up the line. A subordinate, for example, is likely to tell the superior what the latter likes to hear and will omit or soften what is unpleasant. By the same token, subordinates are anxious to cover up their own weaknesses when talking to a person in a higher position. Thus, a supervisor often fails to pass on important information because he or she believes that such information would reflect unfavorably on his or her own supervisory abilities. After two or three selective screenings of this sort by different echelons of the administrative hierarchy, you can imagine how the message is likely to be considerably distorted.

Resistance to Change

Most people prefer things as they are and do not welcome changes in their working situation. This natural resistance to change can constitute a serious barrier to communication because often a message intends to convey a new idea to the employees, something that will change either their work assignment, position, or daily routine. Many employees resist such a change, feeling that it is safer to leave the existing environment in its present state. Ultimately each of us lives in our own little world; although it may not be a perfect world, we sooner or later learn to make peace with it and live within it more or less happily.

Consequently, a message that will change this world is greeted with suspicion and the listeners' receiving apparatus works just like a filter, rejecting new ideas if they conflict with what they already believe. They are likely to receive only that portion which confirms their present beliefs and ignore anything that conflicts. Sometimes these filters work so efficiently that in reality the receivers do not hear at all. Even if they hear, they will either reject that part of the message as false, or they will find some convenient way of twisting its meaning to fit their preconceived ideas. Ultimately, the receivers hear only what they wish to hear. If they are insecure, worried, or fearful in their position, this barrier to receiving communication becomes even more powerful.

As a supervisor, you may have been confronted with situations in which it appeared that your subordinates only half listened to what you had to say. Your employees were so busy and preoccupied with their own thoughts that they paid attention exclusively to the ideas they had hoped to hear. They simply selected those parts of the total communication that they could readily use. The information your employees did not care for or considered irreconcilable was just conveniently brushed aside, not heard at all, or easily explained away. The selective perception of information constitutes a serious barrier to a supervisor's communications, particularly when the message was intended to convey a change, a new directive, or anything that could conceivably interfere with the employees' routine or working environment. If your listeners are worried, insecure, or suspicious, this barrier becomes even more effective. A supervisor must be aware of such possible reactions.

Additional Barriers

In addition to the above-mentioned barriers, many other roadblocks to communication arise in specific situations. For example, there are obstacles due to emotional reactions, such as deep-rooted feelings and prejudice, as well as obstacles because of physical conditions, such as inadequate telephone lines, lack of a private place to talk, heat, or noise. Or it may be indifference, the "don't care" attitude, that stands in the way of communication. In such a case, the message may get through, but it is acted on only halfheartedly or not at all. Or complacency on the subordinate's part may prevent the message from getting across.

All of these and many other barriers form serious roadblocks to good communication. Unless managers are familiar with such blocks, they are in no position to overcome them. Supervisors should not just assume that the messages which they send will be received as intended. It may be more realistic, although discouraging, to assume the opposite. Since the effectiveness of the supervisory job depends largely on the accurate transmission of messages and orders, managers must do everything possible to overcome these barriers and improve their chances for mutual understanding.

Overcoming Barriers to Communication

Major communication barriers can be prevented and overcome in numerous ways. Familiarity and utilization of these techniques will increase the likelihood for successful communication.

Adequate Preparation

The first step toward overcoming communication barriers is to know exactly what you want to communicate. You must think the idea through until it becomes hard and solid in your mind; do not just proceed with imprecise thoughts and desires that you have not bothered to put into final form. Only if you understand your ideas can you be sure that another person will understand your instructions. Therefore, know what you want to communicate and plan the sequence of steps necessary to attain it.

For example, if you want to make a job assignment, be sure that you have analyzed the job thoroughly, so that you can explain it properly. If you are searching for facts, decide in advance what information you will need, so that you can ask intelligent, pertinent, and precise questions. If your discussion will entail disciplinary action, be certain that you have sufficiently investigated the case and have enough information before you reprimand or even penalize. Do not initiate communication before you know what you are going to say and what you intend to achieve.

Feedback

Feedback is probably the most effective tool for improving communication. Managers must always be on the alert for some signal or clue indicating that they are being understood. Merely asking the receiver and getting a simple "yes" is not usually enough. Most of the time more feedback is required to make sure that the message is received as intended and that understanding is actually taking place.

The simplest way to obtain such reassurance is to observe the receiver and judge the responses by nonverbal clues, such as a facial expression of bewilderment or understanding, the raising of an eyebrow, or a frown. This kind of feedback is, of course, only possible in face-to-face communication, which is one of the outstanding advantages of using it.

Another way of obtaining feedback is for the senders to ask the receivers to repeat in their own words the information that has just been transmitted. This is much more satisfactory than merely asking the receivers whether or not they understand or if the instruction is clear, both of which require only a yes answer.

If the receiver can restate the content of the message, then the sender will really know what the receiver has heard and understood. At the same time, the receiver may ask additional questions that the sender can answer immediately. This direct feedback is probably the most useful way to make certain that a message has gotten across. Additional feedback can be obtained by observing whether or not the receivers behave in accordance with the communication. If direct observation is not possible, such as with a written message, the senders must watch for responses, reports, and results. Without being aware of it, you as a supervisor have probably already been using the principle of feedback in daily communications with subordinates.

Direct and Simple Language

Another helpful way to overcome blocks in communication is for the manager to use words that are as understandable and simple as possible. Long, technical, complicated words and jargon should be avoided, unless both the sender and receiver are comfortable with them. As mentioned before, the single, most important question is not whether the receiver should have understood it, but, rather, did he or she understand it?

Effective Listening

By spending more time for listening effectively to the receiver, the sender has an additional means for overcoming barriers to communication. Because of different backgrounds, such as education or religion, the world of the subordinate is often significantly different from that of the superior. Yet some common ground is necessary for understanding. Therefore, you must give the other party a chance to tell what is on his or her mind. The only way you can convince the other party of your interest in and respect for his or her opinions is to listen carefully and completely. Good listening means more than a mere expression of attention. It means to put aside biases and to listen without a fault-finding or correcting attitude and to listen to the meaning of the idea, rather than to mere words. (See Figure 5-2.)

The supervisor who pays attention and listens to what the subordinate is saying learns more about the employee's values and relationships to the working environment. Understanding, not agreement, is essential. It may even be advisable for the supervisor to state from time to time what has been expressed by asking the common question, "Is this what you mean?" The listener must patiently listen to what the other person has to say, even though it may seem to be unimportant. Such listening will greatly improve communication, since it will reduce misunderstandings. Careful listening allows a speaker to adjust the message to fit the responses and world of the receiver. This adjustment opportunity is another advantage of oral communication over written messages.

Actions Speak Louder Than Words

Supervisors must realize that they communicate by actions as much as by words. In fact, actions usually communicate more than words. Therefore, one of the best ways to give meaning to a message is to behave accordingly. Managers who fail to bolster their talk with action fail in their job as a communicator, no matter how capable they are with words. Whether the supervisor likes it or not, the supervisor's superior position makes him or her the center of attention for the employees, and the boss communicates through all observable actions, regardless of whether or not it was intended. Verbal announcements backed up by appropriate action will help the supervisor overcome barriers to communication. However, if the supervisor says one thing,

Figure 5-2. Effective listening guides.

1 Stop talking!
You cannot listen if you are talking.
Polonius *(Hamlet):* "Give every man thine ear, but few thy voice."

2 Put the talker at ease.
Help a person feel free to talk.
This is often called a permissive environment.

3 Show a talker that you want to listen.
Look and act interested. Do not read your mail while someone talks.
Listen to understand, rather than to oppose.

4 Remove distractions.
Don't doodle, tap, or shuffle papers.
Will it be quieter if you shut the door?

5 Empathize with talkers.
Try to help yourself see the other person's point of view.

6 Be patient.
Allow plenty of time. Do not interrupt a talker.
Don't start for the door or walk away.

7 Hold your temper.
An angry person takes the wrong meaning from words.

8 Go easy on argument and criticism.
These put people on the defensive, and they may "clam up" or become angry.
Do not argue: even if you win, you lose.

9 Ask questions.
This encourages a talker and shows that you are listening.
It helps to develop points further.

10 Stop talking!
This is first and last, because all other guides depend on it.
You cannot do an effective listening job while you are talking.

• Nature gave people two ears but only one tongue,
which is a gentle hint that they should listen more than they talk.

• Listening requires two ears,
one for meaning and one for feeling.

• Decision makers who do not listen
have less information for making sound decisions.

From Keith Davis, *Human Behavior at Work,* 6th ed. (New York: McGraw-Hill Book Company, 1981), 413. Reprinted by permission of the publisher.

but does another, sooner or later the employees will "listen" primarily to what the boss "does." For example, the director of nursing services who says she or he is always available to see a subordinate with a problem will undermine the verbal message if the door to the office is kept closed all the time.

Repetition

It is also advisable for a supervisor to repeat the message several times, preferably using different words and means of explanation. A certain amount of redundancy is especially advisable when each word is important or when the directives are complicated. The degree of redundancy will, of course, depend both on the content of the message and the experience and background of the employee. But the sender must be cautioned not to be so repetitious that the message may be ignored because it sounds overly familiar. If in doubt, a degree of repetition is safer than none.

Summary

To perform the managerial functions effectively, a supervisor must realize the importance of good communication. Without it, objectives cannot be achieved. Communication means the process of passing information and understanding from one person to another, from the sender to the receiver. As long as two people understand each other, they have communicated, although they may not agree. Agreement is not necessary for communication to be successful.

Throughout every organization, there are formal and informal channels of communication. They carry messages downward, upward, sideward, and diagonally. The formal channels are established mainly by the organizational structure and authority relationships. The position of the supervisor plays a strategic role in the communication process in all of these directions. He or she is a vital link in every dimension.

Although words are the most significant media of communication, we must not overlook the importance of pictorial language as another meaningful medium in which to communicate. In addition, action is a communication medium that often speaks louder than words. In the health care field, the written word is a major medium of communication. But of all media, oral face-to-face communication between supervisors and employees is still the most effective, since it provides some sort of immediate feedback.

There are many reasons why messages frequently become distorted or do not come across. There are roadblocks to communication because of language, status and position, and normal resistance to change. The supervisor must be aware of these potential barriers and make an effort to either prevent or overcome them. Feedback is the most effective remedy. The use of direct and simple language will also help. Furthermore, the supervisor must be an effective listener by tuning in on the world of the receiver. Since a supervisor communicates not only by what is said but also by what is done, it is necessary that actions bolster the words and do not contradict them. Often a certain degree of redundancy will also help in preventing and overcoming roadblocks.

In addition to the formal communication channels, there is an informal network, usually referred to as the grapevine. It is a natural outgrowth of the informal organization and the social interactions of people. It serves a useful purpose in every organization. The grapevine spreads information with great speed but without a definite pattern or a stable membership. The supervisor should accept the grapevine as a natural outlet of the employees; he or she should tune in on it, and at times even feed it, cultivate it, and put it to good use.

Legal Aspects of the Health Care Setting

Carolyn A. Haimann, JD

All persons involved with the operation of a health care institution are cognizant of the importance and effect of law in health care delivery. All have occasion to apply laws and legal principles in their daily routines, and legal aspects have become of major importance. This is true with the problems faced not only by the members of the board, by administrators, physicians, and surgeons but also by all supervisors, department heads, and possibly everyone involved in health care delivery in a private health care setting.*

The contents of this chapter are intended to provide very general and basic information in lay language and should in no way be used in lieu of the advice or consultation with legal counsel. The purpose is to give department heads and supervisors an overall general perspective of some of the legal aspects of their positions. The reader should be aware that problems of hospital liability evolve from court decisions based on principles of common law and vary from jurisdiction to jurisdiction. As with all aspects of law, hospital law and court decisions applying these principles evolve and change on a continuous basis.

For example, for a long time the courts protected hospitals and other charitable institutions from lawsuits which might infringe upon the assets of a charitable institution. This was generally known as the doctrine of charitable immunity. As discussed later in this chapter, nearly every state has now established the doctrine that charitable organizations have the obligation for compensation for injuries caused by them.

Liability

This is a word and a problem that has become increasingly familiar to hospital administrators, supervisors, and employees in recent years. Hospital managers and employees at all levels are constantly being reminded of the potential for liability and its resulting costs to the institution permeating their

---

*Our discussion does not cover situations in hospitals operated by the Veterans Administration, Army, Navy, Air Force and Public Health Services.

everyday activities and decisions. Hospital in-house legal counsel, risk managers, consent forms, incident reports, and numerous requirements for documentation are constant reminders of the litigious environment within which the health care team works. Liability is on everyone's mind and the burgeoning number of multimillion dollar judgments against hospitals and their staffs has become an albatross around the necks of hospital management and physicians. This chapter will discuss some of the various aspects of liability for the hospital, the supervisor, and the employee in relation to the patients.

The Hospital's Direct Responsibility

While liability is frequently imposed on hospitals for negligence resulting in injuries to visitors and employees, most lawsuits filed against hospitals involve patient injuries and allegations of negligent care. Therefore, let us turn our attention to the hospital's liability for injuries to its patients and its responsibility for the medical care rendered by its physicians.

The law requires that any organization, such as a hospital, that through its actions allows the public to rely on it for its safety, has a duty to exercise ordinary care to prevent injury. The duty owed by the hospital to its patients varies to some degree from jurisdiction to jurisdiction and also varies depending on the particular circumstances involved. But generally speaking in most jurisdictions a hospital owes a duty of due care to its patients to provide that degree of skill and care and diligence that would be provided by a similar hospital under the same or similar circumstances. More specifically, a hospital has a legal duty to provide its patients with, among other things, premises kept in a reasonably safe condition, appropriately trained and skilled staff, reasonably adequate equipment, and proper medications. Whether the hospital has breached any of its duties to the patient in a particular situation will be decided, in most cases, by a jury. If a jury finds that a hospital has failed to meet the various standards of care owed to its patients thereby breaching its duty, then the hospital will be found negligent.

Respondeat Superior

As discussed, the hospital is directly responsible for its actions in relation to the patient. But in addition to this, the hospital is indirectly liable for patient injuries in that it is legally responsible for the actions of those persons, employees and staff, over whom it exercises control and supervision. This vicarious liability arises from the doctrine of respondeat superior. Under the doctrine of respondeat superior the hospital-employer is legally responsible for the negligent or wrongful acts of the employee even though the hospital itself committed no wrong; the negligence of the employee is imputed to the employer. If a hospital employee commits a negligent act which is the direct cause of injury to a patient, then the hospital-employer may be liable for the damages awarded to the injured party. The doctrine of respondeat superior applies only to civil actions and an employer is not responsible for the criminal actions of its employees.

In order for the hospital to be liable under respondeat superior, it is necessary that the employer have the right to control the actions of the employee in the performance of the employee's duties. If the jury determines that the employer has the right to control the actions of its employee (that is, the method, time, and manner of work performance), and that the employee (or agent) was acting within the scope and course of employment, then the hospital will be liable. An act will generally be considered within the scope of employment where the employee is acting on behalf of or perceives himself or herself to be acting for the benefit of the hospital.

But the theory of respondeat superior does not absolve the employee of liability for his or her wrongful act and does not eliminate the employee's own liability for the negligent act. The employee, as well as the employer, may be found liable in damages to an injured third party. Under the law, the employer may pursue indemnification from the employee for damages paid on his or her behalf under respondeat superior; in other words, the hospital can seek recovery for the financial loss from the employee where the latter's actions caused the hospital to be responsible for the loss.

ications to the patients. Joe fails to carefully check the order for patients, Mrs. Jones and Mrs. Brown, and administers the medication ordered for Mrs. Jones to Mrs. Brown instead. As a direct result of the wrong medication being administered to her, Mrs. Brown suffers a severe and sudden drop in blood pressure resulting in shock. Mrs. Brown recovers but not until after an extended hospital stay in the intensive care unit. Mrs. Brown sued the nurse and the hospital for negligence. The jury found the nurse liable for negligence and found the hospital vicariously liable because it was the employer. The jury awarded a single sum of money, $50,000, against both the hospital and the nurse jointly even though the nurse was negligent and the hospital's responsibility was based solely on the theory of respondeat superior. The hospital paid the $50,000 to Mrs. Brown and in accordance with its policy, did not exercise its right of indemnification and did not ask Joe Smith to pay the hospital $50,000.

In this example, the employer-employee relationship existed; Joe Smith was a salaried employee, his hours of work, type of duties, and procedures for carrying out those duties were all controlled by his employer, the hospital. Further, the wrongful act, giving the wrong medication to the wrong patient, occurred while Joe was on his assigned shift performing his assigned duties, and thus the act was "within the scope and course of his employment."

Just as the hospital in the above example was responsible for the acts of its nurses, so is it responsible for the acts of all other employees, professional and nonprofessional, over whom it exercises the requisite degree of control. Thus a hospital will be liable for the negligent acts of technicians, orderlies, transporters, housekeepers, and dietary personnel, etc.

The *"borrowed servant"* theory and the related *"captain of the ship"* doctrine are often mentioned in connection with the principle of respondeat superior. The "borrowed servant" doctrine applies in certain situations, where it is clear that a private physician has the right to control and direct a hospital's employee in the performance of a duty or task. Here then, the physician and not the hospital-employer will be liable for that employee's negligent acts. The "captain of the ship" doctrine, a narrower concept than the "borrowed servant" theory, applies in the operating room setting. Under this doctrine, the surgeon is considered the "captain of the ship," that is, he or she has complete and total control and supervision over the hospital personnel assisting him or her. Thus, the surgeon is responsible for the employee's negligent acts which occur during the procedure. The "captain of the ship" doctrine does not apply outside the operating room setting. It is important to note that the "captain of the ship" doctrine has been increasingly rejected by the courts in various jurisdictions and the current trend is to hold the hospital, rather than the surgeon, responsible under respondeat superior for the actions of its operating room personnel.

In both the "borrowed servant" and "captain of the ship" situation, the key element is the extent and right of control the physician has over the hospital employee whose acts caused the alleged injury. Courts carefully examine and juries decide whether or not a hospital employee truly has become the "borrowed servant" of the physician before vicarious liability can be imposed on the physician for the employee's negligent acts. Generally speaking, in nonoperating room settings, a physician will not be held liable for negligence of a hospital employed nurse in her carrying out his order in the regular course of her duties.

The concept of respondeat superior also plays an important role in the question of the hospital's responsibility for actions of certain members of its medical staff. The hospital is liable under respondeat superior for the actions of those physicians who are employed by the hospital or are under the hospital's direct control and supervision. Interns and residents in a training program are considered hospital employees; they are salaried by the hospital to render care to its patients, they do not have private patients, and they are under the control and supervision of the hospital usually via a physician in chief who is a hospital employee. Because interns and residents fall within the "employee category," because they do not contract privately for services with their patients, and because the hospital has a right of control over them, hospitals are almost always held vicariously liable for their actions.

However, for the most part, hospitals are not held liable for the actions of its private physicians practicing in the hospital or other physicians who act as "independent contractors" and over whom the hospital has no direct control. The private physician is considered an independent contractor because he or she has an independent relationship with the patient apart from the hospital. They make independent judgments regarding care of the patient. The private physician is merely making use of the hospital facilities and support staff for the benefit of the patient and the hospital has no right of control over the medical doctors' actions regarding their patients.

There is, however, an exception to this. A recent trend has emerged where in some settings the hospital has been held vicariously liable for the actions of an independent contractor physician where no employer/employee relationship exists. In these situations, the courts have held that if it appeared to the patient that the physician rendering care to him or her was a hospital employee, and if the patient did not choose the physician himself or herself, then the hospital will be held responsible for the physician's acts under the theory of "ostensible agency."

This principle is most often applied in circumstances where a group of private physicians has contracted with the hospital to render special services, such as anesthetic, radiologic, or emergency room coverage. These physicians are considered independent contractors, and not hospital employees. But some courts have held that patients who come for treatment to the emergency room of a hospital that uses these contracted services do not know that the physicians are not the employees of the hospital and do not choose which physician they want to attend them. In fact, the courts hold, it appears to the patient that the physician is the hospital's employee. The same applies where a hospitalized patient is taken to the radiology department for tests staffed by private physicians who have contracted for the providing of services with the hospital. In the majority of cases, the patient does not select an individual radiologist to conduct the test. The patient accepts treatment from the radiologist assigned and who, although a private physician and an independent contractor, appears to the patient to be a hospital employee and provided to him or her by the hospital to render care.

Hospital Responsibility for Medical Care and Treatment Rendered to Its Patients

Traditionally, hospitals were not considered legally responsible for the negligent actions of those private physicians, chosen by the patients themselves, who utilized the hospital facilities. The hospital was considered to be merely the provider of the physical premises where the physician carried out his or her work. The hospital did not "practice medicine," only the physician did. But the hospital's legal responsibility for the quality of care rendered by private physicians in its facility has expanded greatly in recent years.

This in part is due to emerging case law beginning in 1965 with the Illinois Supreme Court case of *Darling v. Charleston Community Memorial Hospital*, 33 Ill.2d 326, 211 N.E.2d 253, 14 A.L.R.3rd 860 (1965), cert.denied, 383 U.S. 946 (1966). In this case, the plaintiff, Darling, sustained a fracture in his leg during a football game and was taken to Charleston Community Hospital for treatment. There the leg was casted, but severe complications arose resulting in the eventual necessity for amputation of the plaintiff's leg. Plaintiff brought suit against the physician and the hospital. The Illinois Supreme Court held the hospital liable for the patient's injuries and held that the hospital owed a direct duty of care to the patient. This is a landmark decision because it imposed on the hospital the duty to monitor the quality of patient care.

The Darling case has been cited, followed, and expanded upon by courts in various other states. The implications of the Darling decision for hospitals has been widely debated. But it can be said with general accuracy that since the Darling decision the trend has been toward holding the hospital directly responsible for the medical care rendered to its patients. The Court in Darling said:

> The conception that the hospital does not undertake to treat the patient, does not undertake to act through its doctors and nurses, but undertakes instead simply to procure them to act upon their own responsibility, no longer reflects the fact. Present-day hospitals, as their manner of operation plainly demonstrates, do far more than furnish facilities for treatment. They regularly employ on a salary basis a large staff of physicians, nurses and interns, as well as administrative and manual workers, and they charge patients for medical care and treatment, collecting for such services, if necessary, by legal action. Certainly, the person who avails himself of "hospital facilities" expects that the hospital will attempt to cure him, not that its nurses or other employees (sic) will act on their own responsibility.

It seems clear at this point that while the hospital is not legally responsible for the negligent acts of its private physicians acting as independent contractors, a hospital must monitor the quality of patient care and monitor the care being given by its private physicians. A hospital will, in most cases, be held directly liable under the theory of corporate negligence for failing to carefully select its medical staff, periodically review the activities of its physicians, and take necessary action against those physicians when the hospital has knowledge or reason to know that he or she is not performing according to set standards or is incompetent or endangering patient welfare.

Negligence and Malpractice

"Malpractice" is a term often used synonymously with "negligence" in reference to the actions or wrongful acts of physicians, nurses, and other medical professionals. In fact, these terms are not identical but are similar. Negligence is defined in *Black's Law Dictionary* as:

> The omission to do something which a reasonable man, guided by those ordinary considerations which ordinarily regulate human affairs, would do, or the doing of something which a reasonable and prudent man would not do.*

Malpractice is the term for negligence of *professional* persons. Malpractice is defined in *Black's Law Dictionary* as:

> Professional misconduct or unreasonable lack of skill. This term is usually applied to such conduct by doctors, lawyers, and accountants. Failure of one rendering professional services to exercise that degree of skill and learning commonly applied

*Black's Law Dictionary, 5th ed. (St. Paul: West Publishing, 1979) 930.

under all the circumstances in the community by the average prudent reputable member of the profession with the result of injury, loss or damage to the recipient of those services or to those entitled to rely upon them. It is any professional misconduct, unreasonable lack of skill or fidelity in professional or fiduciary duties, evil practice, or illegal or immoral conduct.*

Any individual may be negligent, such as when one drives carelessly and strikes another vehicle, or when a homeowner fails to rope off a hole in his front walk which is not easily visible. But only a professional person, such as a physician, can commit malpractice.

To determine what is or is not negligence the law has developed a measuring scale called the "standard of care." Generally speaking, this "standard of care" is determined by what a reasonably prudent person would do under similar circumstances. This "reasonably prudent person" is more specifically, a hypothetical person with average skills, training, and judgment. This is the yardstick for measuring what others should do in similar circumstances. The person's performance which is being accused of being negligent is then measured against what the reasonable prudent person would have done in similar circumstances. If someone's performance fails to meet the standard, then there is negligence. And if it was foreseeable that failure to meet that standard would cause injury and if the negligence was the direct and proximate cause of injury, then liability will be imposed.

Elements of duty of due care, breach of duty, foreseeability, causation, and damages apply in any situation where a medical professional's acts are challenged as wrongful or negligent by a plaintiff. The standards of care which medical professionals must meet are higher than those imposed upon laypersons. An example of how these elements of negligence apply in the hospital setting in reference to a professional person will be helpful.

Let us assume Jane Doe is a registered nurse in a jurisdiction that permits recovery against nurses for malpractice. Ms. Doe is assigned to give medicine to Mr. James, a patient she is caring for. She misreads the order, which is for 40 mg of Gentamicin, an antibiotic, and instead gives him 400 mg of Gentamicin. This drug is extremely potent and Ms. Doe knows that an excessive dose can cause renal problems. Mr. James suffers renal shutdown and has to be hospitalized for several more weeks. Applying the elements as outlined above, Nurse Doe has a duty to the patient to possess that degree of skill and learning ordinarily possessed by nurses. She also has the duty to meet the standard of care for nurses in this same situation; that is to act as a reasonably prudent nurse would have acted. Here, specifically, to meet that requisite standard of care she should have given the ordered medication to the right patient, in the ordered dose, at the ordered time, and by the ordered mode of administration. This is what a reasonably prudent nurse would have done in this same situation. Ms. Doe deviated from the standard of care (breaching her duty) by failing to give the correct dosage and was thus negligent. If her negligence was the proximate cause of harm to the patient then she will be liable for damages. The burden is on the plaintiff to prove the

*Ibid. 864.

standard and deviation from that standard. It is up to the jury to decide whether the negligent act was in fact the proximate cause of the injury.

But it is important to recognize that not all bad results or unexpected outcomes are the result of negligence or mean liability for the person committing the act. Let's assume Jane Doe gave the correct dosage of medication to the patient. Let's assume further that Mr. James had never taken that medication before and upon inquiry had said he had no known allergies to any drugs. Five minutes after he received the medication he suffered a severe, unanticipated allergic reaction resulting in a cardiac arrest. Here although the medication caused injury to Mr. James, Ms. Doe will not be liable. She met her duty of care. She gave the correct dose to the right patient, at the right time, in the correct manner of administration. She had no reason to know that Mr. James would have an allergic reaction. She did not breach her duty; she was not negligent. Without committing negligence, she cannot be found liable.

It is also important to know that one may be negligent but not held liable if the negligent act does not result in harm to the other party. If Jane Doe gave the wrong dose of medication to Mr. James but he suffered no ill effects, she is still negligent. But because her negligent act caused no harm, she probably will not be held liable for damages.

We have taken a brief look at some of the various types of liability for the hospital, corporate negligence and respondeat superior. General reference has also been made to the employee's own liability for his or her acts. Let us now turn our attention to the liability of the supervisor.

Supervisor's Liability

The health care professional as we have seen can be held personally liable for his or her actions. Many members of this group are supervisors by title and supervise others as a regular part of their job duties. What about that aspect of their job? Can the supervisor be held personally liable for his or her negligent actions *as a supervisor* as well?

The supervisor is not liable for the acts of those supervised on the basis of respondeat superior because the supervisor is not the employer of those he or she supervises. The hospital is the employer and the supervisor has only administrative responsibility for those he or she directs. A supervisor is also not liable just because someone under his or her supervision acts negligently and causes injury to a third party.

But a supervisor's performance will be measured against the standard of care for a reasonably prudent person in the same or similar supervisory position. And if a supervisor fails to meet the standard he or she might be held liable as a supervisor for the harm caused. If a supervisor permits or directs someone to perform a duty which the supervisor knows or reasonably should know that that person is not trained to perform, then the supervisor may be held liable for negligent supervision if that person causes harm.

Let's assume Betty Green is a head nurse in Hospital X, and Hospital X has a provision which states that no nurse employed less than three months shall be allowed to do endotracheal suctioning on her or his own unless the head nurse is familiar with and has reviewed and approved the new employee's performance of that task. Let's say Ms. Burnside, a new employee, has been working under Ms. Green's supervision for one month and Ms. Green has observed Ms. Burnside help another nurse to suction a patient; and the head nurse concluded that Ms. Burnside does not perform the task adequately and needs some additional inservice training. Mr. Kane, a patient, has an order to be suctioned, if needed, and Ms. Green tells Ms. Burnside to suction Mr. Kane. Ms. Burnside does so, but incorrectly, causing injury to the patient's tracheal wall. Ms. Green will probably be held liable for negligent supervision. She had reason to know that Ms. Burnside could not yet adequately and skillfully perform suctioning on a patient on her own.

Liability for the nursing supervisor frequently arises as a result of the actions of nursing students under their direct control and supervision. Supervisors need to exercise particular care in not permitting nursing students and others in training to perform tasks and duties for which they are not yet trained or do not have adequate skill, information, or experience.

Remember the example given earlier where Joe Smith gave the medication intended for Mrs. Jones to Mrs. Brown? Here, Joe had worked on his floor for five years with a good record and no incidents of poor performance or faulty nursing judgment. His head nurse, or supervisor, would not be liable for Joe's negligent act. Since she is not his employer, she is not liable under respondeat superior. And she is not liable as a supervisor because she had no reason to think Joe was not able to properly perform the task of passing out medications. If on the other hand, Joe had made ten similar mistakes in the past several months and the supervisor was aware of this and took no action to counsel or make sure Joe was performing properly, then the supervisor might be held liable for negligent supervision.

Additional Potential Causes for Liability

There are many other areas of hospital activities which have potential for liability of the hospital, its supervisors and its employees. These include obtaining informed consent from patients; following proper admission and discharge procedures to avoid charges of false imprisonment, negligent failure to render treatment or abandonment of care; and careful handling of patient information so as to avoid breach of privacy or patient confidentiality. Hospitals and personnel must also deal with controversial issues fraught with philosophical, moral, legal, and ethical complexities such as abortion and sterilization, the right to die with dignity and many others. But a discussion of these and other issues is beyond the scope of this chapter.

Summary

The hospital's legal responsibility for what occurs on its premises is increasing rapidly and is cause for concern by administrators, supervisors, and employees alike. So too, are the professional members of the health care team being held to stricter and higher standards of care and held liable for their negligent acts. Those practicing in the health care field are well advised to familiarize themselves with the various aspects of their job which could result in liability to themselves or their institution, and exercise caution and care in the performance of their duties.

Part Three

Planning

7

Managerial Planning

Planning is the primary managerial function and the primary task of every manager. It precedes all other functions and is the framework for organizing, staffing, influencing, and controlling. It begins with decision making—the process of selecting from alternatives. Planning is deciding in advance what is to be done in the future. Logically, planning must come before any of the other functions because it determines the framework in which the other functions are carried out. Modern health care centers operate in an environment that is always changing in ways they can neither control nor predict precisely. This increases the need for planning. The only way they can survive is to plan rationally and prepare for change.

Every organization must plan ahead because it dare not face the future unprepared. In planning, management is concerned with formulating strategy, establishing the objectives to be achieved, and determining how to achieve them. Planning information is assembled, the external and internal environments are studied, planning premises are set out, and decisions are made to reach organizational goals. These decisions made in planning provide the other functions with their objectives and standards against which performance is measured.

Thus, when the manager plans a course of action for the future, an attempt is made to achieve a consistent and coordinated structure of operations aimed at the desired results. Of course, plans alone do not bring about these results; to achieve them the operation of the health care center is necessary. But without plans, random activities will prevail, producing confusion and possibly even chaos.

The Nature of Planning

Planning as a Continuous Mental Process and Primary Function

Planning is mental work, and for many managers it is therefore quite difficult to perform. But there is no substitute for the hard thinking that planning demands. It is necessary to think before acting and base actions on facts

70

rather than guesses. For this reason, planning is the primary function that must come before the manager can intelligently perform any of the other managerial functions. Only after having made the plans can the supervisor organize, staff, influence, and control. How could a supervisor properly and effectively organize the workings of the department without having a plan in mind? How could the department head effectively staff and supervise the employees without knowing which avenues to follow and without knowing what the objectives are? And how could the activities of the employees possibly be controlled? None of these functions could be performed without having been planned first.

However, planning does not end abruptly when the supervisor begins to perform the other functions. It should not be a process used only at occasional intervals or when the manager is not too engrossed in the daily chores. Rather, planning is a continuous process that must be used consistently every day. By day-to-day planning, the supervisor realistically anticipates future problems, analyzes them, determines their probable effect on the activities, and decides on the plan of action that will lead to the desired results. In other words, it was decided in advance which of the alternative courses are to be followed, which policies, procedures, and methods will be used as the basis of operations.

Planning as a Task of Every Manager

The question often has been raised as to who does the planning. It is the managers who do the planning, and it is the job of every manager whether that person is the chairman of the board, chief administrator of a hospital, or supervisor of a small department. By definition, all of them are managers, and therefore all of them must do the planning. As noted in Chapter 2, however, the importance and magnitude of plans will depend on the level on which they are determined. Naturally, planning on the top level of administration is more fundamental and more far reaching. In the supervisory levels of management, the scope and extent of planning become narrower and more detailed. Thus, the chief administrator is concerned with the overall aspects of planning for the entire health care center, for example, construction of new buildings, adding new specialties, enlarging the emergency facilities, and so on. Planning for new facilities encompassed most of the long-range planning during the 1960s. Today's long-range planning must make certain that the health care center's services are appropriate and necessary; it probably will also include plans for shared services and linkages with other health care providers. In descending the managerial hierarchy, an example of long-range planning for the nursing director includes writing objectives for patient care, setting priorities, and determining activities to fulfill these objectives. The supervisor is concerned with plans for getting the job in the department done promptly and effectively each and every day.

Although planning is the manager's function, this does not mean that others should not be called on to give advice. A supervisor may feel that certain areas of planning require special knowledge, such as those areas dealing with personnel policies, accounting procedures, or technical aspects. In such instances, the supervisor must feel free to call on specialists within the organization to help with the planning responsibilities. In other words, a manager should avail himself or herself of all possible help to plan effectively. But in the final analysis, it is still the manager's personal responsibility to plan.

Planning as a Cost Saver

Planning is important because it makes for purposeful organization and activities, which in turn minimize costs. Deciding in advance what is to be done, how and by whom, where it is to be done, and when promotes efficient and orderly operations. All efforts are directed toward a desired result. Hap hazard approaches are minimized, activities are coordinated, and duplications are avoided. A minimum amount of time is needed for the completion of each planned activity because only the necessary amount of work is done. Facilities are used to their best advantage, and guesswork is eliminated. Thus, planning by its very nature is a cost-saving activity that no manager can afford to neglect.

Effective management demands optimal use of the organization's resources. As a supervisor you are entrusted with the management of both employees and physical resources of the department. You have to work with people and factors, such as space, equipment, tools, and materials. How all these resources are utilized is your primary responsibility and the basis on which your managerial performance is judged.

Only by planning will you be able to make the best possible use of these resources. Only by planning will you as a supervisor be able to bring out the best in your employees, the most valuable resource you have. Plans for the proper utilization of physical resources are also essential because of the capital investment that the hospital has made in them. Even in the smallest department, the total investment in working space, equipment, tools, materials, and supplies is substantial. Only by planning can all of these resources be utilized most effectively.

The Major Planning Considerations

The Planning Period

For how long a period should the manager plan? Usually a distinction is made between long-range, intermediate, and short-range planning. The exact definitions of long-range and short-range planning depend on the manager's level in the organizational hierarchy, the type of institution, and the kind of activity in which it is engaged. For all practical purposes, however, short-term planning can be defined as planning that covers a period of up to 1 year. Long-term planning usually involves a considerably longer interval of time. In recent years, there has been an increasing trend to plan for 5, 10, or even 20 years ahead. The board and the administrator must plan along these lines, in addition to making short-term plans. Planning for 1 to 5 years is often called intermediate planning.

It is likely that the supervisor's planning period will be short range, that is, planning for 1 year at the most, or maybe for 6 months, 1 month, 1 week, or perhaps even just for 1 day. There are activities in certain departments for which a supervisor can definitely plan 3, 6, 9, or 12 months in advance; for instance, the planning of preventative maintenance. On the other hand, with certain activities in a health facility, supervisory planning will be for a shorter time, namely, a week, a day, or only a shift. Such short-range planning is frequently needed in nursing services. It is more desirable if the supervisor is able to make longer range plans, but for all practical purposes, proper attention must be given to seeing that the work of each day gets accomplished. Such short-range planning for the day is always necessary. It requires the supervisor to take the time to think through the nature and amount of work that is to be done each day by the department, who is to do it, and when. Furthermore, this daily planning must be done ahead of time; many supervisors like to do it at the end of the day or shift, when they can size up what has been accomplished to formulate plans for the following day or shift.

There are occasions when a supervisor will also be involved in long-range plans. For example, the boss may want to discuss planning of other future objectives for the institution. A supervisor may be informed of a contemplated expansion or the addition of new facilities and will be asked to estimate what the department can contribute or what will be needed to achieve the new objectives. Or if the hospital has plans for a day surgical center, the director of nursing, as well as the operating room supervisor, will be involved in such a plan.

From time to time the supervisor might also be requested by the administrator to project the long-run trend of a particular departmental activity, especially if it is apparent that such activity will be affected by major breakthroughs in medical science and technology or by increasing mechanization. Much time and effort will then be spent by the supervisor in making these long-range plans, and even more time will be needed to carry them out once they are made and approved.

Nevertheless, it is important for the supervisor to participate in such long-range planning because the plans may require the reassignment of some of the employees or provide opportunities for employees to acquire additional skills. Or the long-range plans may indicate that subordinates with completely new skills and education are needed and that a search for them must start. Or training in new procedures and new techniques might be necessary as a result of new equipment that will be introduced. In these situations, it is necessary for the supervisors to participate in long-range planning. But most of the time their primary planning period will be of a shorter duration.

The Integration and Communication of Plans

It is always necessary that the short-range plans made by the supervisor be integrated and coordinated with the long-range plans of the top administration. It is wrong to look at long-range planning as an activity separate from short-range planning. Rather, it is essential for the top administration to keep all its managers well informed of the new and existing long-range plans and objectives of the institution and to make certain that the short-range plans of lower level management are in accordance with them. The better informed the supervisors or lower level managers are, the better they will be able to integrate their short-range plans into the overall plans of the health care institution.

All too often, however, there is a gap between the knowledge of top management and lower level management as far as planning is concerned. This gap is often justified by the claim that many of the plans are confidential and cannot be divulged for security reasons. Of course, most employees know that very little can be kept secret in any organization. Therefore, internal security cannot always be used as an excuse. On the other hand, supervisors should realize that there are some limitations and that the top administration does not have to disclose all of its plans as long as lower level managers are made aware of those plans which will directly affect their particular activities.

To this extent, then, plans should be communicated and fully explained to subordinate managers so that they are in a better position to formulate derivative plans for their departments. And by the same token, supervisors should always bear in mind that their own employees will be affected by the plans that they make. Since employees are needed to execute whatever has been planned, the supervisor is well advised to take them into his or her confidence and explain in advance what is being planned for the department. The supervisor may even want to consult the employees and ask for suggestions, since some of them may even be in a position to make helpful contributions. The supervisor should also bear in mind that well-informed employees always are better employees who appreciate the fact that they have not been kept "in the dark."

Different Types of Plans

Objectives

The first step in planning is to develop a statement of the goals or objectives of the institution. They must be expressed clearly and communicated fully so that all managers have a common understanding around which to coordinate their activities. Effective management is always management by objectives. This holds true for the chief executive officer of a hospital, as well as for the supervisor on the firing line, and for all managers on the levels in between. Formulating objectives should therefore be foremost in every manager's mind. Additional plans, such as policies, procedures, methods, rules, and performance standards, are then derived from the objectives. Moreover, the objectives will largely determine how the managers go about their organizing, staffing, and influencing functions. And, of course, controlling would be meaningless without objectives as guidelines.

Primary Objectives

The very first step in planning is a statement of the overall, or primary, objectives to be achieved by the enterprise. Every member of the organization should be familiar with this statement of objectives, because it outlines the goals and end result toward which all plans and activities are directed. The objectives constitute the purpose of the health care center, and without them no intelligent planning can take place. Setting these overall objectives is a function of the top administration, the board together with the chief administrator. In other words, top administration must clearly define the primary purpose for which the undertaking is organized.

Broadly speaking, in many hospitals we find such primary objectives as providing primary, secondary, or even tertiary care to the sick and injured; research; advancement of medical knowledge; help in the prevention of sickness; education; and training in all the professional and nonprofessional activities customarily associated with a hospital.

In addition, a health care facility can have many other overall objectives, for example, maintaining a fine reputation among hospitals, practicing the best possible medicine, creating a good image in the community, discharging the numerous social and charitable responsibilities, cost effectiveness, and cost containment. Moreover, another essential objective of even not-for-profit health care facilities is to ensure fiscal integrity, operate within available financial resources, and balance a preset budget. There are also other, less tangible, objectives toward which a health care facility will strive. For instance, in relation to their own employees there is the goal of being a good employer. The objective here is to establish the reputation of being a good place for people to work.

Of course, in any organization there is a multitude of objectives, and the real difficulty lies in ranking and balancing them. This is especially true for health care facilities. Although it would go beyond the confines of this book to discuss all of the objectives of the different types of health care facilities, the above examples show sufficiently well the multiplicity and complexity of objectives and why top administration has a continuous challenge in balancing and achieving them. All of the above and many more are important objectives of a health care enterprise, and achieving a proper balance is a demanding and sensitive task for top administration. If the chief executive would choose a single objective to the exclusion of all others, the effectiveness of the hospital's overall performance could be jeopardized. All of this is becoming increasingly difficult because all health care organizations must function in a continuously changing environment, making it necessary to reexamine and review old objectives and add new ones.

Secondary or Departmental Objectives

Although the goals established for an institution as a whole are called the primary objectives, those set up for each of the institution's various departments can be called secondary, supportive, or derivative objectives.

Since each department or division has a specific task to perform, it follows that each must have its own clearly defined objectives as a guide for its functioning. Of course, these secondary goals and objectives of the departments must stay within the overall framework set by the primary objectives and must contribute to the achievement of the overall institutional objectives.

Because they are concerned with only one department, however, the secondary objectives are necessarily narrower in scope. Whereas the overall objectives are broad and general, the objectives of a department have to be much more specific and detailed to serve as specific guides for subordinate units. They enable departmental managers to operate at their own discretion, although always within the limits of the overall hospital goals. For instance, the objective that "the welfare of the patients is the foremost concern in our institution" will permeate all of them.

This may become clearer if we use as an example the stated objectives of the hospital's medical records department, also known as medical information services. The objective is to provide management of total medical information systems and analysis of data generated by those systems. This medical record is compiled during the treatment of each patient and preserves all information about a person's illness or injury as noted by the medical team that has contributed to the patient's health care. This is to be used as a permanent record in case of future illness, an aid in clinical and statistical research, an administrative tool for planning and evaluating the hospital's programs, and a legal protection for the patient, hospital, and physician. An additional objective is to collect, analyze, and publish various hospital and diagnostic statistics. Furthermore, the medical information services are to review in retrospect the quality of care and be concurrently involved in utilization review.

In another example, the nursing department's objectives could state that its mission is to provide superior patient care within selected specialties in which it has demonstrated ability; that this includes primary care,* secondary care, and possibly tertiary care; that this care is provided in the context of a medical education program, and possibly in an academic medical center setting. Figure 7-1 illustrates the objectives and philosophy of a large teaching hospital.

Obviously, these departmental objectives are quite specific, but their fulfillment contributes significantly to the achievement of overall hospital goals. As a matter of fact, the primary hospital objectives could not be achieved if these and all other departmental objectives were not fulfilled.

Integration Between Objectives and Review

It is essential for all supervisors and their employees to clearly understand not only the objectives of their own department but also those of the entire institution. The two sets of objectives must be carefully defined and stated, so that they can be integrated, coordinated, and explained on the

---

*Primary care means ambulatory, emergency, and initial physician contact; secondary care refers to high-morbidity, low-mortality, inpatient care provided by specialists; and tertiary care means high-mortality, low-morbidity, and highly sophisticated and specialized inpatient care.

Figure 7-1

Barnes Hospital Nursing Service Philosophy
(1 of 1)

Documentation Number _____ ii _____
Implementation Date _____ 1/84 _____
Replaced Document Number ____ 2 (8/78) ____
New Policy _____
Revised Policy _____ X _____
Next Review Date _____ 10/84 _____

Nursing is the individualized process of caring for and supporting patients as they progress through the changing levels of health.

We are committed to the development of patient-centered nursing care and the accountability of individual professional nurses for specific patient care through the nursing process. This process includes assessment of patients' health care problems, planning for and instituting goal-directed nursing activities and critically evaluating the effectiveness on a continual basis.

We support the dignity of the individual and believe that patients have the right to respectful care. We believe that nurses are patients' advocates, who participate in communications relative to the various aspects of patient care and the coordination of that care. Collaboration with other health care professionals and support of therapeutic medical treatment is recognized as essential throughout the process of care. We believe that patients and/or their important others should be included in the development and evaluation of their care.

We are committed to health teaching which promotes an optimum level of functioning. We believe that discharge planning, which provides for the transition from hospital to community, is an integral part of the patients' plan of care.

We believe that professional growth of nurses is related to the development of competency in nursing practice and the acceptance of responsibility for one's own actions and judgments. We provide experiential and educational opportunities which support professional growth and recognize that research activities are necessary to the continued development of nursing practice.

In response to expressed health needs of the community, we accept the responsibility to share relevant knowledge and information. We recognize that the community has the right to expect care to be provided in a manner which demonstrates concern for cost effectiveness.

Reprinted with special permission from Barnes Hospital, St. Louis.

departmental level. The supervisor must bear in mind that the successful completion of a task depends on the full understanding of its purpose by those who have to carry it out. It is therefore good management to make certain that all employees at all levels are thoroughly informed and indoctrinated about the objectives to be achieved.

Since every health care center operates in an ever-changing environment, contingencies will arise that might necessitate a change in the thrust of the enterprise. This can create the need for change of the objectives. Therefore, reviewing the hospital's objectives from time to time is a managerial duty.

Management by Objectives

To achieve specific results from these departmental objectives so that the organizational overall goals are fulfilled, more and more organizations are

using a process called *management by objectives (MBO).* The term and concepts
were first introduced by Peter Drucker* in the early 1950s and have become
very popular since then. Managers in health care organizations should be
familiar with the MBO concept, since its use in their activity is increasing.

MBO is an integrative management concept, containing elements of
the planning function, together with participative management, motivation,
and controlling. It demonstrates the interrelationships of the managerial functions and the systems approach to management. Therefore, MBO will also be
discussed in other appropriate sections of this text. At this time, however, we
are primarily concerned with the meaning of MBO in connection with setting
and achieving departmental objectives.

MBO is a process whereby a manager at any level and that individual's
immediate subordinate jointly develop goals, in accordance with the overall
organizational goals. Once the latter are clarified, the manager and the subordinate together should develop and agree on the subordinate's goals to be
achieved during a stated time period. To be operational, these performance
objectives set must be *specific, measurable (quantifiable),* and realistically *at-
tainable* by the subordinate within the frame established. This means that
each objective must provide a plan showing the work to be done, the time
frame, and the individual who will accomplish it. There must be quantitative
indicators to measure the work achieved. To be realistic it should be possible
to carry out the activity within the time frame set, a frame long enough to get
the objective done, but short enough to provide timely feedback and still permit intervention if necessary.

The important point is that these goals are jointly established and
agreed on ahead of time. At the end of the period, both participate in the
review of the subordinate's performance to see how results for the period
compare with the objectives he or she set out to accomplish. If the goals were
achieved, new goals will be set for the next period. If there is a discrepancy,
efforts are made to find steps to overcome these problems, and new goals for
the next period are agreed on. It is obvious that MBO is a powerful tool in
achieving involvement and commitment of subordinates. In addition to these
motivational aspects, MBO also helps in the manager's controlling function.

Additional Types of Plans

Once the objectives have been determined, managers can make the
rest of the plans necessary to implement them. A number of different types of
plans are devised to implement objectives: policies, procedures, methods,
rules, programs, projects, and budgets. All of these plans must be designed to
reinforce one another, in other words, they must be integrated and coordinated. Since every manager will probably have to devise or at least use each
type of plan at some time, he or she should be familiar with the meaning of all
of them. Of course, the major plans are formulated by the chief executive, but

*Peter F. Drucker, *The Practice of Management* (New York: Harper & Row, Inc., 1954); John W.
Humble, *Management by Objectives in Action* (New York: McGraw-Hill Book Co., 1970); and
George S. Odiorne, *Management by Objectives* (New York: Pitman Publishing Corporation, 1965).

all department supervisors will have to formulate their own departmental plans accordingly. The purpose of these plans is to ensure that the thinking and actions taken on different levels and in different departments of the institution are consistent with and contribute to the overall objectives.

The different kinds of plans referred to above can be divided into repeat-use plans and single-use plans. Objectives, policies, procedures, methods, and rules are commonly known as repeat-use, or standing, plans because they are followed each time a given situation is encountered. In other words, they are used again and again. They are applicable whenever a situation presents itself that is similar to the one for which the standing plan was originally devised.

The opposite of repeat-use plans are those plans which are no longer needed once their objective is accomplished. They are known as single-use, or single-purpose, plans. Once the goal is reached, the plan is used up. Within this single-use plan category, we find programs, projects, and budgets.

Repeat-Use or Standing Plans

Policies

Among the various plans a manager must devise and depend on, policies are probably the most frequently used and mentioned. *Policies are broad guides to thinking.* They are general statements that channel the thinking of all personnel charged with decision making. Although they are broad, policies do have definite limitations. As long as a supervisor stays within these limitations, he or she will make an appropriate decision, one that conforms to the policy. Thus, policies serve to keep decision makers on the right track, and in this way they facilitate the job of both managers and subordinates. Policies ensure uniformity of decision making throughout the organization.

The Flexibility of Policies

Defining a policy as a broad guide to thinking implies a certain amount of flexibility. Although policies must be consistent to successfully coordinate the activities of each day in a modern health care center, they must also be flexible. Some policies even have flexibility explicitly stated by such words as "whenever possible," "whenever feasible," or "under usual circumstances." For instance, one of the most commonly used policies today is the following: "Our hospital believes and practices promotion from within whenever possible." If these clauses are not built in, then the manner in which the supervisor applies the policy will determine its degree of flexibility. The supervisor must intelligently adapt the policy to the existing set of circumstances. Such flexibility, however, must not lead to inconsistency; policies must be administered by supervisors in a consistent manner. Anything else would defeat the basic purpose of a policy, namely, its effort to provide subordinate managers with a uniform guide for thinking.

Policies as an Aid in Delegation

By issuing policies, top administration sanctions in advance the decisions made by subordinate managers, as long as they stay within the broad policy guidelines. After having set policies, a superior manager should feel reasonably confident that whatever decisions the subordinate managers make will fall within the limits of the policies. In fact, the subordinates will probably come up with just about the same decisions that the superior manager would have made. Hence, policies make it easier for the superior to delegate authority to the subordinates. By the same token, policies are a great help to the subordinate managers also. They provide specific guidelines for their thinking that facilitate decision making and at the same time ensure uniformity of decisions throughout the enterprise. Therefore, the clearer and more comprehensive the policy guides are, the easier and better it will be for the superior managers to delegate authority and for the subordinate managers to exercise authority.

The Origin of Policies

Obviously, policies do not come about by chance. They are determined by management, particularly by the higher administrative levels. Indeed, to formulate policies is one of the most important functions of top management. The top manager is in the best position to establish the various types of overall policies that will enable the enterprise's objectives to be achieved. Once the broad policies have been set by the top administrator, they in turn will become the guides for various policies covering divisions and departments, for example, nursing policies. Such divisional and departmental policies are originated by the various managers lower in the managerial hierarchy. This type of policy formulation, originated by the top administrative level and pursued by the lower levels, is the most important source of policies.

There are occasions, however, when a supervisor may have a problem situation for which no policies appear to exist. In such a dilemma, the supervisor has only one choice; that is, to go to the boss and simply ask whether or not any of the existing policies are applicable. If none applies, then the supervisor will appeal to the boss to issue a policy to cover such situations. Suppose, for instance, that one of your employees asks for a leave of absence. To make the appropriate decision, you would like to be guided by a broad policy, so that whatever decision you arrive at would be in accord with all other decisions regarding leaves of absence. You may find, however, that the administrator never issued any policies on granting or denying a leave of absence. Instead of making an individual decision, you ask your boss to issue a policy, a broad guide for thinking to be applied whenever leaves of absence are requested. It is not likely that you will have to make such a request very often because a good administrator usually foresees most of the areas in which policies are needed. On occasion, however, you may have to appeal to your own boss, stimulating the formulation of what is known as *appealed policy*.

In addition to originated and appealed policies, there are a number of policies that are *imposed* on an organization by external factors, such as the government, accrediting agencies, trade unions, trade associations, and so on. The word imposed indicates compliance with a force that cannot be avoided. For instance, to be accredited hospitals and other health care facilities must comply with certain regulations issued by the accrediting agency. These regulations must be translated into hospital policy, and all employees must abide by them. Another example of an externally imposed policy is the policy of being an equal opportunity employer. Unless the health care center had and practiced such a policy clearly stated before fair employment legislation was promulgated, such a policy statement today can be looked on as one that was externally imposed on the hospital. Any policy forced on the enterprise in this manner is known as an *externally imposed* policy.

Clarity of Policies

Because policies are such a vital guide for thinking and thus for decision making, it is essential that they be stated simply and clearly and communicated so that those in the organization who are to apply them will fully understand their meaning. This is no easy task. It is difficult to find words that will be understood by all people in the same way, since different meanings can be attached to the same word. Although there is no guarantee that even the written word will be properly understood, it still seems desirable that all policies be written. This at least will avoid the added ambiguity of spoken words.

In addition to the benefit of comprehension, many more benefits are derived from written policies. The mere process of writing policies requires the top administrator to think them out clearly and consistently. The subordinate managers can then read them as often as they care to. Moreover, the wording of a written policy cannot be changed by word of mouth because the written policy can always be consulted. Furthermore, written policies are especially helpful for new managers who need immediate help in solving a problem.

Although these advantages are significant, there is one disadvantage connected with written policies. Once they are written down management may become reluctant to change them. Thus, many enterprises prefer to have their policies communicated by word of mouth because they feel that this is more flexible, allowing the verbal policies to be adjusted to different circumstances with greater ease than written policies. But the exact meaning of a verbal policy might become scrambled, making it difficult to apply the policy properly. Thus, written policy statements are generally considered far more desirable.

The Supervisor and Policies

For the most part supervisors do not actually have to issue policies. Instead, they are called on primarily to apply existing policies in making their daily decisions. It is also the supervisors' job to interpret and explain the meaning of policies to the employees of their departments. Although supervisors seldom have to issue policies, they must continuously use them. Therefore, it is essential that they clearly understand the policies and that they learn how to apply them appropriately.

A manager who heads a major department, for example, the director of nursing service, which normally comprises 50 percent of the hospital employees and has several subdivisions within it, may find it necessary to issue and write policies for the department. As a matter of fact the Joint Commission on Accreditation of Hospitals (JCAH) will examine the "Nursing Policies." All of them must reinforce and be in accordance with the overall policies of the entire health care center. Among them we are likely to find a nursing policy stating that the welfare of the patient is the foremost concern of the nursing service and that it takes precedence over all other considerations. In all likelihood the hospital's overall policy of fairness and nondiscrimination will show up in a nursing policy. It may say that patients shall be accorded impartial access to treatment or accommodations, to the extent that they are available and medically indicated, regardless of race, color, creed, or national origin; also that the patient's right to privacy shall be respected, consistent with medical needs, etc.

The director of the nursing service certainly will see that there is a policy for cardiopulmonary resuscitation, also referred to as "code," "no code," or "DNR." This policy in some health care centers will simply state that cardiopulmonary resuscitative measures must be initiated on all patients experiencing cardiac arrest unless a "no code order" has been written by the attending physician. In some hospitals the policy will be broader by reaffirming the traditional role of the physician who, with appropriate regard for the wishes of the patient and concerned family, may determine that heroic resuscitative measures, contrary to the principles of human dignity and humane medical care, should not be carried out. (See Figure 7-3.)

Periodic Review of Policies

Regardless of how well thought out the policies were when originated, policies must change when the organization or environment changes. Because of changing contingencies, the thrust of the enterprise may be changed, and this will create the need for a change in policies. It is therefore necessary to periodically review and appraise policies to see whether they ought to be changed, modified, or completely abandoned. Such an investigation may uncover practices that are a complete contradiction to current written policies. Or it may uncover policies that have become so outdated that no one follows them. In such cases, the top administration must either rewrite or abandon the questionable policies, because an institution certainly cannot afford to let its various subordinate managers decide whether policies are still current or whether they should be observed any longer. Hence, it is absolutely essential for policies to be periodically reviewed by top management and revised if needed.

Figure 7-2. The relationship of policies, procedures, and methods.

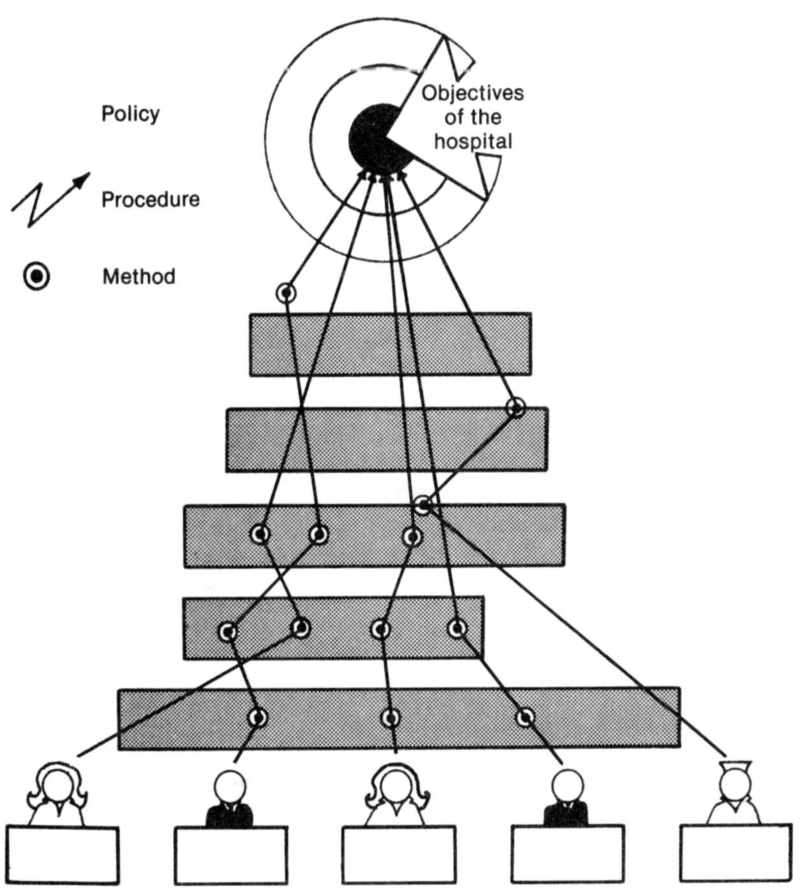

Adapted from Theo Haimann and William G. Scott, *Management in the Modern Organization* (Boston: Houghton Mifflin Co., 1970), 105. Reprinted with permission of the publisher.

Procedures

Procedures, like policies, are also standing plans for achieving the institution's objectives. Procedures are derived from policies. But they are much more specific than policies. Procedures are a *guide to action,* not a guide to thinking. Procedures show the sequence of definite acts. They define a chronological order for the acts that are to be performed. (See Figure 7-2.) Procedures specify a route that will take subordinates between the guideposts of the policies and lead them to the final objectives. In brief, procedures pick a path toward the objectives.

For example, let us recall the policy that stated "Our hospital promotes from within whenever possible." The purpose and objectives of this policy are clear. The procedure designs the steps to be taken in a chronological sequence to fulfill the meaning of the policy. These steps might be stated as follows:

1. Every opening in the hospital must be posted on the employee's bulletin board at the employee's cafeteria for 2 weeks.
2. The potential candidates must be able to obtain a job description from the manager in whose department the job is open.
3. Potential candidates must inform their present boss before arranging for an interview.
4. An interview between the applicant and the head of the department where the opening is will be arranged with the assistance of the personnel department.

There are literally hundreds of procedures in a health care center. Just think of the amount in the nursing service alone, for example, the procedures for medications, intravenous medications, x-ray, examination of critically ill patients, epidermal injections, discharge of patients, and so on.

Or consider, for instance, the need for cardiopulmonary resuscitation in connection with the nursing policy that resuscitative measures must be initiated on all patients who have experienced cardiac arrest unless a "no code order" has been written by the attending physician. Such a procedure is shown in Figure 7-3.

Although supervisors will not have much opportunity to issue policies, there will be many occasions for them to devise and issue procedures. Since supervisors are the managers of the department, they are the ones to determine how the work is to be done. If supervisors were fortunate enough to have only highly skilled employees under their direction, they could depend on them to a great extent to select an efficient procedure. But this is very unlikely, and most employees look to their supervisor for instructions on how to proceed. And, of course, effective work procedures designed by the supervisors will result in definite advantages.

One of these advantages is that the mere process of preparing a procedure necessitates analysis and study of the work to be done. The supervisor is therefore more likely to assign work fairly and to distribute it evenly among the employees. Moreover, once a procedure has been established, it assures uniformity of action. Procedures give us a predictable outcome. In addition to these benefits, procedures provide the supervisor with a standard for appraising the work of the employees. And since a procedure specifies the sequence of actions, it decreases the need for further decision making. This makes the supervisor's job, as well as that of the employees, easier. Naturally, a good supervisor will spend considerable time and effort in devising efficient procedures for the department. From time to time, of course, it will be necessary for the supervisor to review and revise all departmental procedures, since they are likely to become outdated, just as policies do. Because of the advances in medicine, frequently new activities are introduced into the department; then the supervisor's first duty is to write appropriate procedures for them.

**Figure 7-3. Barnes Hospital Nursing Service
Cardiopulmonary Resuscitation (CPR)**

(1 of 3)

Cardiopulmonary Resuscitation (CPR)

Documentation Number ____1C____
NSAB Approved____1/84____

Implementation Date ____1/84____
Replaced Document Number__1C (3/78)__
New Policy ____
Revised Policy ____X____
Next Review Date ____10/84____

I. *Policy*
  A. *Principles to be followed for restriction, limitation, or cessation of therapy:*
    1. The patient's own desires, if willing or able to express them, or as understood by concerned, responsible family members take precedence.
    2. The attending physician bears the ultimate responsibility for the management of his/her patient.
  B. *Recommended procedures for restriction, limitation, or cessation of therapy:*
    1. Recognizing that the care of critically ill patients, including those who are severely impaired and terminally ill, is a group effort and that the ethical, emotional, and legal implications and responsibilities for all of the group are legitimate issues, a review of the therapeutic plan in such situations can be properly initiated either by the attending physician, by the intensive care unit director, via the head nurse, or by other attendants.

    After thorough review and discussion, which should include discussion between the attending physician and the patient, if possible, and with the immediate family and, if uncertainty exists after obtaining additional appropriate consultation when indicated, the planned restrictions, limitations, or cessations of therapeutic measures should be outlined in the hospital record and the necessary orders written by the attending physician.
    2. In order to clarify as precisely as possible for the professional staff the intent and scope of the planned therapy, the Committee recommends that the medical record indicate as precisely as possible what measures are to be excluded; e.g.:
      Cardiopulmonary resuscitation (Standard "CPR")
      Endotracheal intubation
      Mechanical ventilation
      Administration of blood products
      Infusion of vasoactive drugs for the purpose of maintaining arterial pressure
      Antibiotics
      Parenteral nutrition
      Dialysis
      Invasive hemodynamic monitoring
      Withdrawal of blood or body fluids for laboratory analysis
      Return admission to the ICU
      Other (Specify)
    3. Because unanticipated improvement in the clinical course occasionally occurs, it is essential that ongoing re-assessment by the involved professional attendants be carried out. Such significant improvements in the clinical course, together with the subsequent necessary appropriate alternations in therapy, should also be documented on the hospital record.
  C. Cardiopulmonary resuscitation will be initiated on all patients who have arrested unless an order has been written by the attending physician stating no cardiopulmonary resuscitation is to be performed.
  D. Annual re-certification in Cardiopulmonary resuscitation (CPR) is required of all RNs.
II. *Procedure*
  A. *Purpose:* To re-establish and maintain a circulation and ventilation in the event of a cardiac or respiratory arrest.

B. *General Information:*
1. Barnes Hospital standards for basic life support (CPR) are those established by the American Heart Association and set forth in JAMA (August 1, 1980: Volume 244, Number 5, pages 453-509).
2. Basic life support measures (CPR) can and should be initiated immediately without additional equipment.
3. Sustained resuscitative efforts in the hospital setting requires the equipment carried on the Emergency Cart.

C. *Procedure:*
1. Determine that the patient has arrested. Signs of arrest include:
   a. Unresponsiveness
   b. Apnea
   c. Absence of a carotid pulse
   d. Cyanosis
2. Call out for help. *DO NOT LEAVE THE PATIENT.*
3. Begin resuscitative measures:
   a. Place patient in supine position on a hard surface.
   b. Establish an open airway. Clear the airway, hyperextend neck, lift chin, and observe for spontaneous resumption of respirations.
      PRECAUTION: Only the jaw thrust maneuver should be used in the presence of neck or possible C-Spine injury. Do not hyperextend neck.
   c. If no spontaneous respirations, ventilate four times using mouth-to-mouth or mouth-to-stoma, as appropriate. *DO NOT WAIT FOR AN AMBU BAG.*
   d. Check for carotid pulse.
   e. If pulse is absent, begin one-person CPR (15 compressions to 2 breaths). If pulse is present, observe for respiratory activity and continue to support as necessary.
4. On arrival, the assisting staff member(s) will:
   a. Summon the arrest team:
      1) Call 2700 and state, "Code 7" and the location.
      2) Outside of patient care areas, call the Emergency Department (ext. 2604) who will also respond.
   b. Bring emergency equipment to the arrest.
   c. Insert an oral airway and begin two-person CPR (5 compressions to 1 breath).
      NOTE: Because of the difficulty in maintaining a seal with the mask, it may not be possible to use an ambu bag with two-person CPR. Use of mouth-to-mouth or mouth-to-mask technique may be required until a third person is available.
5. On arrival, the arrest team will implement further measures:
   a. The patient's managing resident will assume charge of the medical aspects of the resuscitation. In his absence, the medical resident on the arrest team will assume control.
   b. The charge nurse will assume charge of the nonmedical aspects. In a nonpatient area, this responsibility passes to the Clinical Director of Nursing:
      1) Assignment of staff
      2) Removal of excess furniture and equipment and nonessential personnel from the area.
      3) Disposition of any roommates, visitors, and other nonstaff people.
      4) Determination that all members of the arrest team (medical resident, surgical resident, anesthetist, respiratory therapist, EKG technician, dispatch) have arrived. (Central Paging, ext. 2666, will call the patient care area to check if all the arrest team have arrived. If not, Central Page will reach those who have not arrived.)
      5) Initiation of call to house staff, if not present, and the attending physician of any private patient.
      6) Assurance of physician's notification of family, if not present.
   c. Other nursing responsibilities:
      1) Set-up of IV fluids.
      2) Preparation and administration of IV medications as ordered.

    3) Maintenance of the cardiac arrest worksheet.

    4) Disposition of specimen.

    5) Supportive care for family members present.

III. *Charting*

A. The nursing note should contain the fact of the arrest, initiation of CPR, and a reference to the cardiac arrest worksheet. A second note should contain the outcome and/or disposition of the patient.

B. The cardiopulmonary resuscitation worksheet should be used to record patient condition, therapeutic interventions, and their outcomes. The "Response to Treatment" section is to be used to note vital signs and other information not recorded elsewhere and to expand upon data charted in other areas. It is to be signed by both the physician and the nurse in charge.

References:

A. Medical Staff Bylaws Rules and Regulations, Rule Number 27, approved by Medical Advisory Committee September 17, 1982.

B. JAMA, August 1, 1980: Volume 224, Number 5, pages 453-509.

Methods

A method is also a plan for action, but a plan that is even more detailed than a procedure. Whereas a procedure shows a series of steps to be taken, a method is concerned only with a single operation, with one particular step. The method tells exactly how this particular step is to be performed. (See Figure 7-2.)

For instance, one of the nursing procedures specifies step by step how narcotics are to be accounted for at the beginning of each shift by a nurse going on duty and a nurse going off duty. For each step in this procedure there exists a method. For example, one method tells exactly what is to be done in case of unavoidable waste or accidental destruction of a controlled substance; this must be recorded on the narcotics form by the nurse involved, and another professional nurse must witness the form. The remnants, if possible, are to be returned to the pharmacy.

For the majority of work done by the employees of a department there exists a "best method," a best way for doing the job. Again, if the supervisor had only highly skilled subordinates, they would probably know the best method without having to be told. But, in most cases, it is necessary for the supervisor to specify for the employees exactly what is considered the best method in their health care center. Indeed, a large amount of the supervisor's time is spent in devising methods. But once a method has been devised, it carries with it all the advantages of a procedure, as cited above, such as uniformity of action, predictability of outcome, standard for appraisal, etc. In determining the best method, a supervisor may occasionally need to enlist the help of a professional, such as a physician, surgeon, pathologist, biochemist, methods engineer, or time and motion specialist if such a person is available in the organization. Most of the time, however, the supervisor's own experience is probably broad enough to allow him or her to design the "best" work methods.

Standard Procedures and Practices

In some activities of the hospital there will be little need for the supervisor to be overly concerned with devising procedures and methods because
the employees will already have been thoroughly trained in standard practices and procedures. For instance, nurses, technologists, technicians, and
medical specialists receive many years of schooling and training, during
which great emphasis is placed on the proper procedures and methods for
performing certain tasks. In managing a department in which such highly
skilled employees are at work, the supervisor's job is simplified. One of the
main concerns is to see to it that good, generally approved procedures and
methods are carried out in a professionally accepted way.

However, even then, most health care centers "do things differently
from everyone else," and, even after many years of experience in other health
care settings, new employees have to become familiar with the procedures,
methods, and idiosyncrasies of the new hospital. The same holds true for recent baccalaureate graduates of nursing programs. Regardless of how much
experience a nurse had in another hospital, and regardless of how much has
been taught in school, almost each health care center has its own way of "doing things," for example, collecting specimens, distributing medication,
handling emergency measures, and so on. Therefore, in all likelihood new
employees will go through an indoctrination program of many weeks to
familiarize them with the procedures and methods of the hospital before they
are placed into permanent positions.

Rules

A rule is different from a policy, procedure, or method, although it is
also a standing plan that has been devised to attain the enterprise's objectives.
A rule is not like a policy because it does not provide a guide to thinking; it
does not leave any discretion to the party involved. It is, however, related to a
procedure insofar as it is a guide to action and states what must or must not be
done. But a rule is not the same as a procedure because it does not specify a
time sequence for the particular action. Rules pertain whenever and
wherever they are in effect. No smoking, for instance, is a rule that could be
made by management, probably just one of a long list of safety rules. This rule
is a guide to action, or more precisely a guide to inaction. But there is no order
of steps involved, it is simply no smoking wherever and whenever it is in effect.

Rules develop from policy; they are not part of it. For example, the hospital's safety policy is to make the facility a safe place for the patients, employees, and visitors. Safety considerations play an important role in all procedures and methods, and the no smoking rule is just an outgrowth of the
original safety policy.

It is the supervisor's duty to apply and enforce the rules and regulations of the health care center uniformly, whether they are defined by higher
management or set by the supervisor. There will be many occasions when

supervisors have to set their own rules. For example, the dress code for the hospital may state that employees must come to work "appropriately attired" for their job. This broad and general rule gives the director of the nursing service the right and obligation to devise a more detailed dress code for the nursing personnel; the operating room supervisor in turn would decide on a special dress code for those working in the surgical areas. Since supervisors have the obligation to see that rules are observed, they should be involved in the design of these rules. Of course, these rules are developed from hospital policies and must reinforce and support them and not contradict them.

Single-Use Plans

In the preceding pages we have discussed a variety of plans, such as objectives, policies, procedures, methods, and rules. They are commonly known as repeat-use, or standing, plans because they are plans that are followed each time a given situation is encountered. In other words, they are used again and again. The opposite of repeat-use plans is single-use plans, plans that are no longer needed once their objective is accomplished. Once the goal is reached, the plan is used up. Within this single-use plan category, we find programs, projects, and budgets.

Programs and Projects

Programs are a complex set of plans to reach a specific major undertaking within the organization's overall objectives. They may have their own policies, procedures, and budgets and may extend over several years. For instance, building a new wing with 100 beds is a major one-time undertaking. Such a program, of necessity, involves a multitude of derivative plans, each of which can be considered a project, such as securing the financing for the new construction, publicity for the local community, information for the local medical society, and recruiting nursing and other needed personnel. A project is an undertaking that can be planned and executed as a distinct entity within the overall program; all projects must be coordinated and synchronized so that the major program will become reality. Programs and projects are single-use plans; once they are achieved, they are filed away. From time to time, someone may look at them again, but very likely only for historical reasons. Once accomplished, these single-use plans have served their purpose and are finished. Planning such a program is usually top administration's concern, whereas supervisors and department heads will be involved in one of its many projects only.

Budgets

Budgets are usually thought of only in connection with the controlling function; but this is too narrow a view. Budgets are also plans, plans that express the anticipated results in numerical terms, be this in dollars and cents, nursing hours, staff hours, kilowatt hours, or tests to be run; materials; or any other unit that is used to perform work or measure specific results. However, since most values are ultimately convertible to monetary terms, and since the overall budgets for the entire institution are expressed in the one common denominator, money, all budgets are eventually translated and expressed in monetary terms. Although budgets are an important tool for controlling, preparing and making a budget certainly are part of the planning function, and, as we know, planning is the duty of every manager. Using the budget and living with it is part of the manager's controlling function, and this will be discussed in Chapter 26.

Since a budget is a plan expressed in numerical units, it has the distinct advantage that the goal is stated in exact and specific terms instead of in generalities. The figures put into a budget represent actual plans that will become the standards to be achieved. These plans are not mere projections or general forecasts, but will be considered as a basis for daily operations. They will be looked on as goals and standards to live up to.

A health care center designs a number of budgets, such as income or revenue budgets, capital expenditure budgets, expense budgets, etc. The expense budget is the supervisor's major concern because it defines the limits of the various departmental expenditures for a stated period of time, usually one year. All of the following comments refer to budgets of this nature because the departmental expenses for salaries and wages, materials, supplies, utilities, equipment rentals, travel, etc., are a challenge and of great concern to the department head.

Because budgets are so important for the daily operations of every department, it is essential for supervisors who have to use them to participate in their preparation. It is only natural that people resent arbitrary orders, and this applies to budgets. Thus, it is necessary that all budget objectives and allowances be determined with the full input of those who are responsible for executing them. Every supervisor should actively participate in the budget-making process for his or her unit, and this should not be mere pseudoparticipation. They should participate in what is commonly known as *grass roots budgeting*. The subordinate managers should be allowed to submit their own budgets. Of course, each supervisor will have to substantiate the budget proposals in a discussion with the boss and possibly with top administration, where the budgets are finalized. Indeed, this is what is meant by active real participation in budget making, and this ensures the effectiveness of the process. Such participation, however, should not be construed to mean that the suggestion of the supervisor will always or completely prevail. The supervisor's budget should not be accepted by the superior manager if the latter believes it is based on plans that are inadequate, overstated, or incorrect. Differences between budget estimates should be carefully discussed by the supervisor and superior manager, but the final decision rests with higher management. Nevertheless, if a budget is arrived at with the participation of the supervisors, then the likelihood that they will live up to it is better than if the budget had been handed down to them by their boss.

In conclusion, it is important to remember that the budget is a single-use plan. It will serve only for the period for which it is drawn up. When the period is over, this budget is no longer valid. A new budget will have to be drawn up, and a new planning period will be established. Last year's budget usually serves as a guideline for next year's budget, unless the health care center practices zero-based budgeting. Zero-based budgeting is a fairly new concept. Instead of accepting current expenditures as a base for the new budget, zero-based budgeting requires that all expenditures—new and existing—must be justified, reassessed, and approved from the very beginning.

Summary

Planning is the managerial function that determines in advance what is to be done in the future. It is the function of every manager, ranging from the top administrator to the supervisor of each department. Planning is important because it assures the best utilization of resources and economy of performance. The planning period on the supervisory level is usually much shorter than the period on the top administrator's level. Nevertheless, the short-range plans of the supervisor must coincide with the long-range plans of the enterprise.

Setting objectives is the first step in planning. Although the overall objectives are determined by the top administration, many secondary objectives must be clarified by the supervisor and must be in accordance with the primary objectives of the overall undertaking. To reach all the objectives, different kinds of plans must be devised. Policies are one kind of plan. They are guides to thinking, and the majority of them originate with the chief administrator. In most cases, the supervisor's concern with policies is primarily one of interpreting them, applying them, and staying within them whenever decisions are made for the department. There may be occasions, however, when the supervisor has to appeal to the boss for the issuance or clarification of certain policies. Although supervisors do not usually originate policies, they will often be called on to design procedures and methods. These types of plans are guides for action, not guides for thinking. The supervisor also will participate in the establishment of budgets, which are plans expressed in numerical terms.

8

Supervisory Planning

Much of the success of a health care center depends to a large degree on the skill of all its managers in foreseeing and preparing for the future. Planning, as we have said, is deciding in advance what is to be done in the future. Although the future is fraught with uncertainties, the manager must make certain assumptions about it in order to plan. These assumptions are based on forecasts of what the future will hold. Since the appraisal of future prospects is inherent in all planning, the success of an enterprise depends in large measure on the skill of management first in forecasting and then in preparing for the future conditions.

Forecasts as the Basis of Planning

Administrative Forecasts

All managers must make some assumptions about the future. The president, however, must forecast the future in a much more far-reaching manner than a supervisor would do. But since both are managers, both must make forecasts. Such forecasts are possible in widely diverse areas. Normally, of course, management confines its forecasting effort to factors that experience suggests are important to its own planning. Thus, the chief administrator of a hospital or related facility would select and use primarily those forecasts which have a direct material bearing on the health care field.

In the endeavor to predict the outlook of things to come, one of the factors the administrator will be concerned with is the general economic and political climate in which the institution must operate during the next few years. This includes government attitudes, government spending policies, and possible future legislation that would ultimately affect the activities of hospitals and other health facilities. The administrator will try to predict the general trends for the delivery of health care as it relates to cost effectiveness and enlightened users' reactions. There will be a concern for the outlook of monetary policy, the overall economic activities within the country, inflationary trends, and so on. The administrator will be vitally interested in forecasts of changes in our population and will pay serious attention to forecasts for, say, the year 2000 when the United States population is expected to range between 245 and 280 million people.* The birth rate is going down and with it the overall population growth. We will see the impact of this on every organized activity because population trends are critical planning premises that affect most organizations' long-range strategies. The breakdown of population figures according to age patterns will be even more meaningful, depending on whether we are planning for a general short-term hospital, long-term health care facility, or nursing home.

All of these environmental, economic, and political conditions will affect the operations of a health care facility. Since the administrator's job is to take the broad and long-run outlook, forecasts in these far-reaching fields are necessary.† Although not directly concerned with making such overall assumptions, lower level managers will ultimately be affected by them.

Supervisory Forecasts

Scientific and Technological Developments

When it comes to departmental forecasts, supervisors will have to make certain assumptions as to what the future will hold. But their assumptions will cover a much narrower field. A supervisor must try to forecast only those factors which may have some bearing on the future of his or her department. For example, it should be determined whether there is a growing trend for simplification of the function overseen or whether this function seems to be of increasing or decreasing significance. It is important to keep abreast of developments in technology and automation. For example, much of the nurses' time formerly was spent in preparing supplies for sterilization or sharpening and sterilizing needles. With the advent of prepackaged, sterilized disposables all this time is now utilized in different endeavors. Based on what has happened in the past, the supervisor should venture some kind of assumption as to what the future will hold in this respect. In making such as assumption, one can look to the sources of supplies and equipment used for assistance. Much can be learned by attending meetings, exhibitions, and so on. Medical advances and technology are progressing so rapidly that in a number of years the department's functions may be significantly different from what they had been or are today. Consider, for instance, the impact of further mechanization in laboratories or the impact of disposable products on the laundry department. Such a projection of the future would be essential for laboratory supervisors and laundry managers in order to plan properly.

---

*U.S. Department of Commerce, Social, and Economic Statistics Administration, Bureau of the Census, "Population Estimates and Projections," *Current Population Reports*, Series P-25, No. 704 (July, 1974).

†Hospital administrators do not, of course, have to actually do the research and statistical analysis for all forecasts themselves. They frequently use already published statistics and forecasts made available by experts in various fields. For example, population forecasts would generally come from studies of the United States Bureau of the Census.

Employees and Skills

Supervisors will also have to make forecasts in relation to the kind of employees who will be working. The need for employees who are better educated and more skilled and whose increasing demands the department must be ready to meet may be in the forecast. This refers both to monetary demands and also to demands that the position offer enough of a continuous challenge. For example, supervisors may find that the current pattern of wages and fringe benefits will not be satisfactory in the future, and they would be well advised to plan accordingly at an early time. Similarly, they should be aware of the noneconomic demands that young people coming out of school, whether it is a university, junior college, vocational training program, or high school, expect to fulfill on their jobs. Meeting both types of demands will be particularly important if supervisors have to look for people who possess skills that up to now have never been required in the department or perhaps anywhere in the hospital. It is conceivable that more knowledge in chemistry, physics, electronics, and mechanical engineering could be helpful to nursing personnel working in specialized fields.

A supervisor may also discover a trend toward the upgrading of changes of certain duties. For instance, the supervisor of the operating rooms might foresee an increasing number of operating room technicians. Plans for the impact that this will have on the position of graduate operating room nurses must be made. Or the director of the nursing services might have to view the future in terms of more nurse specialists, more physicians' assistants, and so forth.

On the other hand, it may very well be that because of increased mechanization, fewer people will be necessary to perform the functions currently performed. Indeed, a supervisor might find that the department he or she is supervising will lose its function altogether. It is conceivable that new discoveries or new means of doing the work may make an entire department obsolete. Although this is not a very pleasant thought, it is better for the supervisor to realize it early instead of being confronted with such an event without having prepared for it. If obsolescence is threatened, the farsighted supervisor should inform the superior manager accordingly. Sooner or later the administrator should think of creating a new supervisory position for the supervisor who has been so farsighted. This person is too valuable an employee to lose and can probably be just as good in the supervision of another department, perhaps a department that previously has never existed. In such a case, the supervisor will probably have to acquire special skills with which he or she has not been familiar up to this time. If so, that person should get busy and learn these particular skills, taking advantage of appropriate assistance. Only in this way will the supervisor be able to plan competently for his or her future, as well as for that of the department. Only in this way will he or she be ready with a plan if and when the forecasted technological events occur.

Benefits of Forecasting

It should always be remembered that at the base of all forecasts lie certain assumptions, approximations, and average conditions. Forecasting is an art and not a science, and as yet there is no infallible way of predicting the future; however, forecasting accuracy increases with experience. As time goes on, making assumptions about the future should become a normal activity for all managers from the administrator down to the supervisor. Managers should exchange ideas, help each other, and supply Information whenever available. In all likelihood, they will act as a check on each other, and their final analysis of what the future holds will probably be quite reliable.

But even if some of the events that have been anticipated do not materialize or do not materialize exactly as forecast, it is better to have foreseen them than to be suddenly confronted with them. Having foreseen these events, supervisors have readied their minds and state of affairs so as to be able to incorporate changes whenever they are needed. Although this may sound like a formidable task for supervisors, all that is asked of them is to be alert to all possible changes and trends. This is the only way they can prevent their own and their employees' obsolescence, so that with hindsight they will not have to recall the time when certain trends were already visible and wish they had taken them seriously at that time.

Tactical Considerations in Planning

While planning, supervisors must keep in mind the impact of the plans. They must realize that they do not plan in a vacuum. Success or failure of planning will depend largely on the reaction of those involved in the plans, be they the employees, supervisors of other departments, their own boss, or top administration. A number of tactical or political strategies are at the supervisor's disposal to help minimize negative reactions and facilitate the success of the plans. One or the other or a combination of these political, tactical considerations can be used, depending on the situation at hand.

Since timing is a critical and essential factor in all planning, the manager may choose the strategy that tells him or her to *strike while the iron is hot.* This strategy obviously advocates prompt action when the situation and time for action are propitious. On the other hand, the supervisor may want to invoke the old saying that *time is a great healer.* This is not an endorsement of procrastination, but it is often advisable to move slowly and create an opportunity for cooling off because many things take care of themselves after a short while. This is also known as the *wait and see strategy.*

When significant changes are involved in planning, the supervisor may use the strategy known as *concentrated mass offensive.* This strategy advocates quick radical action all at once to have immediate results. On the other hand, the supervisor may prefer to just *get a foot in the door.* This tactic implies that it may be better to propose merely a portion of the plan in the beginning, especially if the program is of such magnitude that its total acceptance would be doubtful.

Sometimes one supervisor's plan may involve changes that could come about more easily if supervisors of other departments would join in the action. It may therefore be advisable to seek allies to promote the change, that is, to adopt the strategy which states that *there is strength in unity.* For example, if a supervisor plans to try to increase the salaries of the employees, it may be expedient to try to get the other supervisors to join the effort in presenting a general request for higher remuneration to the administrator. This may involve another strategy that is well known in politics: *You scratch my back and I'll scratch yours*. This tactic of reciprocity is practiced not only in political circles and in the activity of purchasing agents, but also among colleagues who wish to present joint action on a particular issue.

There are, of course, many other political strategies that can frequently be of help in initiating and carrying out plans. Mentioning these tactics, however, should not be construed to mean that they are always recommended. The choice and application of these political tactics will depend on the people involved, situation, urgency of the objective, timing, means available, and a number of other factors. But properly applied, they can minimize difficulties and increase the effectiveness of the supervisor's planning.

Planning the Utilization of Resources

As we already know, every supervisor is entrusted with a large number of valuable resources to accomplish the job. It is the supervisor's duty to plan specifically how to utilize the resources available so that the work of the unit can be carried out most effectively. This means that detailed plans must be made for the utilization of the equipment, appliances, instruments, space available, materials and supplies, and, last but not least, the supervisor's and employees' time.

Utilization of Equipment, Appliances, and Instruments

The supervisor must plan the full utilization of the equipment, appliances, and instruments provided for the department. The equipment frequently represents a substantial investment that the institution has made. Therefore, plans for its efficient use must be made to ensure the proper return on the investment. It is the supervisor's job to see that employees respect the equipment and instruments and treat them carefully.

Furthermore, it is the supervisor's duty to see that the equipment of the unit is properly maintained. Equipment that is poorly maintained and does not function properly, for example, the side rails on the patient's bed, could possibly lead to an incident ending up in a patient's lawsuit for damages. The head nurse or team leader, on learning of such a malfunction, should immediately determine whether the employee is operating the equipment properly and if there is a maintenance problem. The proper steps to remedy the malfunction should be taken at once. Supervisors should work closely with the maintenance department and plan for periodic maintenance checkups.

It is the supervisor's job to ascertain if the equipment serves its purpose and if better facilities are available for doing the work. This does not mean that a supervisor must always have the very latest model available; but, on the other hand, plans should be made to replace inefficient equipment.

Once the decision is reached to replace equipment, supervisors must plan such replacements very carefully. They must read professional journals and literature circulated by hospitals and related associations, listen to sales presentations of equipment and instruments, and keep themselves aware of the general development within their fields. Only with this type of background can the supervisor submit intelligent plans and alternatives for the replacement of tools and equipment to the immediate superior or to the administrator. The recommended changes should be well substantiated and supported, but the final decision remains with higher management. Even if the request is turned down, the supervisor has demonstrated that he or she is on top of the job, planning for the future. In the long run, the plans for replacing equipment probably will be accepted, and the administrator will realize that the supervisor planned for the proper utilization of the department's equipment with foresight.

Work Methods and Procedures

In discussing the planning process, it was pointed out that the supervisor is deeply involved in designing, developing, and writing procedures and methods. Indeed, the supervisor should continually review and, if need be, revise them and make plans concerning improved work methods and processes in the department. The difficulty is that many supervisors work under considerable pressure and find little time for this type of planning. Moreover, the supervisor is often so close to the jobs performed in the department that he or she believes the prevailing work methods are satisfactory and not much can be done about them. Nevertheless, to maintain high efficiency and the best possible patient care, it is necessary from time to time to study the operations performed so that improvements can be planned. If the department begins doing something that has not been done before, then the supervisor has to write a whole set of new procedures and methods for this new activity. For example, if heart catheterizations are to be performed in our hospital, the manager of that unit has to develop a whole range of new procedures and methods for this new activity. Or, if the hospital changes from the old procedures of simple blood transfusion to the transfusion of blood components, new procedures must be discussed and worked out.

The supervisor should try to look at all of the department's operations from the point of view of a stranger coming into the department for the first time. In other words, he or she should look at the operations with a detached point of view, observing all methods and processes objectively. The supervisor should question if each operation is really necessary, what the reason for it is, and if it could be combined with something else. Are the various steps necessary? Are they performed in the best possible sequence? Are there any avoidable delays? In this effort to devise more efficient work methods, it may be possible for the supervisor to enlist the help of a staff specialist, such as a nurse clinician, systems analyst, or methods engineer, who may be available within the hospital. The supervisor should also seek ideas from employees who are doing the job, since they often can make valuable suggestions for improved methods and procedures.

Safety

Health care centers have traditionally been very much aware of the need for safety of the patients, employees, and visitors; after all, hospitals are the place where many accident victims ultimately end up. This makes every employee in a health care center doubly aware of the importance of safety. It is also true that a safe environment for patients and employees of a health care center is an ever-present consideration in the training and education of most health care professionals.

Although almost all health care facilities have a safety committee, or even a safety department, it would be wrong to believe that this absolves managers and supervisors of their obligation to create and maintain a safe environment for clients, visitors, and employees. The recent flood of liability and damage suits against hospitals has put additional emphasis on the need for safety.

A hospital patient is entitled to expect the hospital to keep its premises reasonably safe. And since hospitals are used by people who are disabled or infirm, "reasonable care" in case of a hospital may require a somewhat higher standard than that required of other public places or for people of ordinary physical condition. The same care must be taken with respect to equipment, instruments, and appliances that are reasonably adequate for use in the diagnosis or treatment of patients. If defective equipment causes injury to a patient, the hospital may be liable. The hospital is not required to provide the latest equipment. Cases against hospitals have involved defective beds, broken thermometers, inoperative patient call systems, improperly calibrated x-ray equipment, and so on.

Another impetus for safety came with the Occupational Safety and Health Act (OSHA) of 1970, an act that places on employers a greater amount of responsibility to provide employees with a safe and healthy work environment. Since OSHA covers far-reaching areas with many ramifications, implications, and changes of interpretations, the supervisor cannot possibly be familiar with all of it or its most important aspects. Therefore supervisors should be in close touch with that person in the health care center who is the expert, for example, the safety director or someone in that office. In any event, this act has added to the supervisor's responsibility for planning and maintaining a healthier and safer work environment.

Although many health care centers have a safety director, safety committee, or committee for claim prevention and loss control, the true responsibility for safety lies with every manager, from the chief executive officer down to the supervisors. The supervisors, being the persons on the spot, must stress safety more than anyone else and plan for it. The supervisors must be alert to unsafe practices, correct them, and in general enforce safety procedures. Safety must be an integral part in everything and uppermost in everyone's mind, the supervisors' and the employees'. Safety must be a continuous consideration in all supervisory planning. It must be integrated in all policies, procedures, methods, practices, directives, etc., so that accidents and incidents do not occur or are significantly reduced, if not completely prevented.

If the health care center employs a safety director, this person can be helpful to the supervisor in planning for safety. But ultimately, it is the supervisor's job to make the employees think and practice safety in everything they do. In the final analysis, people cause far more accidents than faulty equipment.

Use of Space

A supervisor must also plan for the best utilization of space. First, it should be determined whether or not the space assigned to the department is being used effectively. Some industrial engineering help, if available, may be called on to make this determination. If it is not available, the supervisor should make a layout chart, showing the number of square feet the department has to work with, the location of equipment and supplies, and the work paths of the employees as they carry out their tasks. Such a chart can then be studied to determine whether the allocated space has been laid out appropriately or whether things need to be rearranged so that the department's work can be done more efficiently.

For example, the chief technologist of the clinical laboratories can show that the annual work load has been increasing by approximately 10 percent annually, which would result in doubling the workload in approximately 9 years. He or she would also point out that 40,000 to 75,000 tests equate to so many square feet and that the laboratories now occupy the same space they had for many years. The chief technologist should also draw up a typical laboratory plan for this size hospital, showing a layout for separate work units for all technical sections—hematology, urinalysis, biochemistry, histology, serology, bacteriology, support areas, etc. At the same time, the supervisor may also want to point out that laboratory facilities should preferably be either in the basement or on the first floor, rather than on the present upper floor location.

This type of layout planning would show the need for additional space and/or a different location. If such a request is placed before the administrator, based on thorough planning of the space currently allotted, then the likelihood that it will be granted is greater. The chief technologist, in this case, must realize, however, that he or she has to compete with many other managers who probably also request more space. Even if the request is denied, these space allocation plans will not have been drawn up in vain. In all probability, they will alert the supervisor to some of the conditions under which the employees are working, and perhaps that information can be used to plan more efficient work methods considering the existing conditions.

Use of Materials and Supplies

The supervisor must plan for the appropriate use, security, and conservation of the materials and supplies entrusted and charged to the department. These would include such supplies as cotton balls, tongue blades, alcohol wipes, syringes, needles, medicine cups, and paper goods at a nursing station.

In most departments, the quantity of materials and supplies used is substantial. Even if each single item represents only a small value, the aggregate of these items adds up to sizable amounts in the budget of a health care facility. Proper planning will ensure that materials and supplies are used as conservatively as possible, without compromising sterility, asepsis, and sanitary requirements. Supervisors must teach their employees proper use, because many of them are careless and do not realize the amount of money involved. By careful explanation, supervisors can call their workers' attention to this fact, pointing out to them that the economic utilization of supplies is to their own advantage because whatever is wasted cannot be used to raise their wages or improve their working conditions. Another problem is the loss and theft of materials and supplies often carried out by the employees themselves. Supervisors must take adequate precautions to minimize this source of loss. Although proper planning for the utilization of materials and supplies will help significantly in performance, it will not prevent all waste.

Time Management

Last, but not least, supervisors must plan the use of time. The old saying "time is money" applies with equal force to the supervisor's own time and to the employees' time. Thus, supervisors must not only plan their employees' time, but they must also consider at least as carefully the management of their own time.

The Employees' Time

When planning for the effective use of the subordinates' time, much will depend on the supervisors' basic managerial strategy and their assumptions about human nature. According to Douglas McGregor,* a well-known author and professor of management, most managers base their thinking on one of two sets of assumptions about human nature, which he calls Theory X and Theory Y. The Theory X manager believes that the average employee dislikes work, will avoid work, and tries to get by with as little as utterly possible. He has little ambition and has to be forced and closely controlled in each and every job. The Theory Y manager operates with a drastically different set of assumptions regarding human nature. He or she believes that most employees consider work natural, that most are eager to do the right thing, will seek responsibility under the proper conditions, will exercise self-control, and do not need to be continually urged. Theory Y further states that external controls and threats are not a good means for producing results. Rather, since work is as natural to people as play or rest, it will not be avoided. Although there may be some situations in which a manager has no choice but to follow Theory X, in all likelihood practice and belief in Theory Y is much preferred. A great deal more will be said about McGregor's theories in Chap-

*Douglas McGregor, *The Human Side of Enterprise* (New York: McGraw-Hill Book Co., 1960), Chapters 3 and 4.

ter 19, but it is appropriate to bring them up now because they are important when planning for the effective utilization of employees' time.

For example, if a supervisor is a Theory Y manager, he or she will expect employees to do the right thing and to turn in a fair day's work. Of course, one cannot expect employees to work indefinitely at top speed. Thus, the plans for their time will be based on a fair output instead of a maximum output. Allowances will be made for fatigue, personal needs, unavoidable delays, and a certain amount of unproductive time during the workday.

In planning employees' time, as in other aspects of planning, the supervisor may be able to get assistance from a specialist employed by the hospital, preferably a motion and time specialist. But, normally, most supervisors can use work methods studies to come up with a pretty fair idea themselves as to what can be expected of their employees. Such reasonable estimates of employees' time are necessary because the supervisor must depend on the completion of certain tasks at certain times. The supervisors themselves may have been given deadlines, and, to meet them, they must have a fairly good estimate or idea of how fast the job can be done. Most supervisors are capable of planning reasonable performance requirements that their employees accept as fair. Such requirements are, of course, based on average conditions and not on emergencies.

There are some situations in hospitals in which the subordinate's time is paced and set by someone other than the supervisor because of the nature of the activity performed. For instance, the time an operating room nurse or technician spends on a case is determined by the speed and skill of the surgeon doing the operation. Furthermore, unexpected complications may add to the time normally necessary to complete the job. In cases of this sort, average time estimates can still be made; but the time allotted must allow for the various contingencies that can arise.

In addition to planning for the normal employee time, it may be necessary to plan for overtime. Overtime should be considered only as an emergency matter. If the supervisor finds that overtime or working a double shift is regularly required, then plans need changing by altering work methods, obtaining better or more equipment, or hiring more employees. The supervisor must also plan for employee absences. Of course, one cannot plan for those instances in which employees are absent without notice. But one can plan for holidays, vacations, leaves of absence, layoffs for overhaul, etc. Plans for this kind of absence should be worked out in advance so that the functioning of the department will suffer as little as possible.

Flexible Work Schedules

Work schedules for many employees in different organizations have become more flexible. The leading thought is that employees should be able to choose the hours during which they would like to work. The plans are designed to give employees greater opportunities to enjoy their life *off*, as opposed to *on*, the job. Flex time enables employees to choose a schedule that fits into their off-the-job activities. It enables working parents or others with responsibilities at home the opportunity to combine work with family life. The concept of flex time has been successfully introduced into various private and public organized activities and in health care centers. It is likely that flexible work schedules will become even more popular in the future, especially for professional and clerical work.

It is well known that some health care professionals, especially nurses,* have left their field of expertise because they were dissatisfied with a number of factors, among which grueling hours and schedules loomed large. There are many nurses who cannot or do not want to work the traditional 5-day, 40-hour week of rotating shifts, 7 to 3 o'clock, 3 to 11, and 11 to 7. Therefore, it was necessary to do away with the traditional pattern of nursing staff scheduling. To alleviate these dissatisfactions, flexible work hours have been introduced and varied plans are available; for instance, 4-40, which means 4 days at 10 hours, or 7 days on and 7 days off, using the 10-hour workday, or 24-hour weekend shifts, or two 16-hour shifts on a weekend, or the 3-day weekend plan, etc.† In this situation, the introduction of flexible work schedules certainly has been a good idea and probably will be expanded.

There is little doubt that flexible working schedules create some additional scheduling and planning problems for supervisors. Furthermore, they cause problems for proper supervision of the employees during different shift arrangements. There also is the real concern that schedules with long hours can potentially cause fatigue and an increase in errors. However, studies show that such deterioration could not be documented and that these initial fears are unwarranted, especially after the employees had been on the new schedules for a few months. These and others are additional challenges for supervisors. But as long as flexible working schedules produce good results, e.g., easier staff recruitment, better staff retention, higher morale, fewer absences, less tardiness, less dissatisfaction, better patient care, etc., supervisors will make every effort to overcome these problems by being better managers.

The Supervisor's Time

Time is one of the most valuable resources that cannot be renewed or stored. The supply of time is inflexible; if supervisors want more time, they have to "make" it themselves. The supervisor's own time is one of the resources for which he or she is responsible. Every supervisor has probably experienced days that were so full of pressures and demands that he or she began to feel as though all the matters that needed attention could never be taken care of. The days and weeks just were too short. The only way to keep such days at a minimum is for the supervisor to plan the time for the most effective use.

---

*The same considerations are applicable to other hospital employees.

†The M. D. Anderson Hospital and Tumor Institute in Houston gives nurse applicants about 30 different work schedules from which to choose. *Time Magazine,* Vol. 118, No. 8 (Aug. 24, 1981): 37; also see "The Demise of the Traditional 5-40 Workweek?" and Elmina M. Price, "Seven Days On And Seven Days Off." *American Journal of Nursing,* Vol. 81, No. 6 (June, 1981): 1138-1143.

Unfortunately, the supervisor's problems come up on a continual basis but without any order of importance. Thus, the first thing the supervisor must do is sort and grade them, that is, decide between those matters which he or she must attend to personally and those which can be delegated to someone else. There are some matters that the supervisor actually cannot delegate, but the majority can be assigned to one of the employees. Every time the supervisor dispenses with one of the duties by assigning it to an employee, time is gained for more important matters. This is worthwhile even if some valuable time must be spent training one of the employees in a particular task. In case of doubt, therefore, the supervisor should be inclined to delegate. Then the available time must be planned so that it is divided among those matters to which the supervisor alone can attend. And these matters again have to be classified according to their urgency.

Unless supervisors distinguish between those matters which *must* be done and those which *ought* to be done, they are inclined to pay equal attention to all matters before them, and the more important ones may not get the attention they truly deserve. But by distinguishing they will be giving priority to those matters which need immediate attention. A supervisor should therefore plan the time so that the most important things to attend to will appear at the top of the schedule. The supervisor must make certain, however, that some flexibility is left in the time schedule because not every contingency can be anticipated. There will be some emergencies to which a supervisor must pay attention when they arise. The flexibility will make it possible to take care of these situations without significantly disrupting the other activities planned on the time schedule.

Many techniques have been devised to help supervisors control their time schedules. One of the simplest methods is to use a desk calendar to schedule those things which need attention, such as appointments, meetings, reports, discussions, etc. The supervisor should schedule these events far in advance, and, in so doing, they will automatically come up for attention when they are due.

Another effective way of planning each week's work in advance and also of knowing what is being accomplished as the week goes on is to keep a planning sheet. Such a planning sheet is prepared at the end of one week for the week to follow. It shows the days of the week divided into morning and afternoon columns and a list of all things to be accomplished. Then, a time for accomplishment is assigned to each task by placing it in the morning or the afternoon blocks of the assigned day. Thus, at a glance the supervisor knows what is planned for each morning and afternoon of the week. As a task is accomplished, its box is circled. Those tasks which have been delayed during the day must be rescheduled for another time by placing them in an appropriate block on a subsequent day. Those tasks which are planned but have not been accomplished during the week (they are still uncircled) must be rescheduled for the following week. Such a record will show how much of the original plan has been carried out at the end of the week and will provide a good answer to the question of where the supervisor's time went. Based on this record the supervisor will then be able to plan the next week and so on. Regardless of whether this particular system is used or another, the supervisor must schedule the time periods each week and have some method of reporting the tasks that are planned and those which have been accomplished. (See Figure 8-1.)

Figure 8-1. Sample planning sheet.

MONDAY 10/23	TUESDAY 10/24	WEDNESDAY 10/25	THURSDAY 10/26	FRIDAY 10/27
AM	AM *work on job descriptions*	AM *Set up Personnel Director Review. Talk to maintenance about new fl. outlets.*	AM *Arrange date for evaluation interviews.*	AM *Work on dress code revisions.*
PM *Check leave of absence policy.*	PM	PM *Read minutes of last meeting of inspection com.*	PM *Start work on new budget.*	PM *Attend management seminar.*

Time-Use Chart

Among the many tools for using time effectively a supervisor should consider what kind of work his or her time is currently spent on. A time-use chart will help. The supervisor should create some broad classifications for daily activities, such as routine duties, regular supervisory duties, special duties, emergencies, and innovative thinking. After each day the supervisor should write down how much time was spent in these categories; having done this for several weeks he or she will learn a geat deal about where the time went.

The supervisor may find that 20 percent of the time was spent on *routine work,* which could and should be assigned to some of the subordinates. A large percent of time was devoted to *regular supervisory duties,* such as checking performance, giving directives and instructions, evaluating and counseling employees, promoting, maintaining discipline, etc. These are supervisory duties which he or she alone should do, and no time can probably be gained from this area. Then the supervisor will find out how much time was spent in *special duties,* for example, serving on committees, attending professional meetings, planning next year's budget, changing the dress code, reviewing procedures, etc. Again, all of this time is probably spent wisely. And then there will be a certain amount of time spent on *emergencies,* a subject that is unpredictable and will demand some of the supervisor's attention. Also, hopefully, some time is open for *creative and innovative thinking,* which is essential for the climate of the department and the progress of the institution. Although the boss evaluates the supervisor on how well the department's job gets done, somehow the supervisor is also appraised as to his or her innovative changes, suggestions, and constructive new ideas.

Such a time-use chart will illustrate where the time went and in which areas a supervisor can "make" some more time. Unless he or she has a clear picture of this, it is likely that routine tasks will creep in and reduce the time available for the truly supervisory duties.

Utilization of Work Force

The employees in a department are the most valuable resource. Therefore, planning for their full utilization must be uppermost in every manager's mind. Although a supervisor must plan for the utilization of equipment and tools, improved work methods and processes, utilization of space, conservation of materials and supplies, and proper use of time, the most important planning of all is that connected with utilization of the work force.

This, of course, does not mean planning to squeeze an excessive amount of work out of each employee. Rather, utilization means giving employees as much *satisfaction* as possible in their jobs. To plan for the best utilization of the work force also means to develop methods for recruiting good employees, to search for all available sources of employees, and for their retention. Furthermore, it means to search continually for the best ways to group their activities. It includes the problems and plans of training, supervising, and motivating employees. Finally, the question of effective utilization of workers means the continual appraisal of their performance, appropriate promotions, adequate plans for compensation and rewards; and at the same time, fair disciplinary measures.

All of these considerations play an important role when the supervisor plans for the best utilization of the department's employees. Only by such human resource planning can a situation be created in which workers willingly contribute their utmost to achieve both personal satisfaction on the job, as well as attainment of the department's objectives. The supervisor may rest assured that the efforts made in this connection will be rewarded amply by the employees. Actually, the matter of planning for the best utilization of employees is at the heart of expert supervision. It is discussed here only briefly, but in reality this entire book is concerned with bringing about the best possible utilization of employees.

Summary

All planning must be done with forecasts of the future in mind. Since the future is uncertain, it is necessary to make various assumptions as to what it holds. Overall forecasts or assumptions are made by the top administrator, and the supervisor narrows these down to forecasts for the departmental activity. Based on such forecasts, the supervisor will then make plans for the department. Plans must be made for the full utilization of all the resources at the supervisor's disposal. More specifically, he or she must plan for proper utilization of equipment and instruments and work methods and processes. There must be plans to effectively utilize the space available and the materials and supplies under supervision, and the efficient use of time must be planned. Even more important, the supervisor must plan for the best overall utilization of the employees in the unit. This means, among other things, seeing that employees are able to find satisfaction in their work. Throughout all planning, the supervisor should be concerned with the effects of these plans on other members of the organization. At times the manager may need to resort to various tactical considerations that will be helpful in getting the department's plans accepted and effectively carried out.

Part Four

Organizing

9

Fundamental Concepts of Organizing

Authority and Span of Management

Organizing means setting up a formal structure of activities and authority relationships. Organizing is closely related to planning. Planning defines the goals and objectives of the institution, the expectations. Organizing defines the activities needed to accomplish these objectives and establishes the relationships among various functions. These activities and functions form subsystems that are synchronized and coordinated into a larger system, called the *formal organization.*

How this structure looks and how it works depends on the organization's objectives and size, state of the arts and science, technology, and many other factors, but not on people. The managerial function of organizing is an impersonal function. Of course, the organization must be a structure that can be inhabited by people, the most valuable asset of any organization. It must be a structure in which people can function and thrive. Naturally, the human element is important, and we will put all of these considerations to work in the staffing and influencing functions. But when the manager designs the structure, it is done without thinking of specific people. Organizing means setting up a formal structure of activities and authority relationships based on major principles.

Formal organization theory rests on several major principles or premises: *authority* is the lifeblood of the managerial position and the *delegation of authority* makes the organization come alive; the *span of management* sets outside limits on the number of subordinates a manager can effectively supervise; the *division of work* is essential for efficiency; the *formal structure* is the main network for organizing and managing the various activities of the enterprise; *unity of command* must prevail; and *coordination* is a primary responsibility of management and is fulfilled by performing the managerial functions properly. These major principles of organization are a primary concern of the chief executive officer. He or she is the one who must translate them into a formal organizational structure so that the institution operates smoothly and accomplishes its objectives.

Since the application of these formal organizational principles involves all levels of management, it is also necessary for you as a supervisor to understand them and know how they are used. This knowledge will help in organizing your own department and in coordinating its activities with those of the rest of the institution. As a supervisor, you will certainly be asked to carry out and may be even asked to help make decisions involving departmentalization or the division of work, the span of supervision, the delegation of authority, etc. And as you move up in the managerial hierarchy, you will probably be called on to participate in more and more such organizational decisions. Thus, although it is the chief administrator who initially applies the formal principles to establish the organization's overall structure and activities, it is the department heads, supervisors, and other middle and lower level managers who must make these principles and the resulting structure work. This is why it is essential for us to discuss the organizing process on an overall, or institutional, basis before we can discuss it on the departmental, or supervisory, level.

The many contingencies facing management are a continuous challenge, and the dynamic nature of organizing enables the manager to bring about change and absorb and accommodate change as the need arises. This will enable the enterprise to pursue and achieve its objectives continuously. Although organizing is a dynamic process, it rests on two fundamental concepts, *authority* and *span of management*.

This chapter will examine these two fundamental concepts of authority and span of management: authority, the right to give orders, is one of the bases through which the manager gets the job done. The span of management deals with another dimension, the scope of supervision.

Authority

A brief reference to the importance of authority to the managerial position was made in Chapter 2, and our discussion of authority at that point merely stated that authority is the lifeblood of the supervisory position and that authority is one of the two characteristics of a manager. And the process of delegation of authority breathes life into an organization. Without it an organization cannot and does not exist. Therefore, we must examine and understand first the concept of authority.

The Meaning of Authority

Authority is a difficult concept; it has many interpretations and meanings, including the one we have used before, that authority is an attribute of the managerial position, the key to the managerial job. In this sense, authority refers to the formal or official power of a manager to obtain the compliance of the subordinates with directives, communications, policies, and objectives. Such authority is associated with the manager's function in the organization. It is vested in organizational roles or positions. As long as an individual holds the position, he or she has the privilege of exercising the authority that is inherent in it. And since positions are meaningless unless they are occupied by someone, we generally speak of the authority of the manager, the authority that is delegated to the manager, and so forth. Although it would be more precise to speak of the authority of the managerial position itself or the authority delegated to that position, rather than to the person who occupies it, the difference is generally regarded as semantic. As long as we understand that authority in this sense resides in the position, we may speak rather loosely of the authority of the manager, supervisor, etc.

Source and Nature of Authority

As stated before, authority is a difficult concept; it has many interpretations and meanings. The definition of authority as "legitimate power" to give orders was first clearly expressed by Max Weber.* The subordinates' compliance rests on the belief that it is legitimate for managers to give orders and illegitimate for subordinates not to obey them. Other writers, such as Fayol, have expressed similar views. This kind of authority is vested in organizational roles and positions, not in the individuals who occupy these positions. As long as an individual holds the position, he or she has the privilege of exercising the authority that is inherent in it. Once a manager leaves an organizational position, he or she loses the authority inherent in it, and the authority will go on to the successor.

While examining the foundation for this organizational authority, Weber identified three bases of authority, *tradition, rules and regulations,* and *charisma.* Traditional authority "rests on the belief in the sacredness of the social order."† For instance, in a patriarchal society the father receives legitimacy through custom. Rules and regulations form a second base. Subordinates will comply with orders because, in a bureaucratic organization, superior-subordinate authority relationships are defined by rules and regulations. In charismatic authority, the compelling personal characteristics and charisma of the leader** makes the subordinates and followers carry out the orders.

In addition to the above explanations of the meaning and sources of authority, other views have been developed and expressed. In reference to the

---

* Max Weber, *The Theory of Social and Economic Organizations,* ed. Talcott Parsons, trans, A.M. Henderson and Talcott Parsons (New York: Oxford University Press, 1974). 324-363

† Max Weber, "The Three Types of Legitimate Rule," trans. Hans Gerth, *Berkeley Journal of Sociology* 4 (1958): 3-10.

** The concept of leadership will be discussed in Chapter 21.

source of authority there are two contradicting views: the *formal authority theory* and the *acceptance theory*. In formal authority theory, authority originates at the top of the organizational hierarchy and is delegated downward from superiors to subordinates. In acceptance theory, authority originates at the bottom of the organizational pyramid and is conferred upward from subordinates to superiors. Let us look at each of these theories more carefully to gain further insight into the difficult authority concept.

Formal Authority Theory

The formal authority theory is the top-down theory. It traces the flow of authority downward from top management to subordinate managers. You can trace your authority directly from your boss, who has delegated it to you. He or she in turn receives authority, let us say, from an associate administrator, who receives authority from the chief administrator, who traces authority directly back to the board of directors, who receive their authority from the owners or the stockholders. In private corporations, therefore, we may say that the actual source of authority lies in the stockholders who are, loosely speaking, the owners of the corporation. These owners delegate their power to administer the affairs of the corporation to those whom they have put into managerial positions. From the top administrator that power flows down through the channel of command until it reaches the supervisor.

Limitations of Authority

There are, of course, limitations to the authority that a manager has by virtue of his or her position in an organization. These limitations can be either explicit or implicit. Moreover, some of them stem from internal sources and others from external sources. External limitations on authority include such factors as our codes, folkways, and life style, along with the many political, legal, ethical, moral, social, and economic considerations that make up our society. For example, laws referring to collective bargaining and resulting contractual obligations, fair employment practices, etc., are specific examples of external limitations on authority.

Internal limitations on authority would be set mainly by the organization's articles of incorporation and bylaws. In addition to these overall internal restrictions, each manager is subject to the specific limitations spelled out by the administrator when duties are assigned and authority delegated. Generally, there are more internal limitations on the scope of authority the further down one goes in the managerial hierarchy. In other words, the lower the rung on the administrative ladder, the narrower the area in which authority can be exercised. This is known as the tapering concept of authority as shown in Figure 9-1.

All of the above would be explicit, fairly obvious restrictions on authority. In addition to these, a number of more implicit limitations, such as biological restraints, exist simply because human beings do not have the

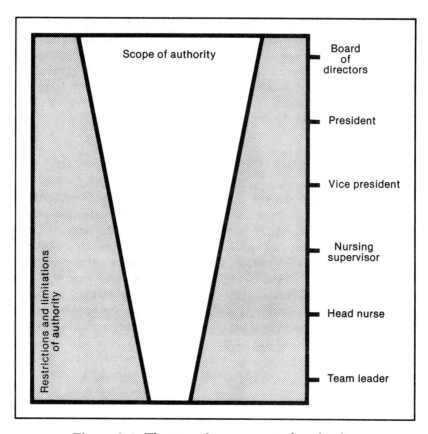

Figure 9-1. The tapering concept of authority.

capacity to do certain things. No subordinate should be expected to do the impossible. Thus, physical and psychological restrictions on authority must be recognized and accepted. In today's society, considerations of this kind significantly limit the scope of authority of every manager.

So far, our discussion has centered on the formal way of looking at the origin of authority as a power that results from our recognition of private property. According to this theory, then, the ultimate source of all managerial authority in America would be the constitutional guarantee of the institution of private property. Since the constitution was created by the people and is subject to amendment and modification by the will of the people, it follows that society is the source from which authority flows.*

This is in agreement with Weber's definition of formal authority, since management's right to give orders is legitimate and the employees are obliged to carry these orders out because they are legitimate. There could be a prob-

* Elmore Peterson, E. Grosvenor Plowman, and Joseph M. Trickett, *Business Organization and Management,* 5th ed. (Homewood, IL: Richard D. Irwin, Inc., 1962), 83.

lem, however, when such an order seems unethical to the employee or outside the limits of the job. This raises the question of whether the subordinate has some say in this matter.

Acceptance Theory of Authority

The acceptance theory of authority addresses itself to the role of subordinates and managerial authority. It is a bottom-up approach in which employees give managers their authority. A large group of writers who do not agree with the formal theory maintain that management has no meaningful authority unless and until subordinates confer it. These writers claim that formal organizational authority is effective only to the extent that subordinates accept it. They state that unless your subordinates accept your authority, you, as a manager, actually do not possess that authority. In reality, of course, subordinates often do not have a choice between accepting authority or not accepting it. The only choice they have is to leave the job. Nevertheless, this is a worrisome thought, indicating that there is considerable merit in looking at authority as something which must be accepted by your employees.

Advocates of the acceptance theory state that in most instances a manager does not have a real problem, since an employee, on accepting a job, knows that the boss of the department has the authority to give orders, take disciplinary action, and do whatever else goes with the managerial position. Whenever an employee decides to work for a hospital, he or she agrees, within the limits of the job, to accept orders given by the organization. But the decision whether an order has authority lies with the persons to whom it is addressed and does not reside in "persons of authority" or those who issue these orders.*

Formal Authority Theory vs Acceptance Authority Theory

To repeat, then, the origin of authority can be considered from two viewpoints: the formal way of looking at authority as something that originates with private property, formally handed down from the owners at the top to the lowest line supervisor; or, in contrast, looking at authority as something that is conferred on the supervisor by the subordinates' acceptance of this authority. It is not the author's intention to go further into this academic argument here. This difference of opinions is discussed because in reality it significantly influences the practice of supervision, the manner and the attitudes with which supervision is approached.

This will become more obvious when we realize that adherence to the acceptance theory does not necessarily rule out the downward delegation of authority from upper to lower levels of management. The acceptance theory can be thought of as merely adding another dimension to the formal concept

---

*Chester I. Barnard, *The Functions of the Executive* (Cambridge, MA: Harvard University Press, 1956), 163.

of organizational authority. That is, in addition to having formal authority delegated from above, managers must also have such authority accepted from below. All managers must be aware that they possess formal authority, and, if need be, they can resort to it as a final recourse. Obviously, in this day and age no one would want to rely exclusively on the weight of this formal authority to motivate workers to perform their jobs. There will be times and occasions, however, when every manager will have to make full use of this authority and power. But hopefully these will be the exceptions and not the rule. And even when the manager does have to invoke this authority, the manner in which it is done will make a difference in whether it is resented or accepted without resentment. If it is accepted graciously most of the time, the manager will know that the subordinates have chosen to recognize and respect the authority which superiors have delegated to him or her formally.

Types of Authority

In the past it might have been sufficient for a manager to rely on authority based on the legitimacy of the social institution, the concept of property rights to get the job done. But this is no longer sufficient for a manager in any organized activity, especially in a health care institution. Therefore, it is necessary to examine the various types of organizational authority, *positional, functional,* and *personal* authority.

Positional authority is based on organizational position and, as stated above, rests on the legitimacy of the manager's position as the agent of a socially valid organization. This authority is vested in the position and in the organization and is impersonal. Positional authority exists in all kinds of organizations: health care, educational, business, military, religious, fraternal, etc. We may not like a particular individual, but we recognize and accept the legitimacy of that person's position and authority.

Functional authority is based on expertise and knowledge. We accept expert advice and recognize that this person is an "authority" in a particular specialty. Functional authority exists in all branches of learning and crafts and comes from specialization. Health care institutions are a prime example of the role and importance of functional authority. The "specialist's" statements and directives are accepted because he or she is the "authority in this field" and carries the weight and power of functional authority. Whereas positional authority is impersonal, functional authority in this sense is highly personal. It adheres to the individual whose knowledge and expertise make him or her the "authority." Whereas positional authority can and must be delegated, functional authority cannot be delegated; it remains with the individual wherever he or she may be and work. Although it is highly personalized, functional authority has some aspects of positional authority because some organizations, especially health care centers, demand that certain positions can only be filled by individuals with special skill and expertise. A hospital abounds in examples and applications of functional authority, probably more than any other organized activity. Functional authority rests on acceptance, but it stems from an individual's knowledge and not from society.

Personal authority is based on an individual's characteristics, magnetism, and charisma. Subordinates and followers accept personal authority because their needs are consistent with the leader's goals. Personal authority motivates the subordinates to work willingly and enthusiastically toward the achievement of the objectives. This concept of personal authority can be equated with leadership, which will be discussed in Chapter 21.

Integrated Approach to Authority

To be an effective manager in a health care institution it is not enough to depend on the weight of positional authority based on legitimacy; there are occasions when this may be the last resort. But it is far more desirable if the manager relies on a combination of all three types, positional, functional, and personal, to manage effectively. This is much more important in the health care field because of the occupational character of the people involved; new fields of scientific advances and new technologies make greater expertise a necessity, leading to more and more functional authority. For instance, the chief medical technologist should not rely on only positional authority as the "chief" of the department, but should also use his or her expertise in this field and leadership ability and charisma. Reliance on all three types of authority will create a highly desirable and motivating organizational climate.

The Span of Management

Span of management, also known as span of authority, span of supervision, or span of control, is a concept that has been a challenge to managers and leaders ever since biblical times. It deals with the scope of supervision, the number of people any one person can supervise effectively. Because this number is limited, we have to create departments of different areas of activities and place someone in charge of each.

The establishment of departments in an organization is not an end in itself. It is not desirable per se because departments are expensive; they must be headed by various supervisors and staffed by additional employees, all of which runs into large sums of money. Furthermore, departments are not desirable per se because the more there are, the more difficulties will be encountered in communication and coordination. As discussed earlier, departments do make possible the division of work. And what is equally important, they allow an organization to incorporate what is commonly known as the *principle of the span of management,* or the span of supervision. This principle states that *there is an upper limit to the number of subordinates a manager can effectively supervise.* This is a very important concept in organizational theory and practice.

The Relationship of Span to Levels

Almost every manager knows that there is a limit to the number of employees he or she can effectively supervise. The problem is caused by the many superior-subordinate relationships that are possible. There are *direct relationships* between the superior and the immediate subordinates, there are *direct group relationships* between the superior and different groupings of the subordinates, and then there are *cross-relationships* among the subordinates. The number of superior-subordinate relationships and cross-relationships that can be handled is limited. Since no one can manage an infinite number of subordinates, the administrator must create departments, distinct areas of activities over which a manager is placed in charge. To this manager, the administrator delegates authority. The manager in turn will redelegate authority to some of the lower subordinates, who in turn will supervise only a limited number of employees. In this manner, not only are departments and subdepartments created, but also the *span of supervision,* or the number of employees under each manager, is established, and the number of managerial *levels* in the organization is determined.

To examine this relationship between the span of supervision and the levels of an organization, imagine a situation in which 81 subordinates report to one chief executive, thus representing one organizational level. Then let us assume that 81 subordinates are too many and that only three should report to the top administrator. Under each of these three associate administrators there would now be 27 employees. By creating associate administrators, however, we have established two levels of organization and have a total of four executives. Now, assuming that 27 subordinates are still too many, and this number is reduced to 9, the organization will require a third managerial level, increasing the total number of managers to 13. Each of the 4 executives on the upper two levels will have 3 subordinates and each of the 9 supervisors on the lowest level will have 9 subordinates. The span of supervision has thus been reduced drastically from the original 81 to a maximum of 9.

This obviously extreme example is illustrated in Figure 9-2, which shows very clearly what occurs when one begins to narrow the span of supervision. The narrower the span becomes, the more levels of management have to be introduced into the organizational setup. As with departments, this is not desirable per se because it is expensive. Every manager costs money, not only in salaries, but also in supporting salaries. Many levels complicate communication, since the dangers of distortion, omission, and misinterpretation are increased. Finally, levels create problems with morale because the addition of levels increases the distance between employees and upper administration. Therefore, there is a constant conflict between the width of the span and the number of levels: the narrower the span, the more managerial levels. The problem is whether to have a broader span of supervision or more levels or vice versa. This problem is one that all managers face throughout their entire career.

Moreover, the problem of span vs. levels is as old as mankind. And we have still not found a pat answer to it. It is simply not possible to state a definite figure as to how many subordinates a manager can have. It is correct to say only that there is an upper limit to this figure. Although we do not know exactly what the upper limit should be, it is interesting that in many enterprises the top administrator has only from five to eight subordinate managers reporting directly to him or her. Descending down the managerial hierarchy,

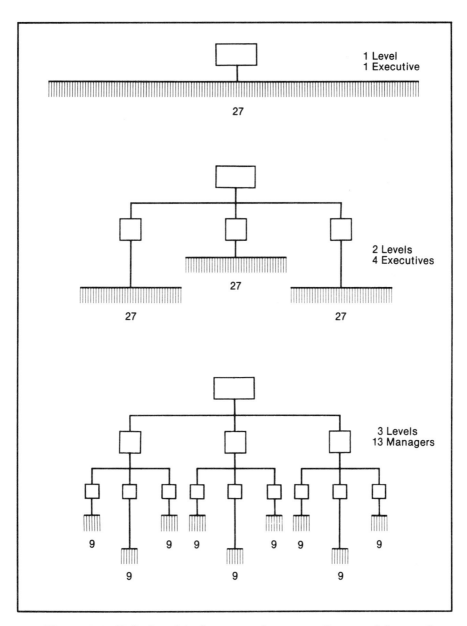

Figure 9-2. Relationship between the span of supervision and the levels of an organization.

we find that the span of supervision generally increases. It is not unusual to have anywhere from 15 to 20 people reporting to the supervisor. On closer inspection, we find that the number of subordinates who can be effectively supervised by one manager actually depends on numerous different contingency factors. These factors determine not only the actual number of relationships but also their frequency and intensity. Therefore, before deciding the proper span of supervision in a particular organization, it is necessary to examine the more important contingencies that influence the magnitude of the span.

Factors Determining the Span of Supervision

One of the factors that influences the magnitude of the span is the *supervisors' competence*—their quality of management, experience, and know-how. Obviously, some supervisors are capable of handling more subordinates than others. Some are better acquainted with good management practices; some have had more experience and are simply better all-around managers. A person who is a "good manager" probably can supervise more employees. But there are still limitations of the human capacity and the amount of time available during the working day.

What the manager does with this time is of utmost importance in determining the span. For example, it takes more time for a supervisor to make an individual decision for every problem that comes up than it does initially to make policy decisions that anticipate problems which might arise later. Clear and complete policy statements reduce the volume of, or at least simplify, the personal decision making required of a manager and hence can increase the span of supervision. The same applies to other managerial processes that determine in advance definitions of responsibility and authority, performance standards, programs, procedures, and methods. Predeterminations such as these reduce the number of decisions the manager has to make and likewise increase the potential span of management. Thus, we can see that one of the important factors in determining the quantity of employees a manager can effectively supervise is managerial competence.

Another factor that will determine how broad a span a manager can handle is the *competence and makeup of the subordinates.* The greater the capacities and self-direction of the employees, the broader the manager's span can be. The training possessed by the subordinates is also of importance. The better their training, the less they will need their supervisor, thus freeing the manager to increase the span.

Another contingency of the manager's span is the amount and availability of *help from staff specialists* within the organization. If a hospital has a range of experts who provide various kinds of advice and service, then the manager's span can be wider. For instance, if the personnel department assists the supervisor with help, advice, and service in recruiting employees, then more time and energy are available to increase the span of subordinates. But if the supervisor has to do all the recruiting, preliminary interviewing, and testing, then obviously that portion of time cannot be utilized for doing something else. Therefore, the amount of additional help available within the institution will influence the width of the span of supervision.

The number of subordinates that can be supervised will also depend on the *nature and importance of the activities* performed by them. If these activities are complicated, highly important, of critical consequences, and/or frequently changing, the span of supervision will of necessity have to be small.

But the simpler, uncomplicated, or more uniform the work, the greater can be the number of persons supervised by one supervisor. If the task to be performed is repetitious, the span may even be as broad as 25 to 30 employees. If the activities are varied and demanding, the span might have to be as small as three to five employees.

Closely related factors that have a bearing on the span of supervision are the *dynamics and complexity of a particular activity.* Some aspects of the hospital routine are most certainly dynamic, whereas others are more stable. In those departments which are engaged in dynamic, critical, and unpredictable activities, like the coronary intensive care unit, the span will have to be very narrow. In those departments which are concerned with more or less stable activities, for example, food production in the dietary department, the span of supervision can be broader.

Another factor that will determine the span of supervision is the degree to which *objective standards* are or can be applied. If enough objective standards are available for subordinates to gauge their own progress, they will not need to constantly report to and contact their boss. Objective standards will result in less frequent relationships, freeing the manager for a broader span.

Although we have now discussed most of the major factors that influence the span of supervision, we still cannot state a definite number of subordinates that a supervisor can effectively manage in each and every instance. It will always depend on the particular circumstances and contingency factors that are operative. The principle of span of supervision tells us only that an upper limit exists.

The solution to this important question is a trade-off, a balance between levels and span. Those who advocate a trend toward a wider span are in favor of a shorter chain of command and of encouraging initiative, self-reliance, and more participation among employees.

Summary

Two basic concepts permeate the organizing function, namely, authority and the span of management. Authority is the right to give orders and directives and to expect that they are carried out. Much has been said and written about the source of authority. The formal top-down opinion looks at authority as coming from the top down from our constitution, social institutions, owners, stockholders, board of directors, higher management, and so on down the line to the supervisor. The opposite view, the acceptance theory, looks at authority as coming from the bottom up. Managers have no authority unless and until the subordinates accept their authority, and they will normally accept only those directives which they perceive to be legitimate. There are several bases of authority: traditional, rules, and charisma. These bases lead to three major kinds of organizational authority, namely, positional authority, which is based on the position in the organization; functional authority, based on knowledge and expertise; and personal, or charismatic, authority, which is synonymous with leadership.

A second basic concept in the organizing process is to determine the number of managerial levels and the span of supervision at each level. The span of supervision is another basic principle of organization which states that there is an upper limit to the number of employees a manager can effectively manage. The actual width of this span is determined by such factors as the capability of the supervisor, previous training and experience of the subordinates, nature and dynamics of the work to be performed, and availability of special staff support. No definite figure can be quoted as the ideal number of subordinates to be supervised by one manager; but the manager knows that whenever the span of supervision is decreased, meaning that the number of employees to be supervised is reduced, an additional supervisor has to be introduced for the excess employees. In other words, the smaller the span of supervision, the more levels of supervisory personnel are needed. This will shape the organization into either a tall narrow pyramid, or, in the case of a broad span of supervision, into a shallow wide pyramid.

10

Division of Work and Departmentalization

As stated earlier, formal organization theory rests on several major principles or premises; two important premises are that the *division of work* is essential for efficiency and that the *formal structure* is the main network for organizing and managing the various activities of the enterprise. In this chapter we will discuss the division of work and the design of the formal structure.

These two major premises of organization are a primary concern of the chief executive officer. He or she is the one who must translate them into a formal organizational structure for the institution. Since the application of these formal organizational principles involves all levels of management, it is also necessary for you as a supervisor to understand them and to know how they are used. This knowledge will help in organizing your own department and in coordinating its activities with those of the rest of the institution. In your supervisory capacity, you will certainly be asked to carry out, and maybe even to help make, decisions involving departmentalization and division of work. And as you move up in the managerial hierarchy, you will probably be called on to participate in more and more such organizational decisions.

Division of Work

The practice of division of work is as old as mankind. From the earliest times we have examples of the practice of specialization in military and civilian activities. In the eighteenth century specialization was tied into efficiency, and ever since then division of work and increased specialization have prevailed with an increasing momentum. The division of work, as stated above, simply means to break down a whole job into smaller, more specialized, tasks. Humans have been dividing work in this manner for thousands and thousands of years because a group of people, each performing a small specialized part of the overall job, could obviously accomplish more than the same size group in which each individual was trying to do the whole job alone. In other words, the division of work results in greater efficiency and higher production.

This is particularly true in health care institutions. The result of continuous advances in medical sciences and technology has been greater specialization of personnel, facilities, and equipment and increased fragmentation of the delivery of care. Because of the proliferation and specialization of medical sciences and technologies, health care centers have become very large and complex organizational structures in terms of differentiation of activities and specialization. They utilize the talents of a tremendous array of people who have developed particular specializations. This proliferation of specialties has clear advantages for patients in terms of scientific care; however, it creates additional problems for the administration of health care institutions, namely, the need for new and varied organizational structures to coordinate the specialties to achieve our objectives. Since the purpose of our organization is to get the job done, specialization and division of work play an important role in designing the kind of structure of task and authority relationships conducive for our desired results.

Departmentalization

It is because the division of work into such specialized tasks produces a much more efficient operation that nearly every organization must departmentalize. By departmentalization, we understand the process of grouping various activities into natural units. A department is such a unit; it is a distinct area of activities over which a manager or supervisor has been given authority and for which he or she has accepted responsibility. Of course, the terminology may vary and a department may be called a division, department, service, unit, an office, or some similar term, but it still represents a closely related set of activities.

For all practical purposes, the major departments in an organization are established by the top administrator. The chief executive officer is the one who groups the various activities and assigns them to be a distinct department. Some of the departments established this way will be small and will require no further subdivision. But in a hospital many of the departments will be of sufficient magnitude that their managers will have to further subdivide, that is, set up subdepartments or smaller units within the overall department. For this reason, it is necessary that every manager become acquainted with the various alternatives available for grouping activities. The process of departmentalization can be done on the basis of functions, process and equipment, territory (location), customer (patient), time, or product. We shall now explore each of the six alternatives more fully.

Functions

The most widely accepted practice of departmentalizing is to group activities according to functions, according to the jobs to be done. This is the guiding thought in the establishment of most departments within hospitals and related health care facilities. All activities that are alike and involve a particular function are placed together into one department under a single chain of command. For instance, a director of nursing services would be put in charge of all nursing activities throughout the center, and a director of dietary services is put in charge of all kinds of food- and nutrition-related activities. (See Figures 10-1 and 10-2.) As the institution grows and undertakes additional work, these new duties are added to the already existing departments. For instance, when a hospital adds an outpatient surgical center, performing surgery on patients who do not stay overnight, this new activity would logically be assigned to the operating rooms department and its supervisor. Such increased activities, however, might necessitate the addition of more levels of supervision within the functional departments, a topic that was discussed in Chapter 9.

To departmentalize by function in this manner is a natural and logical way of arranging the various activities of any enterprise and certainly in hospitals. It takes advantage of specialization by putting together the functions that belong together and are performed by the same specialists with the same kind of education, background, equipment, and facilities. Each supervisor is concerned with only one type of work and all of his or her energy is concentrated on it. Functional departmentalization also facilitates coordination, since one manager is in charge of all of one type of activity. It is easier to achieve coordination in this way than it would be in an organization where the same function is performed in several different divisions. Another advantage of functional departmentalization is that it makes the outstanding abilities of one or a few individuals available to the enterprise as a whole. Because functional departmentalization is a simple method and one that has been successful over the years, it is the most widely used method of setting up departments.

Process and Equipment

Activities can also be grouped around the equipment, process, and technology involved. This way of departmentalizing is often found in hospitals because they usually operate certain equipment and handle certain processes that require special training and expertise. Everything involving the use of the particular equipment and technology would be referred to its special department. It is important to note that this kind of organizational structure is similar to functional departmentalization, the major difference being the emphasis on person-machine relationships. For instance, in an x-ray department, specific equipment is used, but also only certain functions are performed. Therefore, departmentalization by function and equipment become closely allied.

Territory (Location)

Another way to departmentalize is according to geographical considerations. Again, this kind of departmentalization is more important in in-

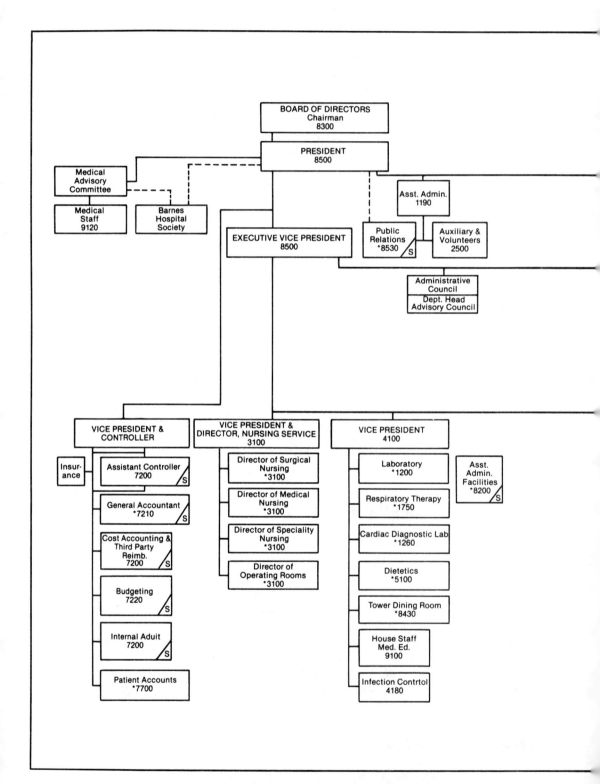

Figure 10-1. Barnes Hospital organizational chart

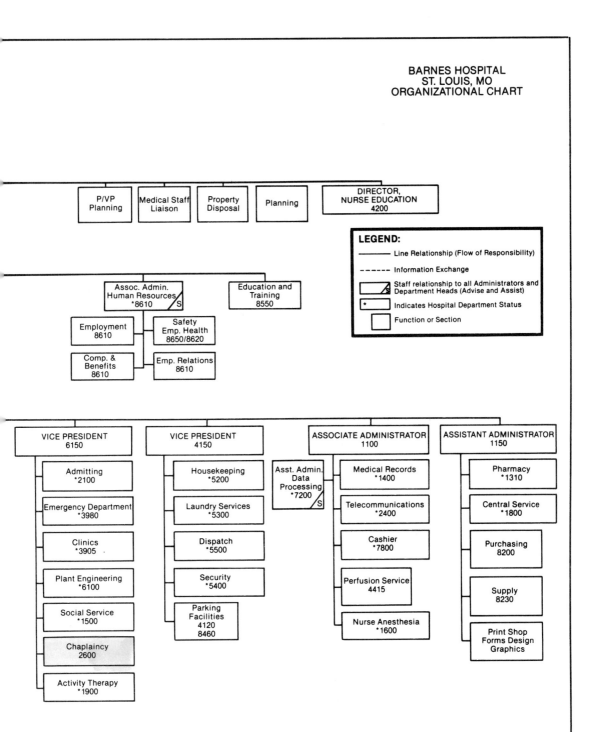

BARNES HOSPITAL
ST. LOUIS, MO
ORGANIZATIONAL CHART

| P/VP Planning | Medical Staff Liaison | Property Disposal | Planning | DIRECTOR, NURSE EDUCATION 4200 |

LEGEND:

——— Line Relationship (Flow of Responsibility)

----- Information Exchange

/S Staff relationship to all Administrators and Department Heads (Advise and Assist)

* Indicates Hospital Department Status

☐ Function or Section

Assoc. Admin. Human Resources/S *8610

Education and Training 8550

Employment 8610

Safety Emp. Health 8650/8620

Comp. & Benefits 8610

Emp. Relations 8610

VICE PRESIDENT 6150

Admitting *2100

Emergency Department *3980

Clinics *3905 .

Plant Engineering *6100

Social Service *1500

Chaplaincy 2600

Activity Therapy *1900

VICE PRESIDENT 4150

Housekeeping *5200

Laundry Services *5300

Dispatch *5500

Security *5400

Parking Facilities 4120 8460

ASSOCIATE ADMINISTRATOR 1100

Asst. Admin. Data Processing *7200 /S

Medical Records *1400

Telecommunications *2400

Cashier *7800

Perfusion Service 4415

Nurse Anesthesia *1600

ASSISTANT ADMINISTRATOR 1150

Pharmacy *1310

Central Service *1800

Purchasing 8200

Supply 8230

Print Shop Forms Design Graphics

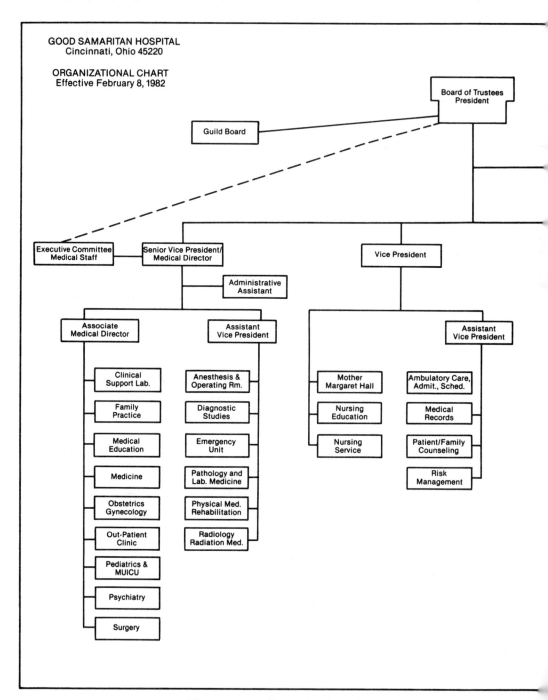

GOOD SAMARITAN HOSPITAL
Cincinnati, Ohio 45220

ORGANIZATIONAL CHART
Effective February 8, 1982

Board of Trustees
President

Guild Board

Executive Committee
Medical Staff

Senior Vice President/
Medical Director

Administrative
Assistant

Vice President

Associate
Medical Director

Assistant
Vice President

Assistant
Vice President

Clinical
Support Lab.

Family
Practice

Medical
Education

Medicine

Obstetrics
Gynecology

Out-Patient
Clinic

Pediatrics &
MUICU

Psychiatry

Surgery

Anesthesis &
Operating Rm.

Diagnostic
Studies

Emergency
Unit

Pathology and
Lab. Medicine

Physical Med.
Rehabilitation

Radiology
Radiation Med.

Mother
Margaret Hall

Nursing
Education

Nursing
Service

Ambulatory Care,
Admit., Sched.

Medical
Records

Patient/Family
Counseling

Risk
Management

Figure 10-2. Organizational chart

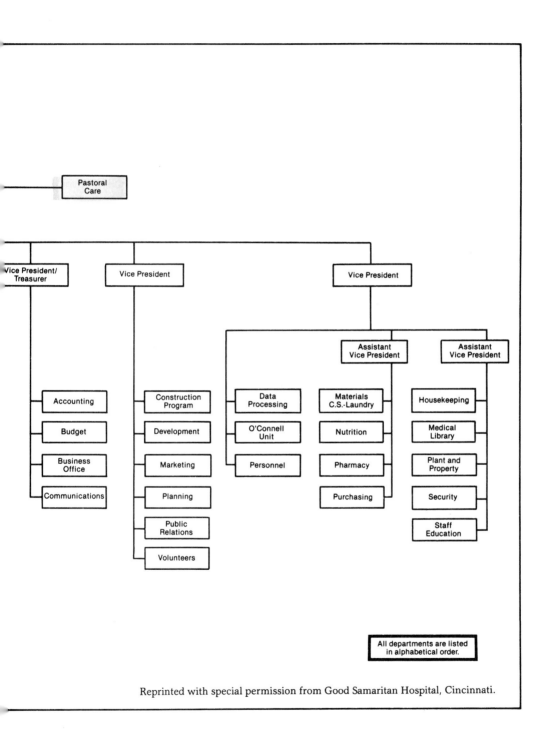

Reprinted with special permission from Good Samaritan Hospital, Cincinnati.

dustrial enterprises, but applications of it are made within a hospital. For instance, a hospital may be confronted with a setup in which there are numerous physically dispersed units. That is, if the same functions are performed in different locations, different buildings, then geographic departmentalization may be feasible. The same considerations are applicable even if all activities are performed in one building, but on different floors and wings, e.g., a medical-surgical nursing unit, third floor, west wing, and fourth floor, south. One of the advantages of territorial departmentalization is placing decision making close to where the work gets done. It has the disadvantage of possible duplications; on the other hand, territorially departmentalized organizations provide opportunities for the development of managerial talent.

Customer (Patient)

At times, management may find it advisable to group activities based on customer considerations. This is commonly known as customer departmentalization, and it means that the organization is structured along consumers' needs and characteristics. Two examples of nonindustrial organizations that have departmentalized along customer lines are a university, in which night programs and day programs comply with the requests and special needs of the "customers," namely, part-time and full-time students; and a hospital, in which certain services and activities are grouped for outpatients and inpatients. In so doing, the health care center delivers its services to more people, especially in supporting services, e.g., the laboratory or x-ray or physical therapy departments. Work referred to the ancillary services on an outpatient basis is on the rise and is a significant factor in a hospital's revenue picture. This is "customer" departmentalization, in which the characteristics of the patient are emphasized.

Time

An additional way to departmentalize is to group activities according to the period of time during which they are performed. An enterprise such as a hospital or public utility, which of necessity is engaged in a continuous process and operates around the clock, must departmentalize activities on the basis of time, at least to a certain extent. In other words, it must set up different time shifts, usually day, afternoon, and night shifts. Usually activities are first grouped on some other basis, such as by function, and then these activities are organized into shifts. Of course, the activities that have to be performed on the other shifts are largely the same as those performed during the regular day shift. Thus, such groupings often create serious organizational questions of how self-contained each shift should be and what relationships should exist between the regular day shift supervisors and the off-shift supervisors.

Product

Industry very frequently invokes the principle of product departmentalization; this principle is not applicable in a health care institution. To departmentalize on a product basis in industry means to establish each product or groups of closely related products as a product line, which is a relatively independent unit within the overall framework of the enterprise. In product departmentalization, the emphasis is shifted from the function to the output, the product. For example, a hospital supply company may have a separate department for furniture, another one for surgical supplies, and a third one for uniforms.

Product departmentalization in a health care facility would involve dividing a hospital into departments based on the "product" turned out, for example, maternity, surgery, intensive care, and dietary. Each such department would have its own supervisor of nursing, its own dietary supervisor, its own maintenance staff, etc. And each such "product" department would have its own boss, the director of surgery, the director of intensive care, the director of maternity, etc. These directors would be in charge of all functions within their "product" departments, including nursing activities, food services, laundry, maintenance, etc.

As you can see, such product departmentalization will result in duplication of effort. Instead of a single director of nursing, there are many, as many as there are departments. Moreover, coordination among all nursing services would be difficult, since each supervisor reports to a different boss. And the same difficulties would, of course, be found in every department. Thus, product departmentalization is not applicable in a health care institution.

Composite Structure (Mixed Departmentalization)

Departmentalization is not an end in itself. In grouping activities, management should not attempt to merely draw a pretty picture. Its prime concern should be to set up departments that will facilitate the realization of the institution's objectives and the coordination of its functions. There are advantages and disadvantages to each method of departmentalization. It is a question of balance and deciding which works most effectively. In so doing, management will probably have to use more than one of the guides for grouping activities, and they may end up with a hybrid structure, mixed departmentalization, i.e., a nursing supervisor (functional) on the surgical unit (subfunction), west wing, third floor (geographical), of the night shift (time). In practice, almost all hospitals have this composite type of departmental structure, invoking function, geography, time, and many other considerations. Any mixture is acceptable, as long as it works and is consistent with the overall objectives of the institution.

"Traditional" Structure

So far our discussion of organizational structure has centered around what is often called *traditional structure*. There are many reasons to discuss and understand this approach first and foremost. It is the most often used structure in all kinds of organized activities in the real world. It is the most studied and researched form of organization, and it has a long history of successful performance. Traditional structure is a contemporary design, it is not "old fashioned." It functions successfully under most prevailing conditions and is capable of producing and accommodating change and of accommodating contingencies as they arise.

Matrix Organization

One of the newer organizational structures building on our traditional concepts is the *matrix organization.* Matrix organization, also known as *project* or *grid* organization, does not do away with the traditional organization, but it simply builds on it and, under certain contingencies, improves on it. It is superimposed on functional organization, creating a matrix that provides horizontal dimensions to the traditional vertical orientation of the functional organization.

During recent years, high-technology industries found a need to create project organizations in order to focus resources and special talents for a given time on a specific project. Management and the customer became increasingly interested in the end result. The essence of matrix management is a compromise between functional and product departmentalization in the same organizational structure. Figure 10-3 shows possible matrix arrangements in a health care institution in which the functional managers are in charge of their professional function with an overlay of project managers who are responsible for the end product—a specific project. The concept of matrix organization gives an enterprise the potential of conducting several projects simultaneously. For example, the president of the hospital sees the need for several projects to be phased into the institution within the next 2 years, a unit-dose pharmaceutical system, a hospital-wide information system, and possibly a third project of getting the hospital ready for accreditation. These three projects could be assigned to three different project managers, and matrix organizations could be established for obtaining these objectives.

By establishing a project organization, better coordination can be achieved than would be possible in a traditional organizational structure. As the project comes along, it is assigned to a project manager from the beginning to its completion, and people from the functional areas needed for this project are assigned either on a full- or part-time basis to this project. The matrix is an overlay on conventional structure. It draws on the latter for the various skills required for this project. The project manager sees the project through from the beginning to the end. When the project is finished, the specialized personnel needed return to their functional departments or are reassigned to a new project; the same happens with the project manager.

There are many advantages to matrix organization. It offers an effective way to phase new projects in and out of operation. It improves coordination and establishes lateral relationships. Matrix organization offers greater flexibility to innovative ideas.

Matrix organization also creates a number of problems. Most of them

Eg. Child Advocacy Team

Bereavement Follow up Program

are due to the ambiguity and role in which the members of the team find themselves while the project lasts. The professional, when assigned to a project, often is faced with duality of command because directives will come from the project manager, whereas conflicting ideas may flow from the functional superior. For instance, the project manager may ask the professional member of the team to perform a task in a way that does not conform to the functional manager's guidelines. While assigned to the project, the professional also may feel isolated from the mainstream of his or her expertise. Further sources of frustration are that the assignment is only temporary and evaluations and possible promotions are usually still vested in the functional department head and not in the project manager. Dual command probably causes the most difficulties.

Most of these problems are caused by poor project preparation and a lack of concise and clear statements of authority; they can be avoided by the chief executive officer at the start of the project. It is important to clarify the authority and responsibility of the functional managers, for instance, those of the chief medical technologist in Figure 10-3 and those of the manager of project A. The project manager should have full authority and responsibility over the integrity of the design and over the budget; he or she must act as decision maker and coordinator for the duration of the project. There must be clear statements of the project manager's frequency of reporting and the scope of the project. The project manager must decide on schedules and work out priorities with the functional managers. The functional managers should be responsible for the integrity of the service or products their departments supply to the project. Statements along these ideas are necessary for the guidance of the project manager and the guidance of the functional managers whose departments are involved in the project.

Despite the best preparations and clarifications, misunderstandings may still arise, for instance, in the matter of priorities between the project managers of two projects who are both vying for a functional manager's services. Provisions to resolve such a dilemma should be made probably by referring such a dispute to higher management for a decision. Thorough preparation and clarifying authority and responsibility when the project is established will minimize most of these problems. But there still might be some borderline cases in which the problems of dual command may come up, especially in questions of accuracy and integrity of the project. Remember that all organizational structures can create some problems occasionally. Matrix organization provides an institution with a contemporary proven method of implementing a complex new task of relatively short duration.

Figure 10-4 is an example of a matrix organization wherein the project involves the computerization of the laboratories. This is a one-time undertaking, a project that is to be completed within a certain time. To phase this project into the organization and have it completed within the allocated period, the administrator decided that a matrix, or project, organization would be the best vehicle to get the job done. After appointing the project manager, a number of functional specialists needed to accomplish this task were assigned to it. A project manager was put in charge of this laboratory computerization project with a clear objective as to what is to be accomplished and when it should

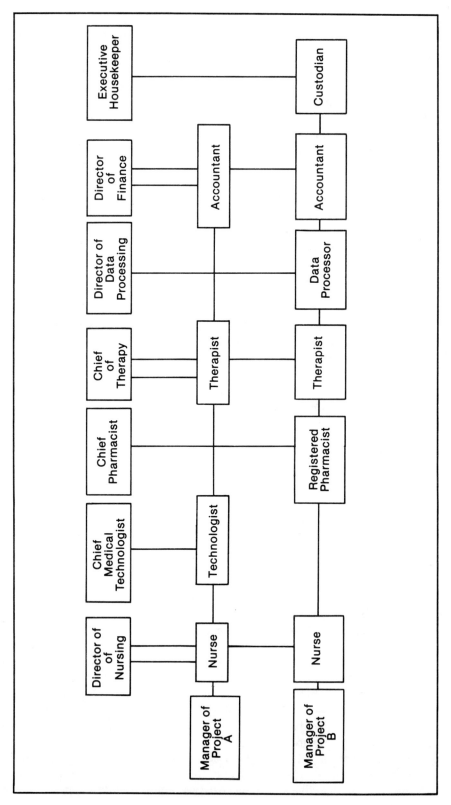

Figure 10-3. Matrix organization.

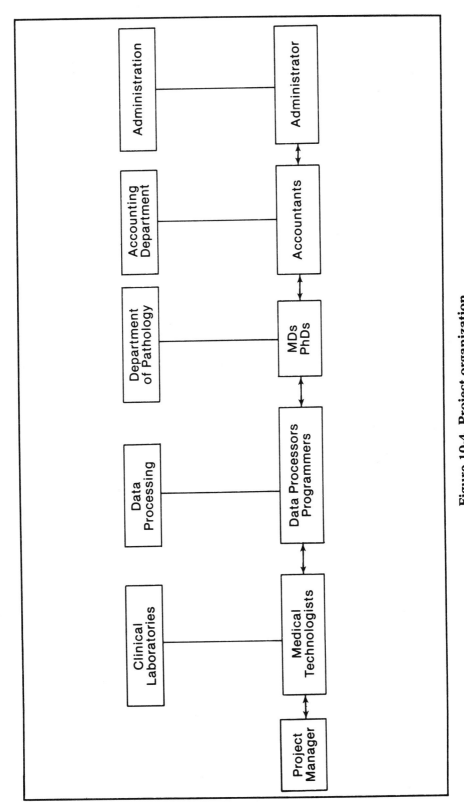

Figure 10-4. Project organization

Project: Introduction of a computer system into the clinical laboratories.

be finished.* To get the job done, it is necessary to have input and coordination from the laboratories, data processing, pathology department, accounting, and administration. These specialized employees work under the supervision and guidance of the project manager; therefore, a number of employees from the functional areas involved are assigned to the project either on a full-or part-time basis. The administrator was able to draft these specialists for the duration of the project and clearly stated that, as far as this project is concerned, the project manager is in charge and is their line superior. The project manager sees the project through from the beginning to the end. On completion the specialized personnel return to their functional departments, as does the project manager, or some of them may go on to another project where their special skills are needed.

Summary

Management's overall organizing function is to design a formal structural framework that will enable the institution to achieve its objectives. The chief administrator establishes this framework initially, using the basic principles of formal organization theory as guidelines, by beginning with the principle that the division of work is necessary for efficiency. This means grouping the various activities of the institution into distinct departments or divisions and assigning specific duties to each. The administrator can approach this departmentalizing task in several ways. The most widely used concept of departmentalization is grouping activities according to functions, that is, placing all those who perform the same functions into the same department. Besides departmentalization by functions, it is possible to departmentalize by process and equipment, geographical (territorial) lines, customers (patients), time (shift), or product. A composite structure made up of several of these alternatives is used most of the time.

These guides lead to the design of an organizational structure that, at times, is referred to as "traditional." This traditional structure is as contemporary as the manager wants it to be. Besides having a long history of successful performance, this form of organizational structure can accommodate contingencies and changes as they occur. One of the more prevalent of new developments in organizational design is the matrix organization structure, which stresses horizontal relationships. It is employed for achieving a special project with a definite result by superimposing a matrix over the traditional organization structure. At the inception, the chief executive officer must clearly state the authority relationships between the project manager who is in charge of this undertaking and the functional personnel assigned to it for the duration and their functional department heads; this is necessary to avoid and minimize possible problems of dual command and various other problems.

* In this discussion we are merely referring to the organizational structural arrangements. The project manager may use a PERT network for the timing of activities and events.

11

Delegation of Organizational Authority

The first task in building the organization is departmentalization based on division of labor and the concept of span of management. The second step is delegation of authority. Without authority the manager's job is meaningless. As stated before, authority is the lifeblood of the managerial position, and the process of delegation of authority breathes life into the organizational structure. The same process of delegation that brings authority to the manager is used to delegate it farther down. As we divide managerial responsibilities, we create additional levels in the chain of command. Decentralization is the degree to which authority is delegated throughout our health care institution; some institutions are highly decentralized and others are highly centralized.

The Meaning of Delegation

Just as authority is the key to the managerial job, so is delegation of authority the key to the creation of an organization. Although the formal structure of an organization may have been meticulously designed by the chief administrator and carefully explained in manuals and charts, the organization will still not have life or body until and unless authority is delegated throughout its entire structure. Delegation of authority makes the organization operative. Through this process of delegation, *the subordinate manager receives authority from the superior.* In other words, if authority were not delegated, there would be no subordinate managers and hence no one to occupy the various levels, departments, and positions that make up the organizational structure. We can truly say that only by delegating authority to subordinate managers is the organization actually created. Only by such delegation can the administration vest a subordinate with a portion of its own authority, thereby setting in motion the entire managerial process.

But delegation of authority does not mean that the boss surrenders all of his or her authority. The delegating manager always retains the overall authority to perform his or her functions. If need be, all or part of the author-

135

ity granted to a subordinate manager can be revoked. A good comparison can be made between delegating authority and imparting knowledge in school. A teacher in school shares knowledge with the students, who then possess this knowledge, but the teacher still retains the knowledge as well.

The Scalar Chain

The line of vertical authority relationships from superior to subordinate is the *scalar chain,* or the *chain of command.* Through the process of delegation, as we have said, formal authority is distributed throughout the organization. It flows downward from the source of all authority at the top, through the various levels of management, to the supervisor, and from there possibly to lower line supervisors. The broad authority necessary to run a private health care center is usually delegated by the board of directors or trustees to the president (also known as the administrator or chief executive officer), who in turn must delegate authority to subordinate managers, who delegate farther down the line, and so forth.

This line of direct authority relationships throughout the organization is commonly known as the scalar chain. It is a clear line from the ultimate source of authority to the lowest managerial ranks. This chain of command must be clearly understood by every subordinate, and it must be closely adhered to or else the risk exists of undermining authority. It is quite possible that by the time this "flow of authority" reaches the supervisory level it has pretty well narrowed down to a discreet "trickle" of delegation rather than a continuous stream. Nevertheless, it can be traced directly upward to the ultimate source. Scalar relationships are based on positional authority as discussed in Chapter 9; they are also based on another important managerial principle—unity of command.

Unity of Command

It has already been stated that delegation of authority flows from a single superior to a single subordinate and each subordinate reports and is accountable to only one superior, namely, that person from whom he or she receives authority. This is known as unity of command, the important organizational principle briefly referred to in Chapter 9. Of course, a superior manager can have a number of subordinates reporting to him or her; for each of these subordinates the one-to-one relationships, unity of command, still prevail.

The scalar chain provides the major route along which the process of delegation moves. Unity of command is a critical organizational concept; it enables the administration to coordinate activities, pinpoint responsibility and accountability, and define and clarify superior-subordinate relationships. Whenever this principle of unity of command is violated or compromised, management must anticipate complications.

The Process of Delegation

The process of delegation, which is the lifeblood of an organization, is something that every manager must be thoroughly familiar with. It consists of three components, all of which must be present. These three components are inseparably related, so that a change in one of them will require an adjustment of the other two. The three components of the delegating process are (1) the assignment of duties by a manager to the immediate subordinates; (2) the granting of permission (authority) to the subordinates to make commitments, use resources, and take all the actions that are necessary to perform their assigned duties; and (3) the creation of an obligation (responsibility) on the part of each subordinate to the delegating superior to perform the assigned duties satisfactorily.

Unless all three of these component steps are taken, the success of the delegating process cannot be ensured. This is true no matter which level of management is doing the delegating. It is important to realize that all managers, from the chief administrator on down to the line supervisors, must do their part in delegating authority throughout the entire organization. The chief administrator does the initial delegation when he or she groups activities, sets up line and staff departments, and assigns them their duties. Then the managers of each department or division must subdivide and reassign these duties within their own section and at the same time delegate the appropriate amount of authority and responsibility to carry them out. It does not matter whether it is the chief administrator who delegates authority to the associate administrators and directors or the line supervisor who delegates authority to the nonmanagerial subordinates, the steps in the process of delegation are the same. In the following discussion of these steps, we will approach the delegation process mainly on the departmental level rather than on the administrative level, because it is for departmental supervisors that this book is primarily written.

Assigning Duties

In the assignment of duties, the supervisor determines how the work in the department is to be divided among the subordinates and the supervisor. All the tasks that must be accomplished in the department will be considered, and it will be determined which of them can be assigned to a subordinate and which the manager must do. Some duties are more routine, and the manager would do best to assign these to the regular subordinates. Other functions can be assigned only to those subordinates who are particularly qualified for them. And then there are remaining functions that a supervisor cannot delegate but must do himself or herself.

In all likelihood, however, a number of duties could fall into any of these groups. In such cases, much will depend on the manager's general attitude and the availability of subordinates. But some logical guidelines can aid the manager when assigning duties. It is better that the assignments be justified and explained on the basis of such logical guidelines, rather than on the basis of personal likes and dislikes or hunch and intuition. This is important because the supervisor will be subject to pressures from different directions when assigning duties. There will be those who wish to acquire more activities and those who believe that they should not be burdened with certain duties. Thus, despite the guidelines, it will often be difficult for the supervisor to decide where best to place a given activity.

One way of doing this is to assign the activity to those employees who will make the most use of it most of the time. Or one may be inclined to assign an activity to employees who are already particularly skilled or primarily interested in it. If there is special interest, it is likely that these employees will carry out the activity in the best manner.

By considering such factors, the supervisor should be able to assign work so that everybody gets a fair share and can do his or her part satisfactorily. To achieve this, of course, the supervisor must clearly understand the nature and the content of the work to be accomplished. Furthermore, one must be thoroughly acquainted with the capabilities of the employees. All of this is not so simple as it might at first appear. The supervisor is often inclined to assign heavier tasks to those employees who are more capable because it is the easiest way out. In the long run, however, it would be far more advantageous to train and bring up the less capable employees so that they also can perform the more difficult jobs. If too much reliance is placed on one or a few persons, the department will be in a bad spot if they are absent or leave the employment of the enterprise. Thus, it is always a good idea to have a sufficient number of available employees who have been trained in the department's most difficult tasks. And the supervisor's problems of assigning various duties will become simpler by building up the strength and experience of all the employees.

Of course, the manner and extent to which the supervisor assigns duties to the employees will significantly affect the degree to which they respect and accept the supervisor's authority. Much of the success of the manager will depend on the skill in making assignments. This function will be discussed further throughout the text. It must be emphasized that the first step in the process of delegating authority is to assign certain tasks or duties to each subordinate; each must have a job to perform in order to warrant a delegation of authority.

Granting Authority

The second component in the process of delegation is granting authority, granting permission to make commitments, use resources, and take all those actions necessary to get the job done. It is advisable to state again at this time that duties are assigned and authority is delegated to *positions* within the institution rather than to people. But unless these positions are staffed by people, this discussion would, of course, be meaningless. That is why one commonly refers to the delegation of authority to subordinates instead of to subordinate positions.

To be more specific, granting authority means that a supervisor confers on the subordinates the right and power to act and make decisions within a predetermined and limited area. It is always necessary for the manager to determine in advance the scope of authority that is to be delegated. The range of delegated authority is usually specific when a task is routine and more general when the task is less formalized.

How much authority can be delegated will, of course, depend on the amount of authority that the delegating manager possesses and on the type of job to be done. Generally, enough authority must be granted to the subordinate to adequately and successfully perform what is expected. There is no need for the degree of authority to be larger than necessary; but by all means it must be sufficient to get the job done. If employees are expected to fulfill the tasks assigned to them and make reasonable decisions for themselves within this area, they must have enough authority to do all of these things.

The degree of authority delegated is intrinsically related not only to the duties assigned but also to the results expected. Whenever management delegates authority, it is necessary to let the subordinate know the results that are expected, for example, how fast the employee is expected to accomplish the job or how "perfect" the work is expected to be. For this purpose, standards of performance are established to provide a basis for judging work done and to facilitate management's control. These standards will be discussed more fully in the control discussion of the book. (Chapter 25.)

At this point, it is enough to say that you as a supervisor must be specific in telling each employee just what authority he or she has and what results are expected while exercising the authority. If this is not stated clearly, the subordinate will have to guess how far the authority extends, probably by trial and error and experimentation. As a supervisor, you may have experienced this when your own boss was not explicit as to how much authority you really had. To avoid this happening to your subordinates, it is necessary that the scope and results of authority be clearly defined and explained. As time goes on, of course, less explanation will be necessary. But bear in mind that if you should change an employee's job assignment, you must at the same time check to see that the degree of authority you have given is still appropriate. Perhaps it is more than is needed. Then you may have to revoke some of the delegated authority. Whenever conditions and circumstances of the job change, additional clarification of the scope of authority also becomes necessary.

Limitations to Authority

As discussed in Chapter 9, there are, of course, limitations to the authority that a manager has by virtue of his or her position in an organization. These limitations can be either explicit or implicit; some of them stem from internal sources and others from external sources. Generally, there are more internal limitations on the scope of authority the farther down one goes in the managerial hierarchy. In other words, the lower the rung on the administrative ladder, the narrower the area in which authority can be delegated and exercised. This is known as the tapering concept of authority as referred to in Figure 9-1.

The Exception Principle

Although the scope of authority clearly delineates the area of decision making, the supervisor may be confronted by a problem beyond and outside of that area. Then the *exception principle* becomes active; these problem situations are exceptions and must be referred to the delegating manager higher up for decision making. The latter must make certain that this is truly an exception since there is a danger that some subordinate managers may refer too many decisions upward when their own authority would be sufficient. In those situations, the superior should refrain from deciding and refer the problem back to the subordinate manager. But, if it is truly an exception, beyond the scope of the subordinate's authority, the superior manager must decide.

Only One Boss

In granting authority the principle of unity of command must be followed. Employees must be reassured that all orders and all positional authority can come only from the immediate supervisor, the only boss they have. It is very important that this principle be constantly stressed, because situations do occur in which two superiors try to delegate authority to one subordinate. Since biblical times it has been pointed out that it is difficult, if not impossible, to serve two masters. This sort of dual command is bound to lead to unsatisfactory performance by the employee, and it definitely results in confusion of lines of formal authority. The subordinate does not know which of the two "bosses" has the authority that will contribute most to his or her success and progress within the organization. Eventually such a situation will result in conflicts and organizational difficulties. It may have to be resolved by revoking some of the delegated authority.

Revoking Delegated Authority

As stated before, delegating authority does not mean that management has divested itself of its authority. The delegating manager still retains authority and the right to revoke whatever part of the authority that was delegated to a subordinate. From time to time, as activities change, there is a definite need to take a fresh look at the organization and to realign authority relationships. Managers frequently speak of reorganizing, realigning, reshuffling, and so forth; what is meant by this is the revoking of authority and reassignment of it elsewhere. Naturally such realignments of authority should not take place too often, since frequent changes create uncertainty, affecting morale. But periodic reviews of authority delegations are not merely advisable, they are necessary in any organization. This applies to top administration, as well as to the lowest level manager.

Creating Responsibility

The third major aspect of the delegation of authority is creating an obligation on the part of the subordinate toward the boss to satisfactorily perform the assigned duties. The acceptance of this obligation creates responsibility. And without responsibility, the process of delegation would not be complete.

Of course, the terms responsibility and authority are closely related to each other. Both terms are often misused and misunderstood. Although it is common to hear such expressions as "keeping subordinates responsible," "delegating responsibility," etc., these expressions do not get at the heart of the matter because they imply that responsibility is handed down from above, whereas in actuality it is accepted from below.

Responsibility is the *obligation of a subordinate* to perform the duty as required by the superior. By accepting a job, by accepting the obligation to perform the assigned tasks, an employee implies acceptance of responsibility. But this responsibility cannot be arbitrarily imposed on a person; rather, it results from a sort of mutual contractual agreement in which the employee agrees to accomplish the duties in return for rewards. Thus, it is clear that although the authority to perform duties flows from management to subordinate, the responsibility to accomplish these duties flows in the opposite direction, from the subordinate to management. This is still another manifestation of the way in which the formal theory of authority and the acceptance theory can be inextricably linked.

It is essential to bear in mind, however, that responsibility, unlike authority, cannot be delegated. It cannot be shifted. Responsibility is something that your subordinate accepts, but which you still have. The supervisor can assign a task and delegate to a subordinate the authority to perform a specific job. But the supervisor does not delegate responsibility in the sense that once the duties are assigned, the supervisor is relieved of the responsibility for them. The delegation of tasks does not relieve the supervisor of responsibility for these tasks. A manager can delegate authority to a subordinate, but cannot delegate responsibility.

It is true that the administrator of a hospital must delegate to the associate administrators a great deal of authority in order for them to oversee the performance of various tasks and services. These associate administrators, in turn and of necessity, have to delegate a large portion of their authority to the supervisors below them; but none of them delegates any responsibility. Each still accepts all the responsibility for the tasks originally assigned. Although subordinates may be granted the authority to actually perform these tasks, the superior is still responsible for seeing to it that the performance is satisfactory. This obligation cannot be shifted or reduced by assigning duties to another person.

Similarly, when you as a supervisor are called on by your boss to explain the performance within your department, you cannot plead as a defense that you have "delegated the responsibility" for such activity to some employee or group. You may have delegated the authority, but you have remained responsible and you must answer to your boss. It is essential that every supervisor clearly understand this vital difference between authority and responsibility. You must understand that when managers delegate the authority to do a specific job, they reduce the number of duties that they have to perform and also conditionally divest themselves of a certain amount of authority that can be taken back at any time if conditions are not fulfilled. But in this process managers do not reduce the overall amount of responsibility originally accepted from superiors. Although subordinates also accept a certain amount of responsibility for duties assigned them, this does not in any way diminish the manager's responsibility. It does add another layer or level to the overall responsibility, thereby creating *overlapping obligations*. Such overlapping obligations provide double or triple insurance that a job gets done and that it gets done correctly and responsibly.

Thus, the fact remains that although responsibility is something you accept, you cannot rid yourself of it. This may be a worrisome thought. After all, delegations and re-delegations are necessary to get the job done. Although as a supervisor you will try to follow the best managerial practices, you cannot be certain that each and every one of your subordinates will use his or her best judgment all of the time. Therefore, allowances must be made for errors, and, in evaluating your performance as a supervisor, some attention will be paid to the degree to which you must depend on your subordinates to get the work of your department accomplished. Although the responsibility has remained with you, your boss will understand that you cannot do everything yourself. In appraising your skill as a manager, some of the following points will be considered: how much care you have shown in the selection of your employees, training them, supervising them continuously, and controlling their activities. All of these matters will be taken into consideration in evaluating your ability in the event that something goes wrong in your department.

Equality of the Three Components

Always bear in mind that the three components of the process of delegation must go together to make this process a success. Authority, responsibility, and duties must be commensurate. There must be enough authority (but not more than necessary) granted to your subordinates to do the job, and the responsibility you expect them to accept cannot be greater than the area of authority you have delineated. Subordinates cannot be expected to accept responsibility for activities if they have not been handed any authority. In other words, do not try to "keep your subordinates responsible" for something that you have not actually delegated to them.

Inconsistencies between delegated authority, responsibility, and assigned tasks will generally produce undesirable results. You may have been in organizations where some of the managers had a large amount of authority delegated to them but had no particular jobs to perform. This created misuses of authority and disturbance. Then again, you may have been in positions in which responsibility was exacted from you when you did not have the authority to fulfill an obligation. When responsibility exceeds authority, it is nearly impossible to do the job. This, too, is a most embarrassing and frustrating situation. Therefore, you must make certain that the three components necessary for successful delegation are of equal magnitude and that whenever one is changed, the other two are changed simultaneously.

There are some rare occasions when responsibility and authority are not equal. For example, in emergencies managers are often inclined and even forced to exceed their authority. Hopefully, this will be an exception and not the normal state of affairs.

Decentralization—The Degree of Delegation of Authority

As discussed earlier, delegation of authority is the key to the creation of an organization. If no authority has been delegated, one can hardly speak of an organization. Hence, from an organizational point of view the problem is not whether or not to delegate authority, but rather *how much* authority will be delegated to the various subordinates on different organizational levels. It is not a question of yes or no, instead it is a question of the *degree* of authority to be delegated.

This question of the degree of delegation is extremely important because it will determine the answer to another highly significant organizational question, that is, the extent to which the organization is decentralized. It is the question of how much of what authority should be given to whom and for what purpose. Variations in the extent of decentralization are innumerable, ranging all the way from a highly centralized structure, in which one can hardly speak of an organization, to a completely decentralized organization, in which authority has been delegated to the lowest possible levels of management. In the first instance, the chief executive is in close touch with all operations, makes almost all decisions, and gives almost all instructions. Hardly any authority has been delegated and, strictly speaking, it cannot be said that an organization has been created. Many small enterprises regularly operate along these lines. Often such one-man shows will collapse if their chief executive dies, becomes incapacitated, or for some other reason leaves the scene.

A much less extreme situation is found in organizations in which authority has been delegated to a limited degree. In such organizations, the major policies and programs are decided by the top manager of the enterprise, and the task of applying these policies and programs to daily operations and daily planning is delegated down to the first level of supervision. There are few or no other levels between the top manager and the supervisors. This kind of arrangement is often found in medium-sized enterprises. It is obviously advantageous in that it limits the number of managers which the general manager must hire, thus keeping expenses down. Furthermore, it is advantageous in that the unusual knowledge and good judgment the general manager possesses can be applied directly. Quite a large number of enterprises in the United States have this type of organization with a limited degree of delegation of authority.

At the other end of the spectrum, we find those organizations in which authority has been delegated to the broadest possible extent and to the lowest levels of management. To find out if an organization is this decentralized, it is necessary to determine the kind of authority that has been delegated, how far down in the organization it has been delegated, and how consistent the delegations are. In other words, one must ask how significant a decision can be made by a manager and how far down within the managerial hierarchy. The more important the decisions made farther down in the hierarchy are, the more decentralization is prevalent. The number of such decisions and the functions affected by them also serve as indicators of decentralization. Furthermore, the less checking that is done with upper level management, the greater the degree of decentralization. The answers to all of these questions will indicate whether or not you are dealing with an organization that has delegated authority to the greatest extent possible. It is likely that most health care institutions find broad delegation of authority and decentralization advisable and necessary because of the nature of the activities involved and the background of the people working there.

It should be pointed out that timing is a very important factor in solving this degree of delegation problem. Although centralization of authority or limited decentralization may be the most logical organizational forms to use in the early stages of an enterprise, later stages will usually require the top administrator to face the problem of delegating more authority and decentralizing the organization to a greater extent. Such decentralization of authority becomes necessary when centralized management finds itself so burdened with decision making that the top executives do not have enough time to adequately perform their planning function or maintain a long-range point of view. This type of situation usually occurs when an organization expands. It should indicate to top management that the time has arrived to delegate authority to lower echelons. In other words, there should be a gradual development toward decentralization of authority commensurate with the growth of the enterprise.

Advantages and Disadvantages of Delegation

You are probably aware by this time that there are numerous advantages to delegating and decentralizing authority. Moreover, these advantages become even more important as the enterprise grows in size. For example, by delegating authority, the senior manager is relieved of much time-consuming detail work. Subordinates can make decisions without waiting for approval. This increases flexibility and permits more prompt action. In addition, such delegation of decision-making authority may actually produce better decisions, since the manager on the job usually knows more pertinent factors than the manager higher up, and speedy decisions are often essential. Delegation to the lower levels, moreover, increases morale and interest and enthusiasm for the work. It also provides a good training ground. All of these advantages serve to make the organization more democratic and more responsive to the needs and ideas of its employees and ultimately will result in delivery of better patient care.

Of course, there are some possible disadvantages to considerable delegation. For example, the supervisor of a department may believe that he or she no longer needs the help of upper level managers and can develop his or her own supporting services. This could easily lead to duplication of effort and waste. Another disadvantage could be a possible loss of control, although the delegating manager can take steps to see that this does not happen. All in all, we must conclude that the advantages of a greater degree of delegation far outweigh the disadvantages.

As stated before, the contingencies of health care institutions are such that to deliver the best possible patient care, authority must be delegated broadly. It is a question of balance, of finding the degree of decentralization that works. No two health care centers are alike. Each has its own tradition, history, problems, challenges, and work force to integrate into an organizational structure that works. This is an ongoing process. We have to continuously monitor and adjust the degrees of delegation and decentralization as the environment and the institution change.

Summary

Earlier we discussed the meaning of authority as that power which makes the managerial job a reality. This definition becomes more understandable when considering the source of authority. One way of looking at the source is to state that all formal managerial authority emanates from the top of the organization. From there, it is delegated downward through an uninterrupted chain of command, beginning with the chief executive officer and ending with the supervisor on the lowest level of the managerial pyramid. According to the formal theory, then, managerial authority is conferred from above.

Good managers must know how to use formal authority and how to delegate some of it to their subordinates. Through the process of delegation of authority, management actually creates the organization. This process of delegation is made up of three components: the assignment of a job or duty, granting authority, and creating responsibility. All three are coextensive and coexistent, and a change in one will necessitate a change in the other two. Since this process of delegation is the only way to create an organization, the question is not whether top management will delegate authority, but rather how much or how little authority will be delegated. If authority is delegated all the way down to the lowest levels of supervision, then the organization is highly decentralized; if most authority is more or less hoarded at the top, the organization is highly centralized. Although centralization might be appropriate when an enterprise is just getting started, there are far greater advantages arising from decentralization or the broad delegation of authority, one of the most important being the increased motivation of subordinates.

12

Line and Staff Authority Relationships

First we divided the work to be done into departments, meaning we organized horizontally. Then we divided the managerial work to be done vertically by delegating authority. Now, as another consequence of specialization, there is the need to add staff to the organization. We are creating lateral and diagonal relationships by adding line and staff relationships.

In hospitals and related health facilities, it is common to speak of the nursing staff, medical staff, dietary staff, administrative staff, etc. In this context, the word "staff" applies to a group of people who are engaged primarily in one activity to the exclusion of others. That is, the word staff is used to define all those people who do about the same thing, e.g., nurses, physicians, and dietitians. In the general field of management and administration, however, the meaning of the word "staff" is very different. "Staff" is spoken of in connection with "line," and both of these terms refer to authority relationships, which shall be discussed below. In this context, any reference to "staff" will mean line/staff, not the meaning to which most people working in health care centers are usually accustomed.

Since no one, not even the chief executive officer, could possibly have all the knowledge, expertise, and information that is necessary to manage a modern organization, staff becomes an essential and critical part of the institution. Staff plays an increasingly important part in all modern organizations. This is even more evident today in the delivery of health care. Line managers retain the administrative and authoritative parts of the activities, whereas staff supplies the scientific, technological, technical, and informational aspects without which the institution could not function properly.

Origin of Staff

The concept of staff is not new; there are applications of it since the days of ancient Athens and Rome, in the College of Cardinals, and in the armies throughout history. Even today we can see examples of the need for

146

and use of staff in the highest office of the country, the Presidency. Today staff plays a major role in all organized activities.

As organizations grow in size and complexity, the duties of the managers increase and they try to do more and more. Then they add subordinate managers by creating departments and delegating authority. But sooner or later their span of management is so large that no more can be added because they cannot pay proper attention to them. At this point they add personal staff, which means one or more assistants to do the work that cannot be delegated. But sooner or later, the assistant's knowledge is too general and the other managers also need the help of experts in many functional areas. This is where organizational staffs are added to advise and support any member of the institution who needs their help.

Line and Staff Organization

Much has been written and said about the concepts of line and staff, and probably no other area in the field of management has evoked as much discussion as these concepts. It is probably also true that many of the difficulties and frictions encountered in the daily life of an organization are due to line and staff problems. Misconceptions and lack of understanding as to what line and staff really are can cause bitter feelings and conflicts of personalities, disunity, duplication of effort, waste, lost motion, and so on.

As a supervisor of a department, you should know whether you are attached to your organization in a line capacity or a staff capacity. You might be able to find this out by reading the job description, and, if that does not clarify it, by asking your superior manager. Line and staff are not characteristics of certain functions, rather they are characteristics of authority relationships. Therefore, the ultimate way to determine whether a department is related to the organizational structure as line or staff is to examine the intentions of the administrator. It is that person who confers line authority on certain departments and places others into the organizational structure as staff. Staff is not inferior to line authority or vice versa; they are just of a completely different nature. As we discuss these differences, keep in mind that the objectives of the staff elements are ultimately the same as those of the line organization, namely, achievement of the institution's overall goals, delivery of the best possible patient care.

Line Organization

The simplest of all organizational structures is the line organization. The line organization depicts the primary chain of command and is inseparable from the concept of authority. Thus, when we refer to line authority we mean a superior and a subordinate with a direct line of command running between them. In every organization, this straight direct line of superior-subordinate relationships runs from the top of the organization down to the

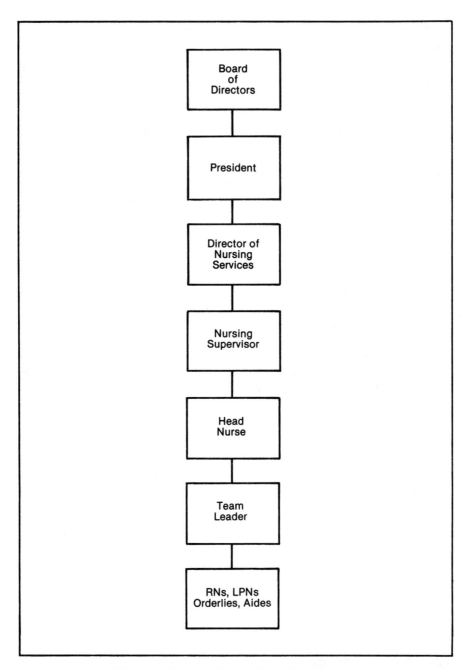

Figure 12-1. A direct line of authority.

lowest level of supervision. Figure 12-1 depicts an example of one direct line of authority running from the board of directors to the president of the institution, to the director of nursing services, to a nursing supervisor, from there to a head nurse, then on to a team leader, and finally to the rest of the nursing employees.

Unity of Command

The uninterrupted line of authority from the administrator to the team leader assures that each superior exercises direct command over the subordinate and that each subordinate has only one superior to obey. This is known as the principle of unity of command. Although this was discussed in Chapter 11, it is advisable to repeat that it is a principle every administrator should follow while arranging line authority relationships. Unity of command means that one person in each organizational unit has the authority to make the decisions appropriate to his or her position. It means that each employee has a single immediate supervisor who is in turn responsible to his or her immediate superior and so on up and down the chain of command. Thus, everyone in the line organization knows precisely who the boss is and who the subordinates are. The individual knows exactly where he or she stands, to whom orders can be given, and whose orders have to be fulfilled.

From what we have said thus far, it is easy to see that line authority can be defined as the authority to give orders, to command. It is the authority to direct others and require them to conform to decisions, plans, policies, and objectives. The primary purpose of this line authority is, of course, to make the organization work by evoking appropriate action from subordinates. Directness and unity of command have the great advantage of assuring that results can be achieved precisely and quickly.

This kind of direct line structure does not answer all of the needs of the modern organization, however. It was adequate at a time when organizations were not as complex as they are today. In most enterprises now, activities have become so specialized and complicated that an executive cannot be expected to properly and expertly direct all of his or her subordinates in all phases of their activities without some additional assistance. Line management today definitely needs the help of others to carry out the job. That is, to perform the managerial functions well, almost every line executive needs someone to lean on, someone who can give counsel, advice, and service. In short, a staff is needed.

Staff Organization

Staff is auxiliary in nature; it helps the line executive in many ways. It provides counsel, advice, and guidance in any number of specialized areas to all members of the organization whenever and wherever there may be a need. Staff cannot issue orders or command line executives to take their advice, however. Staff can only make recommendations to the line. That advice can be accepted, rejected, or altered by the line. Because staff is an expert in its specialty, the advice is usually accepted; but it does not have to be. When the line accepts the staff's suggestion this suggestion becomes a line order. Line authority is based on superior-subordinate relationships; it is positional and managerial, whereas staff's authority is based on expertise; it is advisory and not managerial. Obviously, staff is not inferior to line and line is not inferior to staff. They are just different, and both are needed to complement each other to achieve overall objectives.

Although the right to command is not part of staff authority, it is present in two instances. First, within each staff division, there exists a line of command with superior-subordinate relationships just like in any other department. But staff's own chain of command does not extend over to the line organization. Rather, it exists alongside of the line organization as shown in Figure 12-2. The second application shows up when staff has been given functional authority by the chief executive officer. This concept will be discussed later in the chapter.

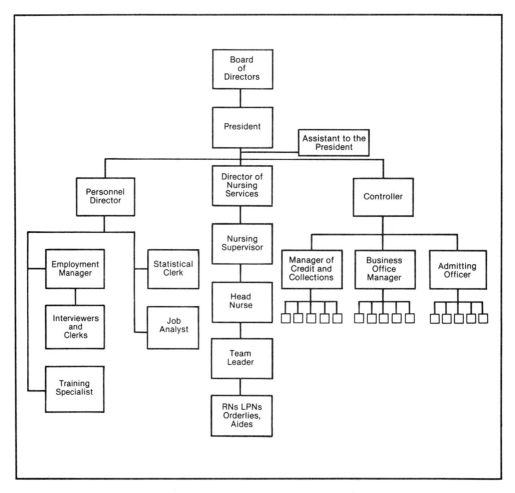

Figure 12-2. Staff's chain of command alongside the line organization.

You can probably now see more clearly why all supervisors must know whether their position is attached to the organization in a line or a staff capacity. They must know this so that they will understand their function and relation to the other members of the organization. If it is staff, then the function is to provide guidance, counsel, advice, and service in this specialized area to whomever may ask for it. But as far as the supervisor's own department is concerned it will not matter whether it is line or staff. Within every department, the supervisor is the line manager. He or she is the only boss, regardless of whether the department is attached to the organization in a staff or line capacity.

At this point, we must distinguish between *personal* staff and *specialized* staff. When executives find themselves in a position where they need a personal aide who will help them in the performance of duties that they cannot delegate, a personal staff position may be created. The person in this position is a staff aide to the particular executive, rather than to the organization at large, for example, the assistant to the president as shown in Figure 12-2. Eventually, however, a personal staff will usually become inadequate because many other managers in the organization also need expert advice and guidance. At this juncture, specialized staffs are introduced into the institution to provide counsel and advice in various special fields to any member of the organization who needs it. Our discussion in this chapter refers to these specialized staff positions.

Relationships Between Staff and Line

From time to time conflict over organizational and operational problems might arise between line and staff, regardless of how well the relationships were defined. This is due to the two kinds of authorities at work: positional and formal on one side and the weight of expertise and knowledge on the other. In most organizations line and staff work together harmoniously; but an occasional skirmish might arise. Harmonious cooperation between line and staff is especially important in a health care institution, since the input of so many specialists is a must for the delivery of good health care. Much will depend on the sensitivity and tact of the staff people and the clarity of organizational arrangements.

It is common practice for certain activities in each organization to be undertaken as staff. But this does not mean that one can assume these activities are always staff. Line and staff, as stated before, are characteristics of authority relationships and not of functions. Thus, even a title will not offer any clue in recognizing line or staff. In industrial enterprises, it is common to find a vice president of engineering, a vice president of industrial relations, and a vice president of production. None of these titles, however, indicates whether the position is line or staff. The little square box on the organization chart does not offer any help either in this dilemma.

The same situation applies in hospitals and related health care facilities. For example, most hospital personnel managers are often known as vice president of human resources, and their departments operate in a staff capacity, although this is not obvious from their titles. The function of a staff personnel department is to provide advice and service on personnel matters to all the other departments of the institution. The personnel department is there to recruit, screen, and test applicants, keep personnel records, help provide reasonable wage and salary administration, advise line managers when difficult problems of fair employment practices or discipline arise, and so on.

Whenever a line manager has a personnel problem, therefore, the specialized services of this staff department should be called on. Certainly, the personnel manager is the one who is best qualified to supply the current advice and information, since this is his or her background and only duty.

But all the personnel manager can do is submit suggestions to the line manager, who in turn can accept, alter, or reject them. If the line manager believes that the suggestions of the personnel department are not feasible, he or she is at liberty to make a decision. But inasmuch as the reason for establishing a staff in most instances is to obtain the best advice, it is usually in the interest of the line manager to follow staff suggestions. After all, staff members are the ones who really ought to know best. For all practical purposes, the "authority" of the staff lies in their thorough knowledge of and expertise in dealing with problems in their specialized field. They will sell their ideas based on their authority or knowledge, not on their power to command. Thus, if any of the suggestions of staff are to be carried out, they are carried out under the name and authority of the line officer and not that of the staff person. A person who acts in a staff relationship must know that his or her task is to advise, counsel, and guide and not to give orders except within his or her own department. It must be understood that if these ideas are accepted by the line executive, the orders to carry them out must be issued by that same line manager following the regular chain of command.

Functional Authority

It is correct in most instances to say that staff provides advice and counsel to line managers, but that it lacks the right to command them. As briefly mentioned previously, one exception to this concept of staff should be pointed out. A staff office may have been given *functional authority*. Functional authority is authority restricted to a narrow area; it is a special right given to someone who normally would not have authority and therefore could not command. Although functional authority is limited to this area, it is full authority and gives this staff member the right and power to command outside of normal authority lines in this limited area. This right is based on expertise in the specialized field.

For example, an administrator decided that for some good reason the personnel director's office should have the final word in cases of dismissal. * In recent years, the laws, regulations, court decisions, and interpretations referring to fair employment practices have become an important area of managerial concern and a specialty that requires daily attention by someone in the organization; probably the personnel department is best suited to keep up-to-date in this area. To avoid such problems for the hospital, the administrator decided to confer the final decisions on separations to the personnel department. In this instance, the administrator has conferred on staff (assuming that the personnel department in this institution is a staff activity)

---

*This type of situation and the difficulties it can cause will be discussed further in Chapter 16 in connection with the supervisor's staffing function and the activities of the personnel director.

functional authority in the special area of dismissals. Now the personnel director has this authority, and it no longer adheres to the line supervisors who would normally have had the authority to do their own firing. This would be an example of functional staff authority.

There is no doubt that functional authority violates the principle of unity of command. This principle, as you will recall, states that the subordinate is subject to orders from only one superior regarding all the functions. Functional authority, however, introduces a second superior for one particular function, such as the discharging of employees in our example. Functional staff orders have to be carried out by the line supervisor to whom they are directed. If the line supervisor should disagree strongly, he or she can appeal to the superior manager up the line. But unless these orders are changed—and this is unlikely—the supervisor has to comply with them.

Functional authority is advantageous because it allows for the maximum effective use of a staff specialist, leading to improved operations. It enables staff to intervene in line operations in situations designated by top management. The price for this intervention, violation of unity of command, is high and may cause friction in some organizations. It is up to the administrator to weigh the advantages versus the disadvantages before functional authority is assigned.

Assistants-to

The assistant-to is a personal staff position belonging to a single executive, e.g., the assistant to the president in Figure 12-2. This person is an extension of the arms, legs, and mind of the manager; he or she does a variety of jobs, such as gather information, do research, relieve the executive of details, and so on. This position is also often used for the training and development of junior managers to acquaint them with how higher level executives function. The assistant-to position has no line authority. More interesting, however, is the role which that individual often plays in the channels of informal communications and the workings of the informal organization.

The Authority of Attending Physicians and Surgeons

At this point, it becomes necessary to discuss another line of internal authority that is found only in a hospital setting, the authority exercised by physicians and surgeons. Here we are not referring to those medical men and women who are full-time chiefs of the medical staff group or full-time chiefs of a medical specialty or members of the resident house physicians group. Let us assume that all the latter are regular, full-time salaried employees of the hospital who do not have a private practice and receive their salary from the hospital. We are not speaking of these types of physicians now. Rather, our reference is to those attending physicians and surgeons who are in the private, fee-for-service, practice of medicine and who have been admitted to practice at the hospital. Only a staff physician, surgeon, or dentist can admit patients to the hospital.

There is a potential for tensions and misunderstanding between administration and members of the medical staff. This is understandable. The administration must consider the entire hospital as an organized activity, its relationships with all its employees, financial viability, its role in the community, etc., whereas the physicians' interests are likely to be geared to the patient and, at times, to the physicians' own economic survival. Members of the medical staff often wonder whether the administrative staff really understands their problems and vice versa. Normally, in most hospitals these frictions are minimal, since both groups strive toward the best results for the health care center. In most situations a natural partnership exists between administration and the physicians, the first providing the necessary facilities and personnel and the latter providing the practice of medicine.

There is little doubt that such outside physicians are in charge of the patients they bring into the hospital. In this connection, they have clinical-therapeutic-professional authority and exercise substantial influence throughout the hospital structure at many organizational levels and in many functions. These physicians admitted to practice at the hospital (usually referred to as the medical staff) are not shown on the hospital organization chart in any direct line or staff relationship under the chief executive officer. They are usually charted in a vague relationship to the board of directors on the organization chart. They practice medicine at the hospital, but they are outside of the administrative line of authority. They are "guests" who are granted practice privileges, yet they have a great deal of authority over various people in the hospital.* Their authority is exercised over the patient and especially over the nursing staff when it comes to the medical issues, but they also give orders to and expect compliance from many other employees of the hospital, for instance, personnel in the radiology department, laboratories, and dietetics.

As a second line of "authority," such orders from a physician or a surgeon clearly violate the principle of unity of command. This may lead to a situation in which nursing personnel in particular are accountable to two "bosses," that is, they must take orders from and are responsible to their supervisor and to the physician on the case. This, of course, can cause great difficulties when orders from the administrative source of authority and the medical professional source of authority are not consistent. Nevertheless, in a hospital the physician can give orders to an employee without being the line supervisor. In other words, the physician constitutes an outside source of authority who can marshal the resources of the hospital without being in the chain of command and without being responsible to the administrator, except for his or her professional responsibility to the medical world and to the medical staff organization of the hospital. Of course, it is assumed that the physician's medical competence warrants the right and authority to remain in practice at the hospital.

This dual command obviously creates administrative and operational problems, as well as human problems. It causes difficulties in communica-

*These remarks of necessity are general. They apply primarily to *general, private, community hospitals.* There are many ramifications in teaching hospitals or in hospitals operated by government agencies in which our statements would not apply or would have to be modified.

tion, discipline, and organizational coordination. Moreover, it can cause considerable confusion in cases in which it is not clear where authority and responsibility truly reside. This can lead to frequent efforts on the physicians' part to circumvent administrative channels. And by the same token, the administration may think that the physicians, through their power and authority, are interfering with administrative responsibilities. In all likelihood, there will be some clarifications in this situation as hospitals' overall legal responsibilities are defined more clearly in the future. Regardless of all the complications inherent in this duality of command, it is an integral part of every general community hospital and exists in most other health care facilities as well. Hospital supervisors and personnel just have to learn to live and cope with the problem of dual authority when it applies to the medical or surgical aspects of the case.

Summary

Management's organizing function is to design a structural framework that will enable the institution to achieve its objectives. First, we divided the work to be done horizontally into departments and then the managerial work was divided vertically by delegating authority. Another result of specialization is the addition of staff to the organization, since no manager could possibly possess all the knowledge, expertise, and information necessary to manage a modern health care institution, or any other organized activity, without the expertise and knowledge of specialists in many functional areas. This leads to the introduction of staff into the organization.

The administrator must decide whether a department is attached to the organization in a line or in a staff capacity. Since line and staff are quite different, it is essential for every supervisor to know in which capacity he or she serves. The supervisor in a straight direct chain of command that can be traced all the way to the top administrator is part of the line organization. The line organization generally follows the principle of unity of command, which means that each member of the organization has a single immediate superior, who in turn is responsible to the next higher immediate superior and so on up and down the line of command. The supervisor who is not within this line of command is attached to the organization as a staff person to provide expert counsel, service, and advice in a specialized field to whomever in the organization needs it. Staff people are not inferior to line or vice versa, rather they represent different types of authority relationships. The line manager has the authority to give orders, whereas the staff manager usually only has the authority to make recommendations that the line manager does not have to accept. The advice can be accepted, rejected, or altered by whomever asked for it. Because staff represents expertise in a specialty, the advice is usually accepted. Staff's authority is based on expertise; it is advisory and not managerial.

But the situation changes in the case of functional authority. There are some cogent reasons why sometimes the chief executive officer may decide to confer functional authority on a staff office, that is, the right to command in a narrow area based on the staff person's expertise in a specific area. Although functional authority is limited to this area, it is full authority and the right and power to command outside of normal lines. Such functional authority violates the principle of unity of command. A similar difficult situation of duality of command is created by the attending physician's clinical-therapeutic authority. These additional channels of command are due to the nature of health care delivery and the presence of many areas of functional authority; they have to be coped with in almost every health care center.

13

Organizing on the Supervisory Level

Most department heads and supervisors will not become involved in the major decisions concerning the overall organizational structure of their health care institution. But they will be concerned with the structure of their own department.

Logically, we could not discuss the organizing process on the departmental level until we understood the basic organizational principles and how they are applied in the creation of the overall structure.

This is why we have discussed thus far the organizing process mainly from an overall institutional point of view. We have outlined how the chief administrator establishes the formal organizational structure and delegates organizational authority. Although the process of delegation was approached more on the supervisory level, we have still not yet focused our full attention on how a supervisor actually goes about organizing and delegating within his or her own department. With this broad understanding, we are ready to approach the organizing function more specifically from the supervisor's point of view of the departmental goals and objectives, daily operations and activities, and existing personnel and resources. In other words, we shall now look at organization on a narrow scale, zeroing in on the microcosm known as the department.

Naturally, it should not be surprising to find that the organizing process is basically the same, whether it is performed by the chief administrator or the lowest line supervisor. It involves grouping activities for purposes of departmentalization or subdepartmentalization on the supervisory level, assigning specific tasks and duties, and, most important of all, delegating authority. In essence, this means that the basic organizational principles must be understood and applied by supervisors when they are setting up their own department, just as they were by the chief administrator when the overall institution was structured. Let us see how a supervisor might actually go about applying these principles, using them on a day-to-day basis so that they are not just abstractions but life-giving parts of a healthy departmental body.

157

Ideal Organization of the Department

Most supervisors are placed in charge of an existing department; only a few will ever have the opportunity to design a structure for a completely new department. When designing or rearranging the organizational structure of the department, the supervisor should conceptualize and plan for the ideal organization. The word "ideal" in this instance is not intended to mean "perfect," rather it is used to mean the most desirable organization for the achievement of stated objectives. It is the supervisor's job to design an organizational setup that will be best for this particular department. In so doing, the principles and guides of organization must be observed. Following these is no guarantee that the department will not have any problems. But a significant number of problems will be avoided because the organizational network has been designed to function smoothly in the majority of cases.

The manager must bear in mind, however, that certain organizational concepts and arrangements which work well in a very large institution may not be applicable to a smaller institution. It is conceivable that in a 50-bed hospital a supervisor may be supervising two different activities, such as purchasing and medical records. In other words, supervisors must not blindly follow the idea that what is good for one enterprise is also good for another. Moreover, it is not essential that the manager's organizational plans for the department look pretty on paper or that the organization chart appear symmetrical and well balanced. Rather, this ideal design should represent the most appropriate organizational arrangement for reaching the departmental objectives. It should be uniquely tailored to suit the conditions under which the manager works, instead of some abstract image of what an "ideal" department should look like.

In planning this ideal, but realistic, organization, the supervisor must consider it as something of a standard with which the present organizational setup can be compared. The ideal structure should be looked on as a guide to the short- and long-range plans of the department. Although the supervisor should carefully plan for the ideal structure on becoming the department's manager, this does not mean that the existing organization should be forced to conform to the ideal immediately. But each change in the prevailing organization should bring the existing structure closer to the ideal. In other words, the ideal organization of the department represents the direction in which the supervisor will move as the organizing function is carried out.

Internal Departmental Structure

At this point, you might be a bit unclear as to exactly how supervisors would go about designing the ideal departmental structure. What does this involve, how is it done, and are supervisors really equipped to do it? In most cases, they are because essentially they are being asked to subdepartmentalize, to establish subdivisions or subunits within their department, just as the chief administrator established the overall divisions or units for the whole organization. Two examples of how a director of nursing service might subdepartmentalize or set up the internal departmental structure are shown in the organization chart in Figures 13-1 and 13-2.*

More specifically, what supervisors are being asked to do is to consider the groupings of activities in the department, the various existing positions, and the assignment of tasks and duties to these positions. Is what he or she finds the best possible arrangement for achieving departmental and institutional objectives? Are all the present positions necessary or could some be eliminated or combined with others? Does each position have a fair assignment of tasks and duties, commensurate with its status and salary? Are the positions related so that there is no duplication of effort and that coordination and cooperation are facilitated? In other words, is the department well organized? Does it function in the most efficient manner? Are there any changes at all that the supervisor would like to see in the internal organizational structure of the department?

If there are any such changes, then these will become the basis for what we have been calling" the ideal organization of the department." They will become the organizational goals toward which the department head will strive when structuring the department.

Of course, if a supervisor is setting up a new department or working in a new institution, much of this ideal structure can probably be implemented at the beginning. This would naturally be the most desirable situation, but is not generally the case. The supervisor is forced to gradually implement organizational goals while working within the existing departmental structure and existing personnel.

Organization and Personnel

It is important to realize that the supervisor should design this ideal organization based on sound organizational principles, regardless of the people with whom he or she has to work. This does not mean that departments could exist without people to staff their various positions. Without people, of course, there can be no organization. The problems of organization should be handled in the right order, however; first comes the sound structure, then the people are asked to fulfill this structure.

If the organizational setup is planned first around existing personnel, then existing shortcomings will be perpetuated. Because of incumbent personalities, too much emphasis may be given to certain activities and not enough to others. Moreover, if a department is structured around personalities, it is easy to imagine what would happen if a particular employee should be promoted or resign. If, on the other hand, the departmental organization is structured impersonally on the general need for personnel rather than on the incumbent personalities, it should not be difficult to find an appropriate successor for a particular position. Therefore, an organization

---

*Also see the various departmental charts and job descriptions in Appendix B.

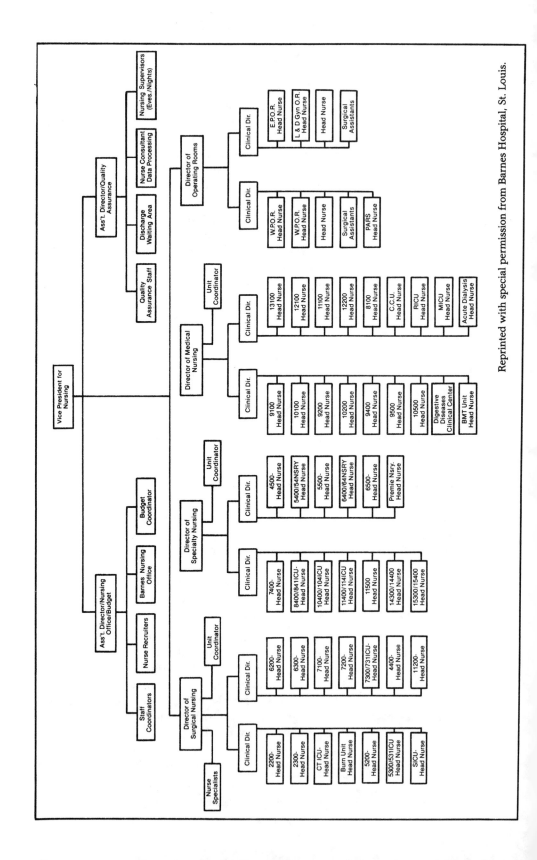

Reprinted with special permission from Barnes Hospital, St. Louis.

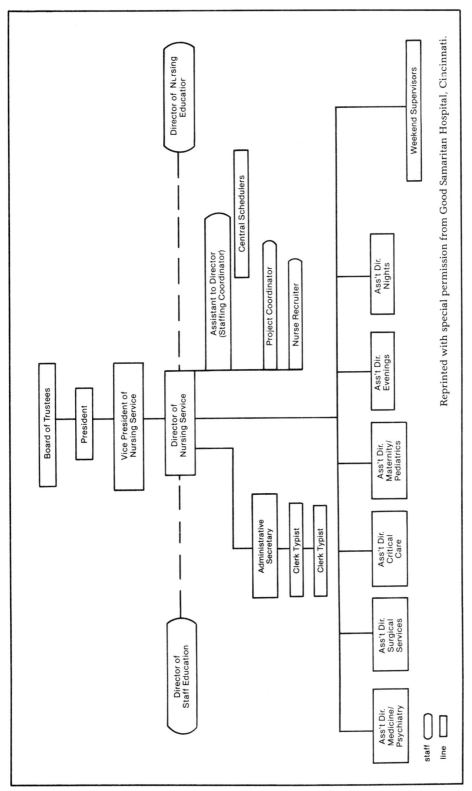

Figure 13-2. Internal departmental structure of a nursing service.

Reprinted with special permission from Good Samaritan Hospital, Cincinnati.

should be designed first to serve the objectives of the department; then the various employees should be selected and fitted into departmental positions.

This, however, is easier said than done. In most instances, the supervisor has been put into a managerial position in an existing and fully staffed department without having had the chance to decide on the present structure or personnel of the department. It frequently happens that the available employees do not fit too well into the ideal structure. Yet they cannot all be overlooked or dismissed. In such cases, the best the supervisor can do for the time being is to adjust the organization to utilize the capacities of the employees he or she has. It should be realized that this is an accommodation of the ideal plan to fit present personalities; it should be regarded as temporary. Such personnel adjustments are sometimes necessary, but fewer of them will be required if the supervisor has already made a plan of the organization he or she would like to have if the ideal human resources were available. Then, as time goes on, the supervisor will strive to come closer and closer to the ideal departmental setup.

Reorganization

It must be kept in mind that organizational structure is not static. The organization is a living institution and therefore needs a certain amount of continuous adjustment. For this reason, the manager's organizing function is also continuous; there is a need for constantly checking, questioning, and appraising the soundness and feasibility of the departmental structure. Organization is not an end in itself, but rather a means to an end, the accomplishment of the objectives of the department. A manager must continuously watch for new developments, practices, and thinking in the field of organization. The supervisor must be willing to *reorganize* the department if these developments warrant it or if it is indicated that the existing structure is too far from the ideal to permit effective functioning.

Of course, the term "reorganization" is used with all kinds of different connotations. In our discussion this term will refer to changes in the organizational structure, departmentalization, the assignment of activities, or authority relationships. From time to time a manager makes such changes because of technological advances, the dynamic and changing nature of the department's activities, a shift of supervisors, or, as noted previously, reorganization may be necessitated by the need to overcome existing deficiencies.

Let us look at an example of reorganization to overcome existing deficiencies. As time went on nurses found themselves burdened with a great amount of secretarial and clerical work that kept them away from actual patient care and bedside nursing. This was an undesirable situation, since the thrust of their education and purpose was the care of patients. Finally, it became apparent that many of these functions could be performed by someone else without a nursing education just as effectively; this led to the creation of positions now commonly known as unit managers, unit clerks, ward clerks, floor clerks, nursing station assistants, and so forth. The care of "things" was assigned to them, whereas the actual care of "people" reverted back to where it should be, the nurses. The job of the ward clerk is to perform general clerical duties, such as preparing, maintaining, and compiling records in the nursing unit. This person copies information from nurses' records, writes requisitions for laboratory tests, dispatches messages to other departments, and so forth. The unit clerk makes appointments for patients' services in other departments as requested by nursing staff and maintains an established inventory of stock supplies on the unit by verifying supplies and making requisitions. There are a multitude of additional duties performed by the floor clerk that heretofore the nursing personnel had to cope with. This was a case of reorganization where duties were reassigned and new authority relationships had to be established between unit managers, clerks, and head nurses.

Once this or any other type of reorganization has been decided on, it can be carried out either as a long-run, gradual, continued change or as a one-time change covering only a short period. The latter approach has commonly been called the "earthquake" technique, indicating that the full shock of the reorganization is felt all at once. The long-run plan, on the other hand, provides for a period of more gradual adjustment to the organizational changes. No doubt this approach is less disturbing and creates fewer upsets than the earthquake approach. It must be kept in mind that changes are always disturbing to those who are affected by them, regardless of how well intended they are. A manager who frequently changes the department's organizational structure runs the risk of damaging the morale of the subordinates. To the supervisor suggesting the reorganization, it might seem trivial, but to the subordinates it will probably appear frightening because it implies changes in their status and security. The wise supervisor will have to learn how to strike a happy medium in the desirable amount of organizational change. In most instances, the supervisor will probably find that most subordinates quickly adjust to changes if they are properly explained and if the need for them is demonstrated. A more detailed discussion of the introduction of change is given in Chapter 19.

As stated briefly in our discussion on delegation of authority, from time to time it is necessary to review the degree of authority that has been delegated. The supervisor may believe that he or she has lost control over certain activities and that it has become necessary to "tighten up" or to *recentralize*. In such a situation recentralization of authority is called for, e.g., authority must be revoked or realigned. This is one form of reorganization that presents a difficult task for the supervisor, since feelings of suspicion, hurt, discouragement, and security on the part of the subordinate are likely to surface. To mitigate these tensions, the supervisor must explain the reasons for this action. Such an unpleasant situation can be avoided or lessened by taking great care in the choice of a subordinate when delegating authority in the first place.

Since organizing is a dynamic process, it should be emphasized that regardless of the difficulties involved, it is necessary for a supervisor to make organizational adjustments from time to time to keep the department as viable as possible.

Delegation of Authority Within the Department

In a Medium or Large Department

Once a supervisor has organized or reorganized the department's internal structure, or at least planned the changes that are needed and recorded them in an ideal organizational design, the supervisor is ready to delegate or redelegate authority in accordance with the organizational structure. We assume that the supervisor has been given sufficient authority and that he or she is in charge of all the activities within this section. Just as any other manager, supervisors are faced with the necessity of delegating some of the authority that has been handed down to them. As mentioned previously, unless this is done an organization has not been created. This is certainly the case when there are very many employees. In other words, the supervisor must assign tasks, grant authority, and create responsibility within each of the subunits and for each of the positions in the department.

Of course, if a supervisor is taking over an existing department probably most of the delegation of authority has already been done. But it is necessary to check carefully to see that it is consistent with the ideal organizational plans. The supervisor should check the amount and type of authority delegated to each position, whether the three component steps in the process of delegation were followed, and whether there is quality and consistency of these three components. In other words, he or she should refer back to the specific procedure outlined in Chapter 11 to see that authority is delegated properly in the department.

In a Small Department

Let us now turn to the situation where the number of employees in the supervisor's department is rather small. Such a department would consist merely of a supervisor and a few employees (three to six). The supervisor may wonder if in these circumstances it is necessary to delegate authority. The answer is yes. Even in a small department the supervisor will need someone who can be depended on to take over if the supervisor should have to leave either temporarily or for any length of time. Even in the smallest department there should be someone who can work as his or her *backstop*. It is a sign of poor supervision when there is no one in a department who can take over when the supervisor is sick or has to be away from the job. It can also happen that the supervisor personally may miss a promotion because there is nobody to take over the unit. So sooner or later every supervisor needs a backstop, understudy, assistant, or whatever this person may be called. It would be appropriate for the supervisor to discuss this intention with his or her immediate boss.

Availability of Suitable Subordinates

Of course, the process of delegation assumes that there is someone available who is willing to accept the increased authority. As a supervisor, you may have wanted to delegate more authority to some of your subordinates and to make one of them your assistant, but you had no one within your department who was willing to accept this authority and to take complete charge of an area of activities. You may not have anyone working for you who is capable of handling more authority. In such a case, authority must be withheld and, for the moment at least, cannot be delegated.

On the other hand, you may find yourself in a vicious circle, complaining that without better trained subordinates you cannot delegate, but without delegating additional authority your subordinates will have no opportunity to obtain the necessary exposure. With additional experience and training, however, their judgment could be improved and they could become more capable subordinates. Although this lack of trained subordinates is often used by supervisors as an excuse for not delegating more authority, the supervisor must always bear in mind that unless a beginning in the delegation process is made, no subordinate capable of being a backstop and of taking over the department, if necessary, will ever be available.

It is the supervisor's duty to develop and train such a person, and in the process it is likely that more authority can be delegated not only to the individual selected as a backstop but to other employees as well. Moreover, this process of training for increased delegation will give the supervisor a much clearer view of his or her own duties, the workings of the department, and the various jobs to be performed. Bringing subordinates to the point where they can finally be given considerable authority is a slow and tedious process, but it is worth the effort. Naturally, in the early stages, the degree of authority granted will be small, but as subordinates grow in their capacities, increasingly more authority can be delegated to them.

Selecting a Backstop

As we have said, this process of greater delegation of authority should include making one particular subordinate into an assistant for the supervisor. The first step here, of course, is to select the right person for the job. No doubt the supervisor knows which employees are more outstanding. These would be the ones to whom the other employees turn in case of questions and who are looked on as leaders. Outstanding employees, moreover, know how to do the job very well, seem to be able to handle problems as they arise, and do not get into arguments. They should also have shown good judgment in the way they organize and go about their own job, be open minded, and be interested in further development and moving into better positions. Without such ambitions, even the best training would not achieve any results. Outstanding employees must have shown a willingness to accept responsibility and must have proven dependability. Sometimes a worker may not have had the opportunity to show all of these qualities. But whatever qualities have remained latent will show up rather quickly during the actual training process.

If the supervisor has two or three equally good employees in the department, training all of them for greater delegations of authority on an equal basis should begin. Sooner or later it will be obvious which one has the superior ability, and this individual will then become the major trainee for the backstop position. Once the selection of a single person is made (or in a large department there could be several assistant backstops), it is not necessary to come out with general formal announcements in this respect. Of course, the supervisor should discuss and explain the intentions fully to the employee chosen. And it is even more important for the supervisor to follow through by laying a thorough groundwork for good training so that the one who has been chosen will work out as an understudy.

Training a Backstop

Although the phrase "training a subordinate" is frequently used, the term "training" is really not appropriate. It would be more fitting to speak of the development or even self-development on the subordinate's part. Understudies must be eager to improve themselves and show the initiative to be self-starters.

The supervisor should gradually let understudies in on the workings of the department, explain some of the reports to them, and show them how needed information is obtained. The supervisor should tell them what is done with these reports and why it is done. The supervisor should also introduce an understudy to other supervisors and other people in the organization with whom they must associate and contact; sooner or later the understudy should contact them himself or herself. It is advisable to take the understudy along to some of the hospital meetings after this person has had a chance to learn the major aspects of the supervisor's job. On such occasions the supervisor should show how the work of the department is related to that of the other departments in the hospital.

As daily problems arise, the supervisor should let understudies participate in them and even try to solve some of them for themselves. By letting understudies come up with some solutions to problems, the supervisor will have a chance to see how well they analyze and how much they know about making decisions. In time, the supervisor should give the understudy some areas of activities for which he or she will be entirely responsible. In other words, gradually more duties and authority should be assigned.

Of course, this whole process requires an atmosphere of confidence and trust. The boss must be looked on by the understudy as a coach and friend, not as a domineering superior. Supervisors should caution themselves that in their eagerness to develop the understudy as rapidly as possible, they do not overload them or pass problems onto them that are beyond their capabilities. The supervisor must never lose sight of the fact that it takes time to be able to handle problems of any magnitude.

Obviously, all of this will require much effort and patience on the supervisor's part. Sooner or later the additional duties should result in some tangible rewards for the backstop. And it is conceivable that just about the time the understudy comes to the point of being truly helpful, he or she may be transferred to another job outside of the supervisor's department. This may be discouraging for the moment, but the supervisor may rest assured that the administrators will give credit for a training job well done.

The Supervisor's Hesitancy to Delegate

Often supervisors do not like the idea of creating a backstop; they may be reluctant to delegate authority because they know that they cannot delegate responsibility. Since in the final analysis responsibility remains with them, they may think it is best to make all decisions themselves. Thus, out of fear of their subordinates' mistakes, many supervisors are not willing to delegate authority and, as a result, continue to overburden themselves. Their indecision and delay may often be costlier than the mistakes they hoped to avoid by retaining their authority. Always bear in mind that there is also a certain likelihood that the supervisor may make mistakes. Moreover, if employees are permitted to learn from some of their own mistakes, they will not resent the supervisor's authority, and they will be more willing to accept greater authority themselves.

As stated above, the supervisors' reluctance in delegating such authority is understandable in view of the fact that they still remain accountable for the results. The old picture of a good supervisor was one who rolled up the sleeves and worked right alongside the employees, thus setting an example by his or her efforts. Such a description is particularly true of a supervisor who has come up through the ranks and for whom the supervisory position is a reward for hard work and professional or technical competence. This person has been placed in a managerial position without having been equipped to be a manager and is faced with new problems that are difficult to cope with. This person therefore retreats to a pattern in which he or she feels secure and works right alongside the employees. There are occasions when such participation is needed, for instance, when the job to be performed is particularly difficult or when an emergency has arisen. Under these conditions, the good supervisor will always be right on the job to help. But aside from such emergencies and unusual situations, most of the supervisor's time should be spent carrying out the supervisory job, while the employees should be doing their assigned tasks. It is the supervisor's job not to do, but to see that others get things done.

Frequently, however, supervisors will still feel that if they want something done right, they have to do it themselves. Often they believe that it is easier to do the job than to correct the subordinate's mistake. And, even if the supervisor lets the subordinate do it, the supervisor may feel a strong temptation to correct any mistakes rather than explain to the subordinate what should have been done. It is frequently more difficult to teach than to do a job oneself. Moreover, supervisors often believe that they can do the job better than any of their subordinates, and chances are they are right. But sooner or later they will have to get used to the idea that someone else can do the job almost as well as they can, and at that point they should delegate the necessary authority. In this manner, they will be able to save their own time for more important managerial jobs, for thinking, planning, and more delegating. If supervisors are willing to see to it that employees become increasingly competent with every additional job, then their own belief and confidence in their employees' work will also grow. This mutually advantageous relationship will permit the supervisor to carry out the basic underlying policy of delegating more and more authority as the employees demonstrate their capability in handling it.

Despite the fact that a certain amount of authority must be delegated to create an organization, some supervisory duties cannot be delegated. The supervisor should always apply and interpret policies, give general directions for the department, take necessary disciplinary action, promote employees, and appraise them. Aside from these duties, however, their subordinates should do most things by themselves.

The Reluctant Subordinate

The delegation of authority and especially the development of an understudy are, of course, two-sided relationships. Although the supervisor may be ready and willing to turn over authority, the subordinates may sometimes be reluctant to accept it. Frequently, subordinates may feel unsure of themselves, unsure that they will be able to handle the job assigned to them. They may be reluctant to leave the security of their job and their co-workers. Merely ordering them to have more self-confidence, of course, will have little effect. The supervisor, as we have said, must create this self-confidence by carefully coaching and training the subordinate to undertake more and more difficult assignments. Then, and only then, will the subordinate be able to accept the increased responsibility that goes along with harder tasks and greater authority.

Naturally, with increased responsibilities there should also be commensurate positive incentives. These may be in the form of pay increases, bonuses, a fancier title, recognized status within the organization, or other rewards of a tangible and intangible nature. Such rewards will, of course, include the self-satisfaction that the subordinate feels when he or she is able to handle increased responsibility and has moved up in the organizational ranks.

Achieving Delegation of Authority

Broader delegations of authority are not always easily put into practice. To be effective, a sincere desire and willingness to delegate must permeate the entire organization. Top management must set the mood by not only preaching but also by practicing broad delegation of authority. Although top management's intentions may be the best, it is still conceivable that at times the desired degree of decentralization of authority is not achieved. For instance, top management may find that authority has not been delegated as far down as it intended because somewhere along the line there is an "authority hoarder," a person who simply will not delegate authority any farther. This person grasps all the authority delegated to him or her without redelegating any of it.

There are a number of reasons why managers might resist further decentralization of authority in this manner. To some, the delegation of authority may mean a loss of status, a loss of power and control. Others may think that by having centralized power they are in closer contact with the administrator. And yet other managers are truly concerned with the expenses involved in delegating authority. Moreover, it is difficult for many managers to part with some of their own authority and still be left with full responsibility for the decisions made by their subordinates.

There are several ways to cope with this problem and to achieve the degree of decentralization that is desired by the top administration. As stated before, the entire managerial group must be indoctrinated with the philosophy of decentralization of authority. They must understand that by carefully delegating authority they do not lose status, nor do they absolve themselves of their responsibilities. One way of putting this understanding into practice is to request that each manager have a fairly large number of subordinate managers reporting to him or her. By stretching the span of management, the subordinate manager has no choice but to delegate authority. Another way to achieve broader delegations of authority is for the enterprise to adopt the policy of not promoting a manager until a subordinate manager has been developed who can take over the vacated position. By doing this, as noted in the discussion of backstops, the manager is encouraged to delegate as much authority as possible at an early stage. Moreover, this process creates an ideal organizational climate in which the subordinates can find maximum satisfaction of many of their most important needs.

Delegation and General Supervision

Now that we have discussed the delegation of authority to employees of a small department who work directly below their supervisor, we have reached the lowest rung of the organizational ladder and further delegation of authority is no longer possible. There is an end to delegation in the strict sense of the word when we reach the point of execution of daily duties, in other words, when we reach the level of employees who are actually doing the work. Since we have reached this level, the question now arises as to how a supervisor can effectively reap the benefits of delegation, how one can take advantage of the motivating factors of delegation in the daily working situation. The answer to this question can be found at the point where the philosophy of delegation takes on the form of what is commonly referred to as *loose*, or *general*, *supervision*.

The Employee's Reaction to General Supervision

Most employees accept work as a part of normal healthy life. Accordingly, most managers display the underlying managerial attitude of McGregor's Theory Y toward their employees. Such managers understand that in their daily jobs employees seek a satisfaction that wages alone cannot provide. Most employees also enjoy being their own bosses. They like a degree of freedom that allows them to make their own decisions pertaining to their work. The question arises as to whether this is possible if one works for someone else, whether such a degree of freedom can be granted to employees if they are to contribute their share toward the achievement of the enterprise's objectives. This is where the ideas of delegation of authority and general supervision can help. The desire for freedom, for being one's own boss, can be enhanced by a delegation of authority that in a working situation means merely giving orders in broad general terms. It means that the supervisor, instead of watching every detail of the employee's activities, is primarily interested in the results achieved. The supervisor permits the subordinates to decide how to achieve these results within accepted professional standards and organizational requirements.

In other words, the delegation of authority in the daily working situation does not amount to more than a general form of supervision whereby the supervisor sets the goals and tells the subordinates what is to be accomplished, fixing the limits within which the work has to be done. But the employees are to decide how to accomplish these goals. This gives each employee maximum freedom within the constraints of the organization and professional standards. This broad general kind of supervision on the employee level has the same results as the delegation of formal authority throughout the levels of the managerial hierarchy.

Advantages of General Supervision

Significant advantages result from this approach to supervision, which are similar to those cited in our discussion of the process of delegation. The supervisor who learns the art of general supervision will benefit in many ways. First of all, the supervisor will have more time to be a manager. If the supervisor tried to practice close detailed supervision and tried to make every decision personally, he or she would probably be exhausted physically and mentally. With delegation, however, the supervisor will be freed from many of the details of the work and will thus have time to plan, organize, and control. In so doing, the supervisor will be freed to receive and handle greater authority and responsibility.

Moreover, the decisions that general supervision allows employees to make will probably be superior to those made by a harried supervisor trying to practice detailed supervision. We have already pointed out that the employee on the job is closest to the problem and therefore is in the best position to solve it. Furthermore, this will give the employees a chance to develop their own talents and abilities and become more competent. It is always difficult for a supervisor to instruct an employee on how to make decisions without actually letting the employee make them. They can really only learn by practice.

This leads us to the third advantage of general supervision; it enables employees to take great pride in the results of their decisions. As stated before, employees enjoy being independent. Repeated surveys reveal that the one quality employees most admire in a supervisor is the ability to allow them to be independent by delegating authority. Employees want a boss who shows them how to do a job and then trusts them enough to let them do it on their own. In this way, the supervisor provides on-the-job training for them and a chance for better positions. Thus, we can see that general supervision allows for the progress not only of supervisors themselves, but also of the employees, department, and enterprise as a whole.

Much more will be said about general supervision when we discuss the managerial function of influencing. Let us repeat that practicing the broad general approach to supervision, instead of an autocratic, dictatorial, detailed approach, provides many of the satisfactions employees seek on the job, which money alone does not cover. Because their needs are fulfilled, employees are motivated to put forth their best efforts in achieving the enterprise's objectives.

Attitudes Toward General Supervision

It seems appropriate at this stage to point out that the broad general approach to supervision and the idea that it is necessary to provide positive motivation for employees were not always as widely accepted as they are today. There was a time when management believed that emphasis on negative authority was the best method of motivating employees. Those who depended on the force of authority as their major means of motivation—and a few may still erroneously believe in this today—believed that managing consisted of forcing people to work by threatening to fire them if they did not. One of their assumptions was that the only reason people work is to earn money and that they will work only if they fear losing their jobs. This approach, of course, ignores the fact that employees want many other intrinsic satisfactions from their work besides the salary. It also assumes that people do not like work, that they try to get away with doing as little as possible. On this basis, the need for close supervision is justified. The supervisor must tell the workers precisely what is to be done every minute of the day and not permit the workers any chance to use their own judgment. The older school of managerial thought was based on Theory X* as its underlying assumption.

Such reliance on the sheer weight of authority has, of course, lost most of its followers. This kind of approach was possible in the early days of the industrial revolution when workers were close to starvation, when they would do anything to obtain food, clothing, and shelter. In recent years, however, employees have begun to expect much more from their jobs. This is particularly so when most of the employees are professionals and when times are good and employment is high. We also find that the educational process of our youth has had a significant influence on recent attitudes. Many years ago children were accustomed to strict obedience toward their elders. But now schools and homes emphasize freedom and self-expression, and it is therefore becoming more and more difficult for the young employee to accept any kind of autocratic management on the job. In addition to this, legislation, regulations, and the impact of unions have made it more difficult for a supervisor to fire an employee.

*Theories X and Y will be discussed fully in Chapter 19.

Perhaps the most important change in current attitudes is the increased awareness that the "be strong" form of "motivation" provides no incentive to work harder than the minimum required to avoid punishment and discharge. Under these conditions, employees will probably dislike work, which, if they are not unionized, can lead to slowdowns, sabotage, and spoilage. Management will probably react by watching workers even more closely. This in turn will encourage the employees to try to outsmart the administration. Thus, a vicious circle is started with new restraints and new methods of evading them. Sooner or later such a circle will produce aggression, arguments, fights, and a general devastating effect on the entire organization.

Summary

In this chapter, we considered the organizing process from the supervisor's point of view. Basically, organizing on the departmental level involves the same general steps as organizing the overall institution, that is, grouping activities or subdepartmentalizing, assigning specific tasks and duties, and delegating authority. The supervisor should supplement these steps, however, by designing an ideal organizational structure specifically for the particular department. Such a structure represents the way the supervisor would organize the unit if starting from scratch with ideal resources and personnel. But in most cases the supervisor comes into an existing department and cannot immediately implement an ideal organizational design. One reason may be that the available personnel do not fit into this model. What must be done instead is to plan changes or completely reorganize the department to make it come closer to the ideal. Such reorganization is a normal and important part of managerial life; however, it should not be so frequent that it undermines the security and morale of employees. Of course, organizational changes can be implemented either all at once or gradually, depending on the imminence of the need for them.

After reorganization has been accomplished or at least planned, the supervisor can proceed to delegate or redelegate authority in accordance with the departmental structure. In a large or medium department, the process of delegation will be that outlined in Chapter 11: assigning duties, granting the authority to carry out these duties, and encouraging employees to accept responsibility for their duties. In a small department, the delegation of authority will take the form of developing a backstop, an understudy who can take over when the supervisor is not there. This is a long and tedious process because it involves careful development and progressively increasing delegations of authority. It is well worth the effort, since it will contribute to high motivation and morale among employees. Moreover, unless the supervisor does train someone to be the backstop and does grant authority to that person, the supervisor will not have created any organization, and the department is bound to collapse if the supervisor has to leave the scene.

This decentralization of authority is not as easily achieved as it might seem. Indeed, management frequently runs into obstacles that must be overcome to achieve broad delegation. These obstacles may be caused by an authority hoarder somewhere down the line, a manager's reluctance to shoulder authority and responsibility, or the unavailability of suitable subordinates to whom authority can be delegated. Somehow or other, this vicious circle should be broken and broader delegation should be instituted.

Of course, there comes a place in the organization where further delegation of authority is not possible. This is at the interface between the supervisor and the nonmanagerial employees as they go about performing their daily tasks. At this level, delegation of authority expresses itself in the practice of a general, or loose, kind of supervision that involves giving employees a great amount of freedom in making decisions and determining how to do their jobs. In other words, general supervision is an application of Theory Y and not Theory X. It enables the employees to use their own judgment, and, in so doing, they will receive greater satisfaction from their jobs. Such general supervision is probably also the best way to motivate employees, whereas dependence on the sheer weight of authority would normally bring about the least desirable results. There might be occasions when the manager must fall back on formal authority, but with the new attitudes and expectations of our society, the general trend is toward more freedom and self-determination in management, as well as in other aspects of life.

APPENDIX A

Formal Organization
Charts and Manuals

Formal Organization
Charts and Manuals

Organization charts and manuals are tools to clarify the organization's structure to everyone concerned. The health care institution's structure is formalized graphically in the chart and in words in the manual. These tools help explain to everyone involved in the organization how it works. To be helpful they must be available all the time and up-to-date, which means changes must be incorporated promptly.

Once the chief executive officer has established the formal structure of the organization by setting up departments and levels, determining the span of supervision, and deciding which functions are to be line and which are to be staff, the entire structure can be depicted graphically in organization charts and in words by using manuals. These are important organizational tools because they provide a clear-cut picture of the overall institution that can be used by all levels of management. For the supervisor, organization charts and manuals can be particularly helpful in understanding the formal organizing process and the goals and intent of the administration. By studying them, the supervisors can see the positions and relations of their own department within the overall structure and learn about the functioning and relationships of all other departments as well.

The responsibility for preparing an organization chart rests with the chief executive officer. A number of individuals, especially those in staff positions, will probably help in the collection of information and preparation of charts, but in the final analysis it is one of top administration's duties. Although the administrator is responsible for preparing charts and manuals for the institution as a whole, it will be necessary for the supervisor to devise some of these organizational tools on a departmental level if they are not available or up-to-date. Thus, we must look more carefully at how such tools are prepared and at the information they supply.

Organization Charts

Organization charts are a means of graphically portraying the organizational structure at a given time; it is a snapshot. The chart shows the skeleton of the structure, depicting the basic relationships and groupings of positions and functions. Most of the time the chart starts out with the individual position as the basic unit, which is shown as a rectangular box. Each box represents one function. The various boxes are then interconnected horizontally to show the groupings of activities that make up a department, division, or whatever other part of the organization is under consideration. They are connected vertically to show scalar relationships. Thus, it can readily be determined who reports to whom merely by studying the position of the boxes in their scalar relationships. For example, we saw in the organization charts on pp. 124-125 some of the scalar relationships that can be found in a typical hospital.

Advantages and Limitations

One of the advantages is the analysis and work that is necessary for the preparation of a chart, whether it is for the overall organization or a department. As the chart is prepared, the organization must be carefully analyzed. Such analysis might uncover structural faults and possibly duplications of effort or other inconsistencies. Or one might uncover cases of dual reporting relationships (one person reporting to two superiors), overlapping positions, and so on. Moreover, charts might indicate whether the span of supervision is too wide or too narrow. An unbalanced organization can also be readily revealed. Charts are also helpful in personnel administration. They can indicate possible routes of promotions for managers, as well as for other employees. In addition, charts afford a simple way to acquaint new members of the organization with its makeup. It is only natural that most employees within the organization have a keen interest in knowing where they stand, in what relation their supervisor stands to the higher echelons, and so forth.

Another advantage of charts is their help for better communications and relations. Charts can also be valuable for future planning purposes. Indeed, a supervisor may want to have two charts for his or her department, one showing the existing arrangements and another depicting the ideal organization. The latter may be used so that all the gradual changes planned fall within the design of the ideal, representing the ultimate organizational goal of the department in the future. Charting shows what is changing and how the change affects the members of the organization.

Of course, there are some limitations to charts, especially if they are not continually kept up to date. It is imperative that organizational changes be recorded at once because failure to do so makes charts outdated and as useless as yesterday's newspaper. Another shortcoming of charts is that the information they give is limited. A chart is a snapshot, not an x-ray film or a CAT scan; it shows only what is on the surface, not the inner workings of the structure. A chart does not show the amount of authority and responsibility. Sometimes people read into charts things that charts are not intended to portray; for example, employees may interpret the degree of power and status by checking how distant a position is on the chart from the box of the chief executive officer. Moreover, a chart does not show any informal relationships or the informal organization. (See Chapter 15.) Despite these shortcomings, charts are still a very useful tool for every manager.

Types of Charts

There are three main types of charts: vertical, horizontal, and circular. Of these the vertical chart is the one used most often in organized activities.

Throughout this text and especially on pp. 124 and 160 the charts shown and referred to are the vertical type. *Vertical charts* show the different levels of the organization in a step arrangement in the form of a pyramid. The chief administrator is placed at the top of the chart and the successive levels of administration are depicted vertically in the pyramid shape.

One of the main advantages of this type of chart is that it can be easily read and understood. It also shows clearly the downward flow of delegation of authority, chain of command, functional relationships, and how those activities relate to one another. One of the disadvantages is that the information conveyed is incomplete; also the vertical chart can convey a wrong impression about the relative status of certain positions. This is because some positions have to be drawn higher or lower on the chart, when in reality they are on the same organizational plane. For example, an incorrect impression can result if one division of an organization has more levels than another. An organizational unit of three levels may show a supervisor on the lowest level, whereas in a five-level unit that person would be on the third level.

In addition to the vertical chart, some hospitals may occasionally prefer a *horizontal chart,* which reads from left to right (Figure 13-3). The advantage of a horizontal chart is that it stresses functional relationships and minimizes hierarchical levels. The left-to-right chart of a matrix or project organization is a combination of these two arrangements. Horizontal relationships are superimposed on the vertical chart.

A *circular chart* can also be used. It depicts the various levels on concentric circles rotating around the top administrator who is at the hub of the wheel (Figure 13-4). Positions of equal importance are on the same concentric circle. This graphic portrayal eliminates positions at the bottom of the chart.

A few hospitals prefer an *inverted pyramid chart,* showing the chief administrator at the bottom and his associate administrators farther up. This type tries to express the idea of the ''support'' given to each manager by the ''superior.''

Organization Manuals

The organization manual is another helpful tool for achieving effective organization. It provides in comprehensive written form the decisions that have been made with regard to the institution's structure. It defines the institution's major policies and objectives. The organization manual, moreover, is a readily available reference defining the scope of authorities, responsibilities of managerial positions, and channels to be used in obtaining decisions or approval of proposals.

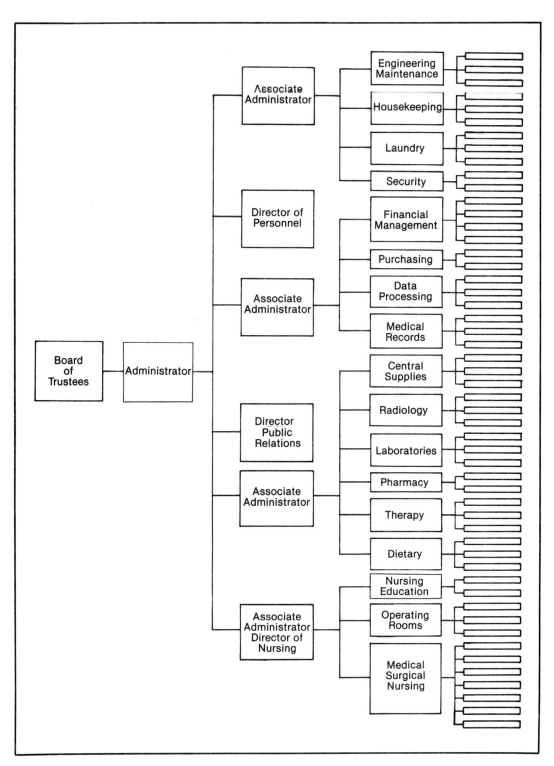

Figure 13-3. Horizontal chart. This chart is merely for illustrative purposes; it is not all inclusive, nor is it a recommended organizational arrangement.

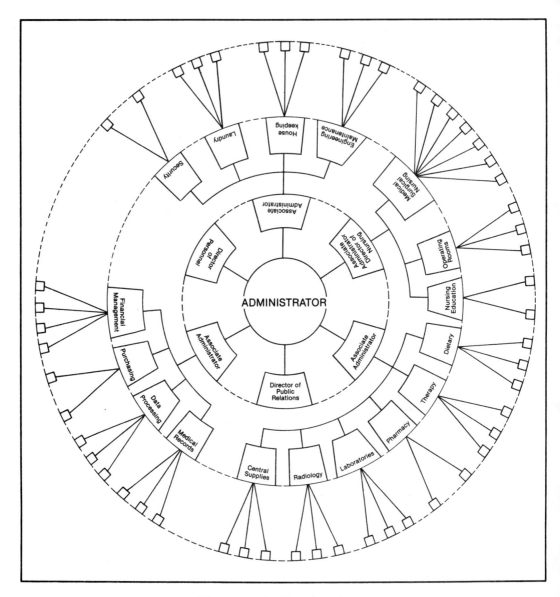

Figure 13-4. Circular chart.

One of the chief advantages of a manual is the analysis and thinking necessary before one can be written. Another advantage is that it will also be of great help in the indoctrination and development of managerial personnel. The manual should clearly specify for each manager what the responsibilities of the job are and how they are related to other positions within the organization. In addition, it reiterates for the individual manager the objectives of the enterprise and of the department, and it provides a means of explaining the complex relationships within the organization. Supervisors will do well to familiarize themselves with the contents of the institution's manual, especially those parts affecting their own department.

Organization manuals are a valuable tool only if they are up to date. Since the manual is written, it is more difficult to change. Unless manuals are kept current and incorporate changes, they are more of a hindrance than a valuable aid. As stated before, another difficulty with a manual is the initial great effort it takes to compile one.

Content

Although the content of the manual varies from one health care center to another, almost all include statements of objectives, overall policies, job descriptions, organization charts of the institution and specific department, and possibly an explanation of titles.

Objectives and Policies

In the manual, as we have said, top management states the major objectives and goals of the institution. It would mention, for example, the hospital's objectives of the education of medical and many other professionals, investigative studies, and possibly research in the fields of medical sciences and services. It may state the objective to be alert and responsive to the changing needs of the community. In the case of a hospital, the manual would state the institution's creed, philosophies, and broad policies in regard to patient care, the quality of medicine practiced, social responsibility, and many other areas of activities; it would also include a statement of overall hospital policies.

Job Descriptions

All manuals contain job descriptions. There is some confusion, however, in the use of the term *job description* as compared to *job specification.* Generally, job descriptions objectively describe the elements of a position, that is, the principal duties and functions and scope and kind of authority. A job description is an accurate, up-to-date record of all pertinent information about a job as performed in a given department. Job specifications, on the other hand, specify the human qualities required, the personal qualifications necessary to perform the job adequately, such as education, training, experience, disposition, etc. In most enterprises, job descriptions are extended to include such human qualities; however, they do not necessarily have to appear in the organization manual. Job descriptions that are supposed to appear in the manual will vary depending on the size of the departments and type of work involved. For instance, in the section for nursing services, all jobs starting with the director of nursing services down to the jobs of aides and orderlies should be described. If a job is particularly complicated or involves

numerous activities, its description will probably be rather lengthy; otherwise, most descriptions are fairly short.* (See Figures 13-5 and 13-6.)

Initially job descriptions should be written by the chief administrator
and his or her staff as they go about the organizing process. If a hospital does
not have job descriptions, the departmental supervisors should see that they
are drawn up. To help in this endeavor, the supervisors should be able to call
on the personnel department, which has the necessary expertise to facilitate
the job. Even when job descriptions are available, it is the supervisor's duty to
become familiar with them to make sure they are realistic, accurate, and up to
date. Job descriptions have a tendency to become obsolete, and this can have
serious consequences. Thus, it is necessary for the supervisor to check with
employees who hold the various positions in the department and compare
their job descriptions with those in the manual. If the manual is outdated or
incorrect, the supervisor must have it revised. Times are changing, and in all
likelihood the content of some jobs has changed without the administrator
being aware of it. Furthermore, requirements for background, education, and
training have undergone significant changes in many cases. All of this should
be recorded on the job description.

If they are kept current, job descriptions will prove invaluable to many
people throughout the organization. For instance, the personnel director will
refer to the job description when requests are made by the supervisor to
recruit applicants for an open position. Someone in the personnel department
will use them in the preliminary interview. The supervisor will also keep the
job description in mind when applicants for positions in the department are
interviewed. And the new employee should, of course, have a chance to see
the description of the job for which he or she has been hired. In many hospitals, it is standard practice to hand new employees a copy of it for them to
keep and study. In this respect job descriptions serve as a basis of common
understanding between employees and management. The job description is
also used when the supervisor evaluates and appraises the employee's performance at regular intervals. For all of these reasons, both the supervisor and
the administrator should be vitally concerned that the content of the job
description is proper and current.

Titles

There is no standard agreement on the use and meaning of titles,
especially in the upper echelons of health care centers. This is because of the
recent trend toward the use of corporate titles for the top person. The role of
the executive head has evolved from superintendent to hospital administrator
to executive director to executive vice president to president. The job of the
top person in larger hospitals is no longer concerned only with the internal
operations of the hospital, but also with the external relations in the larger
field of community health responsibilities. Although it is probably not yet a
common practice, the title of president is gaining acceptance, and, in the
future, the chief executive officer of the health care center will be known as

*Also see the departmental charts and job descriptions in the Appendix B.

POSITION: _____ Staff Nurse _____   DATE: _____ January 22, 1984 _____

DEPARTMENT: _____ Nursing Service _____   NEXT REVIEW DATE: _____ December, 1984 _____

SECTION: _____ 3100-3840, 3925, 3980, _____   JOB GRADE: 15

4405-4413, 4420-4440

REPORTS TO: _____ Head Nurse or other _____   JOB CODE NO.: 126

Registered Nurse

JOB DUTIES: Provides direct and indirect patient care activities and professional nursing services required in the nursing care of patients.

Utilizes nursing process to: admit patients, obtain medical histories, identify nursing care priorities, assess patients' problems, develop patient care plans and assign patients appropriately. Implements the care plan: evaluates patients' responses to medical and nursing care.

Assumes charge nurse responsibility and accountability as assigned for various nursing service personnel. Demonstrates leadership ability and takes corrective actions as situations arise with follow through to the appropriate personnel. Acts as a role model and maintains professional demeanor. Assists in orientation of staff members. Maintains effective relationships with patients, visitors, and other hospital personnel.

Observes patients; remains continuously aware of patients' conditions, reports and records observations, symptoms and pertinent information to physicians and to appropriate nursing personnel. Institutes appropriate measures in emergency and crisis situations.

Administers and records medications, cognizant of reactions and reports harmful side effects to physicians. Performs complex nursing activities utilizing sophisticated equipment and invasive instrumentation. Adheres to Nursing Service Policies and Procedures in the performance of patient care activities.

Initiates and participates in health care teaching for patients, families, and/or important others. Develops and implements the patients' discharge plans, seeking assistance from other health care members as necessary.

Documents in the patients' medical records nursing observations and care provided according to the Problem-Oriented Medical Record (P.O.M.R.) System.

Participates in continuing education programs and research for the improvement of patient care whenever opportunities are present. Performs job related duties as directed.

TRAINING, EDUCATION, EXPERIENCE, OR OTHER REQUIREMENTS: Graduate of a state approved school of nursing and possesses current RN licensure with the Missouri State Board of Nursing or current RN Missouri temporary work permit. Required to work rotating shifts.

PHYSICAL DEMANDS: Stands and walks most of time on duty. Lifts and pushes patients on stretchers and in wheelchairs. Usually works in a clean, air-conditioned area.

REPLACES JOB DESCRIPTION(S): Nurse, Staff, dated 5-19-80.

Reprinted with special permission from Barnes Hospital, St. Louis. This description is for illustrative purposes only.

Figure 13-5. Position description

the hospital president just as his or her counterpart in industry. This will assist those who are not familiar with hospital operations to properly identify the president's organizational role. Before too long, the term president for the health care center's chief executive officer will be the most appropriate designation.* This title will communicate to patients, relatives, visitors, physicians, and the general public that the president is the top person in the organization.

---

*Throughout this text the terms president, chief executive officer, and administrator have been used interchangeably.

POSITION: _____ Head Nurse _____   DATE: _____ January 22, 1984 _____

DEPARTMENT: ____ Nursing Service ____   NEXT REVIEW DATE: ___ November, 1984 ___

SECTION: _____ 3140, 3220-4440 _____   JOB GRADE: _____ UG _____

REPORTS TO: ____ Assistant Director II, ____   JOB CODE NO.: _____ 122 _____
_____ Nursing Service _____

POSITION PURPOSE: To manage the delivery of nursing services and to coordinate other services to an assigned patient population on a 24-hour basis.

DIMENSIONS: Accountable for the management of a specific patient care area(s) or Operating Room service(s), including staff, supplies, and equipment.

NATURE AND SCOPE: The Head Nurse reports to an Assistant Director II, Nursing Service. Directly reporting to the incumbent are assistant head nurses/clinical nurses, staff nurses, LPNs, nurse assistants, unit clerks, and technicians.

The incumbent interviews, selects, evaluates, and terminates registered professional nurses, licensed practical nurses, nurse assistants, clinical nurses/assistant head nurses, technicians, and unit clerks. The Head Nurse performs these activities within the stated guidelines of Nursing Service and the policies and procedures of Nursing Service and the Department of Human Resources. This position controls work time for all employees, assigns staff to work duties and makes appropriate adjustments. This responsibility in his/her absence is delegated to the Assistant Head Nurse. The incumbent is responsible for the practice of nursing as indicated by professional standards, by the Nurse Practice Act for the State of Missouri, and by the Nursing Service Policy and Procedure Manual.

The incumbent is responsible for the coordination of all other services to the patients.

In conjunction with the budget/unit coordinator, unit manager, or operating room manager, the Head Nurse establishes supply standards, recommends capital expenditures, and maintains budgetary standards.

The incumbent maintains a close working relationship with the medical staff on the assigned area, Dietetics, Pharmacy, Laboratories, Radiology, Respiratory Therapy and other service areas related to the specialty of the patient care area. This position also has frequent contact with Admissions in regard to admitting, discharging and transferring patients.

This position serves on committees that recommend policy, procedure or standards of patient care delivery or operational methods. Such committees are: Policy and Procedure Committee, Total Head Nurse Group, Nursing Audit Committee (or sub-committee), Safety Committee and ad hoc committees as appointed.

The Head Nurse must have graduated from an accredited school of nursing and be licensed to practice professional nursing in the State of Missouri. Advanced education is preferred. Past nursing experiences must have demonstrated leadership ability, good interpersonal relations and the ability to apply sound principles of administration and supervision. In addition, 2 to 5 years of professional nursing practice in a hospital setting (preferably with a minimum of 1 year in the specialty area) is necessary. Previous experience as a Head Nurse, Assistant Head Nurse, or comparable position is desired.

PRINCIPAL ACCOUNTABILITIES:
1. Ensure that hospital policies and procedures for patient care are observed through regular and frequent evaluation of care delivered, and by frequent contact with the staff.
2. Ensure that patient care is provided through the application of policies and procedures and recognized nursing practices.
3. Coordinate patient care efforts between departments by interdepartmental consultation and problem solving.
4. Maintain adequate staffing schedules to provide consistent levels of and competent nursing care to patients.
5. Ensure adequate, well-trained and competent nursing personnel through on-going educational and professional development programs.
6. Maintains open and accurate communications upward and downward on a regular consistent basis.
7. Ensure establishment of goals and evaluates these goals periodically to assure feasibility and compliance.

REPLACES JOB DESCRIPTION(S): Nurse, Head, dated December, 1982.

Reprinted with special permission from Barnes Hospital, St. Louis. This description is for illustrative purposes only.

Figure 13-6. Position description

Following corporate usage of titles, this would lead to a number of vice presidents on the next level, for instance, vice president of patient care (nursing), vice president of fiscal affairs, vice president of professional services, vice president of human resources, environmental affairs, etc.

Although the titles of the upper echelons vary trom one health care institution to another, there must be internal consistency. Within a health care institution titles must be clear and consistent. The best way to do this is to use a basic title, for instance, director, and then add adjectives to indicate the rank and area of activity (associate or assistant director, nursing, medical and surgical; or chief technologist, radiology, outpatient section).

The supervisor's job will be greatly facilitated by having these organizational tools available. Charts and manuals properly maintained and updated explain to everyone involved in the organization how it works and how the individual department fits into the overall organization.

14

Committees as an Organizational Tool

The continuous growth in size and specialization makes the administration and coordination of a large institution by the chief executive officer and associates increasingly difficult and, at the same time, more necessary. One method to cope with this difficulty is to establish committees and turn over to them specific problems. We find committees, boards, task forces, commissions, and teams everywhere, in business, government, schools, churches, agencies, and certainly in health care organizations. Committees are an organizational tool that, if utilized properly, can be of great help in the smooth functioning of an enterprise. *A committee is a group of people who function collectively by working together.* It differs from other units of management insofar as committee members normally have regular full-time duties in the organization and devote only part of their time to committee activities in addition to their regular job.

Yet the amount of time spent in committee activities is increasing. There is definitely a growing emphasis on committee meetings within today's organizations. This is true for several reasons. First, since most enterprise activities have become more complex and specialized, there is an increased and more urgent need for coordination and cooperation. Conferences and meetings have proven to be a good means of answering this need. Another reason for the emphasis on meetings is the growing realization that people are more enthusiastic about carrying out directives and plans that they have helped to devise than those which are handed down from above. Thus, committees are an additional means for effectively combining the formal and the acceptance theories of authority, giving employees more freedom and greater delegations of authority, and motivating them. In other words, committees are another proven tool for carrying out the general approach to supervision.

As we know, the job of a supervisor is to get things done through and with the help of the employees in the department. Skill in establishing, running, and participating in committee meetings will significantly help in achieving this objective. Although a common complaint is that there are too many meetings and that they take up too much time, committees are still a widely used device in all organizations, especially in health care centers. They seem to have no substitutes. Without committee meetings it would be almost impossible for an organization of any size to operate efficiently and effectively. Of the many ways of obtaining ideas and opinions on how to handle certain problems, there is really no better way than by holding a meeting. The real criticism of meetings is probably not that there are too many, but that the results produced often do not warrant the time and effort invested.

No doubt you have sometimes been annoyed at being tied up in a meeting in which the chairperson was allowed to amble along in all directions, "covering the waterfront" without any purpose whatsoever. In the meantime, more important work was accumulating on your desk. It is very likely that the chairperson had not properly prepared the meeting, and that the performance did not increase your respect for his or her managerial ability. After an experience of this type, you can quickly see how important it is for supervisors to acquaint themselves with committee meetings and with committee or conference leadership techniques. In other words, supervisors should learn how to run committees well and how to obtain effective participation. Meetings will then become increasingly interesting and stimulating because the participants will have the satisfaction of knowing that the meeting is accomplishing something.

It must be pointed out that with the growing importance and number of committee meetings, it will not be just the occasional supervisor who comes in contact with them. All supervisors must familiarize themselves with the workings of a committee. There may be occasions when the supervisor will find it necessary to establish an intradepartmental or interdepartmental committee or to chair a committee. At other times, the supervisor may only be an ordinary member of the committee. And there will definitely be many instances when the supervisor will have to act as a conference leader or chairperson of a committee made up only of employees of the department.

The Nature of Committees

Definitions

A committee is a group of people to whom certain matters have been committed. They meet for the purpose of discussing those matters which have been assigned to them. As stated above, committees function collectively, and their members normally have other duties, making their committee work merely a part-time assignment. Because committees function only as a group, they differ considerably from other managerial devices.

Committees can be found at all organizational *levels* and the chances are that at some time or other a committee exists or existed for every organizational activity.

Committees can be *line* or *staff*. The committee works on the problem assigned to it. When a solution is reached, a committee that has line authority will make a decision. But if the committee is acting in staff capacity, it will merely make a recommendation after having analyzed and debated the problem.

Committees can be classified as *standing* or *temporary*. A standing committee has a formal permanent place in the organization. Typically, it deals with recurring problems; in a hospital, for instance, the medical staff, tissue, infection, safety, and joint committees and many others would be considered standing committees. A temporary committee, on the other hand, is one that has been appointed for a particular purpose and will be disbanded as soon as it has accomplished its task. This type is also known as an *ad hoc committee.* A lecture to a large audience is not a committee, nor is a spur-of-the-moment meeting.

Functions of Committees

The Committee as a Place to Inform or to Discuss

Most committee meetings may be described as either informational or discussional. In an *informational meeting* the leader or chairperson does most of the talking to present certain information and facts. Assume, for example, that a supervisor wants to make an announcement and a meeting is called as a substitute for posting a notice or speaking to each employee separately. It may be expensive to take the whole work force away from the job, but, on the other hand, it guarantees that everyone in the department is notified of the new directive at the same time. Such a meeting also gives subordinates a chance to ask questions and discuss the implications of the announcement. Care should be taken, however, that questions from participants are largely confined to further clarification of the supervisor's remarks so that the meeting will not stray from its purpose.

In the *discussional meeting,* the chairperson encourages more participation of the members to secure their ideas and opinions. The supervisor could ask the individuals singly for suggestions on how to solve a problem, but it is probably better to call a meeting to allow them to make recommendations. Although it is up to the supervisor to make the final decision and to determine whether or not to incorporate some of the employees' suggestions, the employees will nevertheless derive great satisfaction from knowing that their ideas have been considered and that some of them may even be used. It is likely that some good suggestions will be offered, and in all probability the implementation of suggestions will be more enthusiastic if the employees of the department have participated in finalizing them. In this case the committee acted in a staff capacity.

The supervisor can also go beyond merely asking for suggestions. A meeting may be called for the sole purpose of having the employees of the department fully discuss and handle a problem themselves, that is, come up with their own decision. As we shall see below, this involves using the committee as a sort of collective managerial decision maker.

Decision-Making Committees

In addition to committees whose purpose is to spread information or merely discuss a matter and make recommendations, there are those committees to which formal authority has been delegated to make decisions. Just as a supervisor can delegate decision-making authority to an individual subordinate, so can a committee be formed and authority delegated to the group to decide on a solution to a problem that involves them all. In these instances the committee has decision-making power, in other words, line authority.

Many questions in a health care center are of such magnitude and affect so many departments that it is far better to have the decision made by a committee consisting of representatives of many functions than by the administrator or one of the associate administrators alone. The same situation can exist within a department. For example, frequently employees are dissatisfied with the allocation of overtime, weekend work, and so forth, regardless of the supervisor's efforts to be fair. Naturally, the supervisor can make a decision for the employees on this matter; but it would be better if they could find a solution themselves. In such a case, management is not really concerned with precisely what decision is made so long as it falls within the limits set, for example, that the time allotted for overtime is not exceeded. By letting the group make this type of decision, they will come up with an acceptable solution. Even if such a solution is only adequate and not necessarily the best, it is still better if it is implemented by the group with great enthusiasm than a perfect decision that meets with their resistance. There are many problems and areas in which management is not concerned with the details of the decision as long as it remains within certain boundaries.

Benefits of Committees

There is little doubt that a group of individuals exchanging opinions and experiences often comes up with a better answer than any one person thinking through the same problem alone. It is an old saying that two heads are better than one. Various people will bring to a meeting a wide range of experience, background, and ability far beyond that of an individual; this would not be available if the subject had been committed to an individual decision maker. Indeed, many problems are so complicated that a single person could not possibly have all the necessary knowledge to come up with a wise solution. The free oral interchange of ideas among several persons will stimulate and clarify thinking, and chances are that the recommendation made by the group as a whole will be better than that made by any single member. This is perhaps the major benefit of group discussion.

Group deliberation can also be a real help in promoting coordination and cooperation. Members of the committee become more considerate of the problems of other employees, supervisors, and administration. They become more aware of the advantages of and the need for working together and seeking cooperative solutions. By being involved in the analysis and solution of a problem, individual members are more likely to accept and implement what has been decided. In reality, it matters little how much a person actually contributed to the plan, as long as this individual was a member of the committee and sat in on the meeting. Probably the most significant benefit of committees in health services organizations is the promotion of coordination and cooperation between the various units of the institution and motivation.

There are a number of additional benefits. Committees produce continuity in the organization; few committees replace all their members at the same time. Furthermore, they are a good environment for junior managers and executives to learn how decisions are made, absorb the philosophy and thinking of the hospital, and see how it functions. Also it gives representatives from the various departments a chance to be represented, heard, and involved in the affairs of the organization.

Limitations of Committees

Despite all these beneficial features, the committee has often been abused. Sometimes committees are created to delay action, and many people have come to think of the committee as a debating society. Jokes about committees are numerous. They have been defined as a group "that keeps minutes but wastes hours," "where the unwilling appoint the unfit to do the unnecessary." Remarks are often made that there are meetings all day long without leaving any time to get the work done. Indeed, one of the most often-voiced complaints about committees is that they are exceedingly *time consuming.* This is true, since each member is entitled to have his or her say, and often certain individuals use up a great amount of time trying to convince other members of the validity of their points of view.

In addition to their costliness in time, committees also cost *money.* It is clear that time spent in committee meetings is not spent otherwise. Hence, every hour taken up by a meeting costs the institution a certain amount of dollars. Furthermore, there might be travel expenses involved and additional expenses for the preparation of meetings. Obviously, a single executive could reach an answer in a much shorter time and at less expense, but the problem is whether this decision would be as good as the one reached by group deliberation.

Another shortcoming of committees is that there are limitations to the *sense of responsibility* that they evoke. When a problem is submitted to a committee, it is submitted to a group and not to individuals. Responsibility does not weigh as heavily on the group's shoulders as it would on one individual's. In other words, the committee's problems become everybody's responsibility, which in reality means they are nobody's responsibility. It is difficult to criticize the committee as a whole or any single member if the solution proves to be wrong, since each person is quick to answer that the "committee" made the decision. Members are willing to settle for less than the best solutions and blame the committee if the solution does not work out. This thinning-out of responsibility is natural and there is no way of avoiding it.

The dangers of a *weak compromise decision and tyranny of the minority* are other shortcomings of committees. It has often become a tradition to reach decisions of unanimity based on politeness, cooperative spirit, mutual respect, and other considerations; however, this often leads to committee action that is a weak, watered-down compromise solution, frequently utilizing the lowest common denominator instead of the optimal solution. It can also happen that in their efforts for unanimous or nearly unanimous conclusions, committees are tyrannized by a minority holding out as long as possible.

Finally, the majority might allow itself to be dominated by such a minority because of lack of time, interest, or sense of responsibility. This may even lead to a strain in working relationships outside of the committee.

Another danger is that committee members may become victims of the *groupthink* phenomenon.* This phenomenon can be characterized as a way of thinking in a group where deliberations are dominated by a desire to concur at any expense, even at the danger of overriding any realistic appraisal of alternative action and of voicing doubts and dissent.

The Effective Operation of a Committee

After considering the various advantages and shortcomings, administration has decided to establish a number of committees. In addition to those which administration deems advisable, a number of committees exist in all health care centers to fulfill the requirements of the Joint Commission on Accreditation of Hospitals. Now it becomes necessary for supervisors to familiarize themselves with the means for ensuring effective committee operation. It is not easy to make committee meetings and conferences a success, because the goals are numerous and difficult to achieve. As we have already suggested, the goals of a committee meeting are (1) to come up with the best suggestions or solutions for the problem under consideration, (2) to arrive at suggestions or solutions with unanimity, and (3) to accomplish objectives in the shortest period of time. It is a challenge for any committee to fulfill these goals, but the task will be made easier if the following remarks are used as a guide for effective committee operation.

Delineating the Committee's Scope, Functions, and Authority

The first thing a committee must have is a mandate, it must know its scope and functions in order to operate effectively. The executive establishing the committee must define the subjects to be covered and the functions that the committee is expected to fulfill; there must be a description of its job. It must also be stated how the committee relates to other units within the organization. This will prevent the committee from floundering around and will enable the manager to check on whether it is meeting the expectations.

In addition to functions and scope, the degree of authority conferred on the committee must be specified. As briefly mentioned before, it must be clearly stated whether the committee is to serve in an advisory (staff) capacity or decision-making (line) capacity. For example, in many hospitals the human research committee—sometimes known by another name—has line authority to make decisions as to whether a proposed research project should be ap-

---

* For further details on this provocative issue read: Irving Lester Janis, *Victims of Groupthink: A psychological study of foreign policy decisions and fiascos* (Boston: Houghton Mifflin Co., 1972); Philip E. Tetlock, "Identifying Victims of Groupthink From Public Statements of Decision Makers," *Journal of Personality and Social Psychology*, vol. 37, No. 8 (1979), 1314-1324.

The Medical Audit Committee shall consist of Active Staff members who have been nominated by their clinical service Chiefs to chair the Medical Audit Sub-committees. Sub-committees shall be established for the following hospital services: Cardiothoracic Surgery, Dermatology, Genitourinary Surgery, Medicine, Neurology, Neurological Surgery, Obstetrics and Gynecology, Oral Maxillofacial Surgery, Ophthalmology, Orthopedic Surgery, Otolaryngology, Plastic Surgery, Psychiatry, Radiology and Surgery. Each sub-committee nominated by the service Chief shall include no less than three members of the Active Staff and one member of the House Staff. The Hospital Medical Care Evaluation Analyst shall be an *ex-officio* member of each Sub-committee and of the Medical Audit Committee. The Director of In-patient Medical Records shall be an *ex-officio* member of the Medical Audit Committee.

The function of each Clinical Service Medical Audit Sub-committee is:

1) To establish criteria for all the discharge diagnoses that comprise 80% of the hospital admission and major outpatient treatment modalities within that Clinical Service. As a minimum, such criteria shall include indications for admission, diagnostic tests recommended, treatment both medical and surgical, the usual length of stay, complications which might extend the length of stay, critical management of such complications, and the indications for discharge.

2) To review all cases within that Clinical Service which have been referred to the committee because they do not meet the criteria outlined in (1).

3) To refer all cases which after review shall fail to meet the criteria outlined in (1) to the Medical Audit Committee. The respective service Chief is to be notified of this action.

The function of the Medical Audit Committee is to review and make recommendations to the Medical Advisory Committee regarding all cases which are referred by Medical Audit Sub-committees. Meetings and reports of all the Sub-committees and the parent Committee shall be monthly.

Reprinted with permission from Barnes Hospital, St. Louis. This statement is for illustrative purposes only.

Figure 14-1. The functions and scope of the medical audit committee.

proved or not. In reaching the decision, this committee, guided by federal rules and regulations governing human experimentation issued by the Department of Health and Human Services and the Federal Drug Administration, clearly has line authority. On the other hand, in most hospitals the medical executive committee—sometimes known as the medical staff committee or a similar term—acts in an advisory (staff) capacity when it deals with a physician's or surgeon's application for hospital privileges. This committee simply makes a recommendation to the board of directors and they will decide. In such an instance the medical executive committee clearly acts as a staff committee.

In the case of a formal standing committee, all such information should be set down in writing in the organization manual. (Figure 14-1.) Documents stating all of this information for the various committees are also usually required by the Joint Commission on Accreditation of Hospitals. For a temporary committee, scope, functions, and authority must also be explicitly stated but perhaps not so formally. It is extremely important that temporary committees only be established for a subject worthy of group consideration. If a topic can be handled by one person or over the phone there is no need to call a meeting.

Composition of the Committee

Since the quality of committee work is only as good as its members, care should be exercised in choosing people to serve on committees. Members should be capable of expressing and defending their views, but they should also be willing to see the other party's point of view and be able to integrate their thinking with that of the other members. Hopefully, they should be independent of each other so that their deliberations will not be complicated by connotations of a direct superior-subordinate relationship. If possible, members should be from approximately the same organizational rank. If committee members are chosen from different departments, the problems of rank are more easily overcome. Sometimes the composition of a committee is dictated by outside regulations.

Indeed, the committee device is a good opportunity for bringing together the representatives of several different interest groups. Specialists of different departments and activities can be brought together in such a way that all concerned parties have proper representation. This will result in balanced group integration and deliberation. The various representatives will feel that their interests have been heard and considered. Of course, administration should see that this concern with proper representation is not carried too far. It is more essential to appoint capable members to a committee than merely representative members. The ideal solution, of course, is to have a capable member from each pertinent activity on the committee.

Number of Members

No definite figure can be given as to the ideal size of a committee for effective operation. The best that can be said is that the committee should be large enough to provide for thorough group deliberation and broad resources of information. It should not be so large, however, that it will be unwieldy and unusually time consuming. Usually smaller committees with about four to seven members seem to work best. If the nature of the subject under consideration necessitates a very large committee, it might be wise to form subcommittees that will consider various aspects of the problem. Then, the entire committee can meet to hear subcommittee reports and decide on a final solution.

Effective Conference Leadership

Adequate Preparation

Successful committee work requires good preparation. First, the chairperson must carefully outline the overall strategy, the agenda, before the meeting. Topics to be discussed should be listed in the proper sequence, and often it is advisable to set up a time limit as to approximately how long the meeting will last. The chairperson may even want to establish for his or her

own guidance an approximate time limit for each item in order to assure better control of the situation. If possible, the agenda should be distributed to the
members before the meeting so that they can better prepare themselves for
the coming discussion. Furthermore, additional background information
should be gathered either by the chairperson, the committee's own staff, or by
the organization's staff services. This kind of factual information should be
distributed to the members before the meeting for their perusal and study.
Meetings should be planned far enough in advance to give the members adequate notice and time. Written minutes of the previous meeting should be
sent along for review and approval. All of this will enable the members of a
health care center, who often belong to a number of committees, avoid
conflicts.

Even after all or most of the above-mentioned requirements are fulfilled, the success of any meeting will depend largely on the chairperson's
ability to handle it. It is necessary for him or her to be familiar with effective
conference or committee leadership* techniques in order to guide the meeting
to a satisfactory conclusion. There is no doubt that the individual members of
a committee bring to the meeting their individual patterns of behavior and
points of view. The chairperson must know how to fuse the individual viewpoints and attitudes so that teamwork will develop for the benefit of the
group. It will take considerable time and patience on the chairperson's part to
create a closely knit group out of a diverse membership, but that is generally
the best way to achieve integrated group solutions. Let us look a little more
carefully at the chairperson's role.

The Role of the Chairperson

The chairperson is the most important member of the committee. This
person is expected to play and succeed in two roles: to bring about the fulfillment of the task and build and maintain successful group interaction. The
committee is made up of individuals, and great skill is required to eventually
fuse these individuals into a rewarding and productive interaction.

It is only human nature for committee members to think first of how a
new proposition would affect themselves and their own working environment. This kind of egotistical thinking can easily lead to unnecessary frictions.
People tend to see the same "facts" differently. Words mean different things
to different people. The first necessity in a group situation, therefore, is to find
agreement on the basic nature of the problem under discussion so that everybody understands what the issues are. The task of the chairperson is to try to
find out what the participants *think* the issues are in order to learn whether or
not they understand the issues as they actually are.

This, however, is easier said than done. A frequent comment about
committees is that the issues on the conference table are really not as difficult
to deal with as the people around the table. Individuals at a meeting will often

---

*The term *conference leadership* is generally used in the literature. We have used it here to be
synonymous with *committee leadership*.

react toward each other rather than toward their ideas. For instance, just because A talks too much, everything he or she suggests may be rejected. Or B might be a person who automatically rejects whatever someone else is for. And then there is C, that member of the committee who keeps his or her mouth shut all the time.

It is the chairperson's job to minimize these personality differences by using the legitimate tools of parliamentary procedure. The speaking time of each participant can be limited so that one person will not monopolize the entire meeting. And one can be especially careful to call on people who seldom speak. Sooner or later, with the help of such leadership techniques, the committee will start reacting toward the content of the meeting, the issues involved, and not the individuals around the table. For a meeting to be successful, it is necessary for the various members to forget about their personalities and outside allegiances and work together as a team in a manner that will move the meeting toward a meaningful solution of the problem at hand. In all of this, the chairperson plays a critical role.

Of course, the quality of the solution will also depend to some extent on the amount of time spent in reaching it. Too much haste will probably not produce the most desirable solution. On the other hand, most meetings have a time limit. If they did not, the members would become bored and frustrated with a meeting that lasts too long. It is the chairperson's job to give every member a chance to participate and voice his or her suggestions and opinions. This is especially important when the committee members are also expected to execute the decisions they make. Then, it may be necessary for the chairperson to use persuasion to induce a minority to go along with the decision of the majority. Or, on other occasions, the majority might have to be persuaded to make concessions to the minority. All of this takes time and may result in a compromise that does not necessarily represent the best possible solution. If the solution has been arrived at democratically, however, the chairperson's leadership abilities will have been demonstrated and the major purpose of the meeting will have been accomplished.

Should the Chairperson Express His or Her Own Opinions?

It has often been stated that the function of a good chairperson is to help the members of the group reach their own decisions, to work as a catalyst to bring out the ideas present among the committee members. There is no doubt that if the chairperson expresses his or her views, the members of the committee may hesitate to argue further or to make known their opinions, especially if they disagree; this is particularly so if the chairperson also happens to be their boss. On the other hand, there are many occasions when it would be unwise and completely unrealistic for the chairperson not to express his or her views. This individual may have some factual knowledge or sound opinion, and the value of the deliberations would be lessened if these were left unknown to the members of the committee.

On the whole, it is best for the chairperson to express his or her opin-

ions and, at the same time, clearly let it be known that they are subject to constructive criticism and suggestions. After all, silence on the leader's part may
be interpreted to mean that he or she cannot make a decision or does not want
to do so for fear of assuming responsibility. On certain occasions, however,
the chairperson must use sensitive judgment as to whether or not or to what
extent his or her own opinions should be expressed.

The Style of Leadership

There also is the question of how much of a formal leadership role the
chairperson should display. The variations of this role can run anywhere from
the one extreme of an autocratic dictator to the other extreme of a democratic
moderator. At times it may be necessary for even a very permissive
democratic chairperson to use tight control over the meeting, although on
most occasions the loosest sort of control will be employed. Indeed, it has
often been found that if the group of participants consists of mature people
from the upper administrative echelons, no formal chairpersonship or little
control and formal chairpersonship are really necessary.

Although this may be true for the higher level committee meetings,
normally on the lower levels there is a need for a stable structure and strong
leadership from a chairperson. If the group has a formally elected or appointed chairperson, the members will naturally look to that person to keep
the meeting moving along so that it will come to an efficient conclusion.
Under most conditions, the formal leadership of the chairperson is necessary
to ensure that group decision making is effective. If the chairperson lacks
leadership ability, some other member of the committee will rise to be the *de
facto* chairperson. This is a natural event in group dynamics.

Working With the Agenda (Task Control)

The best means of keeping a meeting from wandering off into a discussion of irrelevant matters is a well-prepared agenda. Although the agenda
designs the overall strategy, it must not be so rigid that there is no means for
adjusting it. The chairperson should apply the agenda with a degree of flexibility, so that if a particular subject requires more attention than originally anticipated, the time allotted to some other topic can be reduced. In other words,
staying close to the agenda should not force the chairperson to be too quick to
rule people out of order. What seems irrelevant to him or her may be important to some of the other committee members. Some irrelevancies at times actually help create a relaxed atmosphere and relieve tension that has built up.

Since it is the chairperson's job to keep the meeting moving along
toward its goal, it is a good idea to pause at various points during the meeting
to consult the agenda and remind the group of what has been accomplished
and what still remains to be discussed. A good chairperson will learn when the
opportune time has arrived to summarize one point and to move on to the next
item in the agenda. If past experience tells the chairperson that meetings have

a tendency to run overtime or not to complete all the agenda items, it might be advisable to schedule them shortly before the lunch break or just before quitting time. This seems to speed up meetings; somehow the participants seem to run out of arguments around those hours of the day.

A Typical Committee Meeting

Now that we are familiar with the guidelines for effective committee operation, we are ready to examine how these guidelines can be applied in a typical committee meeting. In other words, we want to see how a diverse group of people can, with the help of an effective leader, hold a meaningful discussion and arrive at satisfactory answers to the questions under consideration.

General Participation in the Discussion

After a few introductory remarks and social pleasantries, the chairperson should make an initial statement of the problem to be discussed. This will open up an opportunity for all members of the meeting to participate freely. Any member should be able to bring out those aspects of the problem which seem important to him or her, regardless of whether or not they seem important to everyone else. Sooner or later the discussion will simmer down to those points which are relevant.

There are always some members at the meeting who talk too much and others who do not talk enough. One of the chairperson's most difficult jobs is to encourage the latter to speak up and to keep the former from holding the floor for too long. There are various ways and means to do this. For example, after a long-winded speaker has had enough opportunity to express his or her opinions, it may be wise to not recognize that member again, giving someone else the chance to speak. It might also help to ask him or her to please keep the remarks brief or arrange the seating at the conference table to a spot where it is easy not to recognize his or her request to have the floor. Most of the time, however, the other members of the committee will quickly find subtle ways of censoring those members who have too much to say.

Of course, this does not mean that all members of the meeting must participate equally. Some people know more about a given subject than others, and some have stronger feelings about an issue than others. The chairperson must take such factors into consideration, but should still do the best possible to stimulate overall participation. In this endeavor, the chairperson's general attitude with regard to participation will be extremely important. It is necessary to accept everyone's contribution without judgment and create the impression that everyone should participate. Controversial questions may have to be asked merely to get the discussion going. Once participation has started, the chairperson should continue to throw out provocative "open-end" questions, those which ask why, who, what, where, and when. Questions that can be answered with a simple yes or no should be avoided.

Another technique that can be used by the chairperson is to start at one side of the conference table and ask each member in turn to express thoughts on the problem. The major disadvantage of this technique is that instead of participating in the discussion spontaneously whenever they have something to say, members will tend to sit back and wait until called on. But the skilled chairperson will watch the facial expressions of the people in the group. This may very well provide a clue as to whether someone has an idea but is afraid to speak up. Then a special effort should be made to call on that person.

If a meeting is made up of a large number of participants, it may be advisable for the chairperson to break it up into small groups, commonly known as *buzz sessions*. Each of the small subgroups will hold its own discussions and report back to the meeting after a specified period of time. In this way, those people who hesitate to say anything in a larger group will be more or less forced to participate and express their opinions. Buzz sessions are usually advisable whenever the number of participants is greater than 20 or thereabout.

Of course, in using all of these techniques to evoke general participation in the discussion, the chairperson should try to stick to the agenda and see that the discussion is basically relevant. It sometimes happens that a chairperson who is inexperienced at holding meetings is so anxious to have someone say something that there will be a lot of discussion for discussion's sake. Most of the time, this is not desirable because it confuses the issues and delays the even more important decision-making phase of the meeting.

Group Decision Making

Once a problem has been pretty well narrowed down and understood in the same sense by all members of the group, it is advisable to get to the facts in as objective a manner as possible. Only by ascertaining all the relevant facts will the group be able to suggest alternative solutions. The chairperson knows that the best solution can only be as good as the best alternative considered. So that no solution is overlooked, the members of the meeting should be urged to contribute as many alternatives as they can possibly think of.

The next step is to evaluate the alternative solutions and discuss the advantages and disadvantages of each. In so doing, the field can eventually be narrowed down to two or three alternatives on which general agreement can be reached. The other alternatives can probably be eliminated by unanimous consent. Those which remain must be discussed thoroughly to bring about a solution. The chairperson should try to play the role of a middleperson or conciliator by working out a solution that is acceptable to all members of the group, possibly even persuading some members that their opinions are wrong.

The best procedure would probably be to arrive at a solution that is a synthesis of the desirable outcomes of the few remaining alternatives. By process of integration, all important points can be incorporated into the most desirable solution. Throughout this process, the chairperson has the difficult job of helping the minority to save face. It is easier to conciliate the minority if the final decision of the group incorporates something of each person's ideas so that everyone has a partial victory. Of course, this can be a long and tedious process and, as we have said, such a compromise may not always be the strongest solution.

Sometimes, however, the group may not be able to reach a compromise or to come to any decision on which the majority agrees. This will frequently happen if the chairperson of the meeting senses that the group is hostile. In such a situation, it is necessary to find out what is bothering the group, to bring their objections out into the open and discuss them. It is not uncommon for participants in a committee meeting to think first of what is objectionable about a new idea rather than to think of its desirable features. A discussion of such objections may dispel unwarranted fears and may allow participants to perceive the positive aspects of a certain alternative. Or, by the same token, the objections may be strong enough to void the proposition. In any case, it is necessary for the group to have a chance to voice negative feelings before a positive consensus can be reached.

Taking a Vote

The chairperson is often confronted with the problem of whether a vote should be taken, or whether the committee should keep on working until the group reaches a final unanimous agreement, regardless of how long this would take. Offhand, many people would say that voting is a democratic way to make decisions. But voting does accentuate the differences among the members of the group, and once a person has made a public commitment to a position by voting, it is often difficult to change his or her mind and yet save face. Also, if this individual is a member of the losing minority he or she cannot be expected to carry out the majority decision with great enthusiasm. Therefore, wherever possible, it is better not to take a formal vote but to work toward a roughly unanimous agreement.

As pointed out previously, one of the disadvantages of reaching a unanimous conclusion is that it can cause serious delay in the meeting. It also is true that the price of unanimity is often a solution that is reduced to a common denominator and may not be as ingenious and bold as it would have been otherwise. Of course, it will depend on the situation and the magnitude of the problem involved whether or not unanimity is desirable. It should be pointed out that in most instances it is not as difficult as one might think to come up with a unanimous decision. The skilled chairperson can usually sense the feeling of the meeting, and all that is necessary is to say that such and such a solution seems to be the consensus of the group. At this point, especially in a small meeting, parliamentary procedure and a formal vote can probably be dispensed with. In a large meeting, of course, unanimity may be an impossible goal and decisions should be based on majority rule.

Follow-up of Committee Action

Regardless of whether a committee was acting merely to come up with a recommendation or whether it has final decision-making authority, its findings need a follow-up. After the chairperson has reported the committee's findings to the superior who originally channeled the subject to the committee, it is the superior's duty to keep the committee posted as to what action has been taken. Indeed, the practice of good human relations and ordinary courtesy will tell the superior that he or she owes the committee some explanation. Inadequate statements or no statements at all from the chairperson will cause the committee to lose interest in its work. Of course, when the committee has had authority to make a final decision, then the problem of carrying out the decision usually belongs to the committee itself. The chairperson will generally be asked to oversee this, or the particular executive who normally deals with the subject matter may execute the decision. In any event, the committee members must be kept informed as to what has happened. From time to time, it is advisable to evaluate the effectiveness of a committee and whether it continues to reach the objectives given to it.

Summary

There is probably no supervisor who has not been involved in committees either as a member or as an organizer. Indeed, committees are becoming an extremely important device for augmenting the organizational structure of an enterprise. They allow the enterprise to adapt to increasing complexity without a complete reorganization. They permit a group of people to function collectively in areas a single individual could not handle. Obviously, the advantages of committees are offset to a certain extent by their limitations and shortcomings, one of the most important being that responsibility cannot be pinned to any individual member of the committee. Despite this and other criticisms leveled against committees, they can be of great value if properly organized and led.

Because the increasing complexities of today's society are making more and more committees necessary, it is essential for the supervisor to familiarize himself or herself with the workings of a committee. Committee meetings are called either to disseminate information or to discuss a topic. If discussion is involved, a distinction should be made between whether the committee is to arrive at a final decision on the question under discussion and take action based on this decision or whether it is to merely make recommendations to the line manager who appointed the committee. A committee can be line or staff.

Regardless of the purpose of the committee, it is likely that group deliberation will produce a more satisfactory and acceptable conclusion than one which was formally handed down from above. Decisions will be carried out with more enthusiasm if employees have had a role in making them or in making recommendations through committees. For group decisions and recommendations to be of high quality, however, it is necessary that the committee members be carefully selected. In the composition of a committee, it is essential that as many interested parties as possible be represented. The people chosen as representatives should be capable of presenting their views and integrating their opinions with those of others. As to the size of a committee, it is advisable that there be enough members to permit thorough deliberations, but not so many as to make the meetings cumbersome.

In addition to these factors, the success of committee deliberations depends largely on effective committee or conference leadership. This means that the chairperson's familiarity with effective group work will make the difference between productive and wasteful committee meetings. The chairperson's job is to produce the best possible solution in the shortest amount of time and, it is hoped, with unanimity. In trying to achieve these goals, the chairperson is constantly confronted with the problem of running the meeting either too tightly or too loosely. If control is too tight, the natural development of ideas may be frustrated, conclusions may be reached before all alternatives have been considered, and in general resentment may be created. If the control is too loose, members of the meeting may get the feeling of aimlessness and confusion. In practice, the chairperson will have to depend on a keen perception of the "mood of the meeting" in order to know exactly how to lead it and bring it to a successful conclusion. Thus, the chairperson will have to sense when there has been enough general participation in the discussion, when alternative solutions have been properly evaluated, and when and if a vote is necessary to arrive at a group decision. In all of these matters, the leadership abilities of the chairperson will be of utmost importance.

15

Informal Organizational Relationships

The formal task structure, organizational goals, and formal organization and its functioning are affected by another element, a social subsystem known as the *informal organization*. Wherever people work together informal relationships exist and become a powerful source of influence on the formal organization. Early scholars maintained that an inherent conflict exists between the goals of the formal organization and informal relationships. Today we know that both formal and informal relationships are essential subsystems of a complex system and that the informal relationships help the functioning of the formal organization by providing individual satisfaction and group morale, which otherwise would be lacking.

The informal organization found in almost all enterprises is closely related to the workings of committees and to the phenomenon of group participation, yet is quite different in origin. The informal organization is a powerful source of influence that interacts with and modifies the formal organization. Although many managers would like to conveniently overlook its existence, they will readily admit that to fully understand the nature of organizational life it is necessary to "learn the ropes" of the informal organization. In almost every institution such an informal structure will develop. It reflects the spontaneous efforts of individuals and groups to influence the conditions of their existence. Whenever people are associated, social relationships and groupings are bound to come about. The informal organization has a positive contribution to make to the smooth functioning of the enterprise, and to this extent the manager must understand its workings, respect it, and even nurture it.

To be more specific, informal organization arises from the social interaction of people as they associate with each other. Such interaction may be accidental or incidental to organized activities, or it may arise from personal desire or gregariousness. At the heart of informal organization are people and their relationships, whereas at the heart of formal organization is the organizational structure and the delegation of authority. Management can create or rescind a formal organizational structure that it has designed; but it cannot rescind the informal organization, since management did not establish it. As long as there are people working together in a department, there will be an informal organization consisting of the informal groupings of employees.

The Informal Group

At the base of all informal organization is the small group,* usually consisting of up to 10 members. And the first question that comes to mind is why people join such groups. We may wonder what advantages they gain from groups, since they are already members of a department where their duties are specifically assigned, channels of communication exist, a line of authority has been established, and they are a significant part of a formal organizational structure. The answer to this question is that employees have certain needs which they would like to satisfy, but apparently the formal organization leaves unsatisfied. One of the needs is for achievement and the other is for emotional satisfaction. People have a basic need to associate with others in groups small enough to permit intimate, direct, and personal contact among individuals. The satisfactions derived from these kinds of relationships generally cannot be obtained from working within a large organization. Thus, the small group provides the individual with satisfactions that are uniquely different from those which can be obtained from any other source.

Benefits Derived From Groups

First of all, group participation provides a sense of *satisfaction.* An individual in a group is usually surrounded by others who share similar values. This reinforces our own value system and our interest; it gives us confidence, since it is always more comfortable to be among people who think the same way we do. There is also the need for *friendship and companionship* that the group fulfills. The employee needs and enjoys the social contact with fellow workers, sharing experiences, joking, and finding a sympathetic listener. The group will, furthermore, fulfill the need for *belonging,* the need to associate with others who have the same purposes and goals.

Another need that is satisfied by belonging to a small group in many instances is the need for *protection,* that is, protection from what the members may think of as an imposition or an encroachment by management, such as protection against increased output standards, changes in working conditions, or reduced benefits. We are all familiar with the old saying that there is strength in unity. In this respect, the small group is a source of *support.* Often when people enter an organization for the first time they have feelings of significant anxiety. The surroundings are unfamiliar and a great deal of uncertainty exists. When several people are in the same circumstance, a small group may arise on this basis alone, providing temporary support in an unfamiliar environment. Whenever people sense the need for protection, they can and do form small groups.

*George C. Homans, *The Human Group* (New York: Harcourt Brace Jovanovich, Inc., 1950).

An additional need that a small group fulfills is the need for *status,* because the group enables an employee to belong to a distinct little organization that is more or less exclusive. It also gives the individual an opportunity for self-expression, a kind of audience before generally sympathetic listeners. Another reason why people join groups is to secure *information* to reduce their uncertainties. The grapevine works very effectively in small groups. Groups tend to form around an individual who seems to be the focal point in a communications network. An individual who has information is able to satisfy the communication needs of others, even though the information transmitted may be false or distorted.

In addition to these emotional needs, there exists the need for achievement, getting things done; groups are a means of getting a *task* accomplished by interacting, communicating, and collaborating. Informal groups help employees to accomplish tasks that may be impossible to accomplish alone. They also serve to bring the goals of these tasks more into the realm of the employee. There are, of course, objectives and goals in the formal organization. But these may appear remote and meaningless to the average employee. It is much simpler to identify with the objectives and goals of one's immediate work group. And often employees will readily forego some of their own goals and replace them with the goals of the group.

It is important for the supervisor of a department to be aware of all of these needs employees want satisfied. Then the supervisor will understand why employees tend to join informal groups, and in the daily supervision an attempt can be made to use these groups constructively rather than being suspicious and trying to destroy them.

Informal Groups and the Informal Organization

Small informal groups, as we said, are at the basis of informal organization, and all small informal groups have the potential to become informal organizations existing in the larger formal structure of the institution. The informal organization develops when small groups acquire a more or less dictinct structure and a set of norms and standards, as well as a procedure to invoke sanctions to assure conformity to the norms. The informal organizational structure is determined largely by the different status positions that people within the small group hold.

Status Positions

Generally, there are *four* status positions: the group's *informal leader,* the members of the *primary* group, the members who have only *fringe status,* and those who have *out status.* (See Figure 15-1.) The informal leader of the small group is the person around whom the primary members of the group cluster; their association is close and their interaction and communication are intense. This is normally considered the small nucleus group of which newcomers would like to become members.

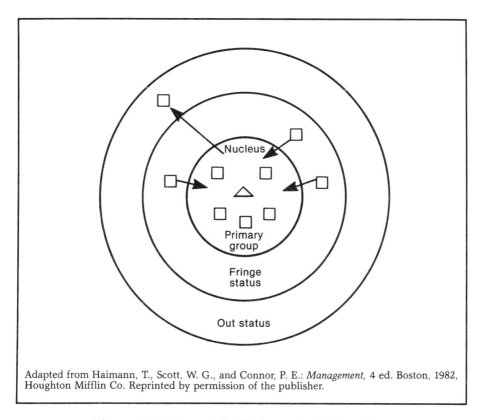

Adapted from Haimann, T., Scott, W. G., and Connor, P. E.: *Management,* 4 ed. Boston, 1982, Houghton Mifflin Co. Reprinted by permission of the publisher.

Figure 15-1. A model of informal relationships.

These newcomers are usually new employees of the department. They remain on the fringe of the group while they are being evaluated by the small nucleus for acceptance or rejection. Eventually these individuals will either move into the nucleus and become a bona fide member of the small group, or they will move into the out shell because they have been rejected.

The people in the out shell are still a part of the department, even though they have not been accepted as members of the core group. Such rejection, however, can have serious behavioral effects, especially if a person wants badly to belong to the nucleus group. This is true because in essence the group represents a system of interaction that causes members to modify their own individual behavior and to have a significant impact on the behavior of persons in the fringe shell or the outer shell. If the rejection is mutual, the person in the out shell can survive very well on his or her own.

Although leadership will be discussed fully in Chapter 21, a few words should be said at this time about informal leadership. The person who plays the role of the *informal leader* is usually the dynamic force of the group. Like the committee chairperson, this individual is the one who crystallizes opinions and sets objectives. This group leader is generally democratically chosen. The leadership role is created by consensus. This leader normally is a dominant personality who functions in such a way as to facilitate the satisfaction of most of the needs of group members. This person usually possesses communicative skills, sensitivity, and intelligence and helps the members achieve their tasks and emotive needs. From time to time, one might find small groups in which the aspects of leadership are shared, in which different leaders perform different functions, sometimes only for a brief period of time. For example, one leader may deal with administration, whereas another may deal with the union, and a third one may try to maintain internal cohesiveness. Most of the time, however, there is only one informal leader with whom the supervisor will have to deal.

Norms and Standards

In addition to status positions, there are norms, standards that regulate group behavior. Norms set the standards for behavior between group members and quality and quantity of work, and many other standards, for instance such things as squealing to management about a co-worker, etc. The standards governing work output are particularly important in almost every informal organization. They tell exactly how many salads a worker in the food production department will fix per hour, how many records will be processed in the medical records department during a day, and so forth. And these norms often are far from what the supervisor would like to have accomplished.

To be admitted to the group, the employee must be willing and eager to comply with such standards in lieu of his or her own. Since groups are capable of granting or withholding the advantages of membership, individuals must modify their behavior so that it corresponds to that of the group. This is why the informal organization has such a significant influence over the behavior of employees who are primary group members. In addition, the interactions between primary group members also influence the behavior of those who are in the fringe shell and even possibly someone in the out shell, since all of them are members of the total system.

Sanctions

Along with norms, there must be an effective procedure for invoking sanctions if a group member does not conform with the standards set. These sanctions can range from being elusive and evasive on the one hand to being quite visible on the other. The most powerful sanction is, of course, that of rejection. Employees who consistently do not comply with the group's norms will soon be on the outside. Their life can then be made miserable, their work can be sabotaged, and eventually they may want to leave the institution completely. But sanctions can also be very mild, perhaps in the form of a friendly admonition or excluding someone from social activities such as lunching together. All of these sanctions of the informal organization, whether subtle or strong, serve to see that group members adhere to the group's idea of correct on-the-job behavior.

Additional Characteristics

One of the reasons people form small groups is the need for information. These groups provide their own unofficial channel of communication, the grapevine. This manifestation of the informal organization has already been fully discussed in Chapter 5. Let it suffice to repeat here that the grapevine is the major connecting link of the informal organization, just as communication through regular channels serves to link the formal organizational structure. As stated above, the informal organization influences the behavior of employees regardless of the status they occupy within the informal group. This is important for a supervisor to remember because one cannot hope to understand individual behavior without understanding the behavior of the organizational forces that shape it.

Another such characteristic of the informal organization is inflexibility, especially *resistance to change.* It resists especially those changes which could be interpreted as a threat to the informal group. Over time, the small group has developed very satisfying social relationships, and any change that may challenge its equilibrium and stability will be greeted with resistance. This resistance can take the form of complaints, work slowdown, excessive absenteeism, reduction in the quality of the job performed, and so on. It is essential for a supervisor to understand the dynamics of these types of group behavior in order to introduce change successfully. This will be discussed further in Chapter 19.

Relations Between Informal and Formal Organizations

Often it might appear that the functioning of the informal organization makes the job of the supervisor a more difficult one. Because of the interdependence between informal and formal organizations, the attitudes, goals, norms, and customs of one affect the other. Informal organizations do frequently give life and vitality to the formal organization. But this is not always the case. Indeed, informal organizations can have either a constructive or hindering influence on the formal organization and on the realization of departmental objectives. In the final analysis, the supervisor's basic attitude will have much to do with whether that influence is positive or negative.

It is important for the supervisor to be aware that these informal groups are very strong, and they may often govern the behavior of employees to an extent that interferes with formal supervision. Sometimes it can even go so far that the pressure of the informal group frustrates the supervisor in carrying out policies which the superior manager expects the supervisor to enforce. The wise supervisor, therefore, should make all possible efforts to gain the cooperation and goodwill of the informal organization and the informal leader and to use them wherever possible to further the departmental objectives.

Both formal and informal relationships are parts of the system and they interact, each modifying the other. As stated before, they may be mutually reinforcing or conflicting. The supervisor should remember that informal groups provide the satisfaction of some needs that the formal organization leaves unsatisfied. Informal relationships make a contribution to the organizational climate; they keep the organization flexible and are a means of getting the departmental job done.

The Supervisor and the Informal Organization

One way the supervisor can put the informal organization to the best possible use is to let the employees know that its existence is accepted and understood. Such an understanding will enable the supervisor to group employees so that those most likely to comprise a good team will be working with each other on the same assignments. The supervisor's understanding of how the informal organization works will also help avoid activities that would unnecessarily threaten or disrupt the informal group. The manager should do his or her utmost to integrate the interests of the informal organization with those of the formal organization.

The supervisor should exhibit such a positive approach because he or she knows that there are positive attributes in a cohesive informal group. Morale is likely to be high, turnover and excessive absences tend to be low, and the members work smoothly as a team. This can make supervision much easier because the supervisor escapes a lot of bickering; it can also ease the burden of communication, since the group provides its own effective, although informal, channels. Therefore, the supervisor should emphasize the positive by "communicating" informal responsibility to the informal leader and by allowing the group, naturally within limits, to go about the job as much on their own as possible.

A supervisor can do even more to bring out the positive aspects of informal groups by sharing the decision-making authority with them, by practicing *group decision making*. In effect, this means turning the informal group into a sort of self-contained committee. As we know, decisions arrived at by a group or committee usually turn out to the advantage of all involved. They enable the group to exercise control over their own activities and to make certain that all their interests are taken into account, with the result that no one comes out a loser. The group has a larger information base and often different and more approaches to the problem. The group decision-making process also produces a broader understanding of the solution, which in turn brings increased acceptance.

Group problem solving has some shortcomings also. Often there is group pressure for conformity and consensus, possibly caused by the dominance of one individual; this at times may lower the quality of the decision. Although these are serious shortcomings, supervisors can reap many advantages by using group problem solving effectively. (See Figure 15-2.)

The supervisor must make sure that certain ground rules for this group decision-making process are established. Otherwise, it could bring about opposite results. First, the supervisor must sincerely believe in group decision making and want it. Second, clear limitations to the area of deliberation must be set. For instance, if the group is to arrange its own vacation schedule, it

Figure 15-2. Assets and liabilities of group decision making

Assets	Liabilities
Groups can accumulate more knowledge and facts	Groups often work more slowly than individuals
Groups have a broader perspective and consider more alternative solutions	Group decisions involve considerable compromise which may lead to less than optimal decisions
Individuals who participate in decisions are more satisfied with the decision and are more likely to support it	Groups are often dominated by one individual or a small clique, thereby negating many of the virtues of group processes
Group decision processes serve an important communication function, as well as a useful political function	Overreliance on group decision making can inhibit management's ability to act quickly and decisively when necessary

Richard M. Steers, *Introduction to Organizational Behavior* (Santa Monica, CA: Goodyear Publishing Co., Inc., 1981), 242. Reprinted by permission.

should be stated how many employees with a special skill must be present, what the time limits are, and so forth. Third, it must be clear whether the group is merely asked for suggestions or whether authority to find a solution and make a decision has been delegated. And last, but not least, the supervisor should choose a problem in which the enthusiastic acceptance and execution are at least as important, if not more important, than the specifics of the decision itself. Under these conditions, group decision making can be an additional means of accentuating the positive aspects of informal organization.

The Supervisor and the Informal Group Leader

It is also important for the supervisors to maintain a positive attitude toward the informal group leader. Instead of viewing this person as a "ring-leader," supervisors will do better to consider this individual as someone "in the know," to respect and work with him or her. In an effort to build good relations with the informal leader, supervisors can pass information on to that person before giving it to anyone else. They can ask for advice on certain problems, and, particularly if a rearrangement of duties or layouts is under consideration, they may want to discuss it with the informal leader first to get some reaction. Or the supervisor may ask the informal leader to "break in" a new employee of the department, knowing full well that he or she would do it anyway.

In taking this approach, however, the supervisor must be careful not to cause the informal leader to lose status within the group because working with the supervisor means working with management. In other words, the supervisor should not extend too many favors to the informal leader, since this would ruin the latter's leadership position within the group at once. Of course, the foregoing discussion assumes that an informal group leader is easily visible in every department. But often it is difficult for a supervisor, and especially for a new supervisor, to identify the informal leader of a group. Observation is probably the best means to find out. The supervisor should look for that person to whom the other employees turn when they need help, the person who sets the pace and who seems to have influence over them. The supervisor must continually and closely observe this because the informal group will occasionally shift from one leader to another, depending on the purposes to be pursued. But regardless of who the leader is, the supervisor should do all possible to work *with* the informal leader instead of against that person.

It would be unrealistic, however, to believe that such a positive approach is the cure for all conflicts between the informal and the formal organizations. No doubt there will be occasions when agreement and harmonious interaction may be impossible. There are situations in which every supervisor must act contrary to the desires of the supervised group. In those instances, the dictates of formal authority will probably be the decisive factor.

Summary

In addition to the formal organization, there exists in every enterprise an informal organization based on informal groups. These groups satisfy certain needs and desires of their members, which apparently are left unsatisfied by the formal organization. For example, an informal group can satisfy the members' social needs. It gives them recognition and status and a sense of belonging. Informal information transmitted through the grapevine provides a channel of communication and fulfills the members' need and desire to know what is going on. The informal organization also influences the behavior of individuals within the group and requests them to conform with certain standards the group has set up. Informal organization can be found on all levels of the enterprise from the top to the bottom. It exists in every department, regardless of the quality of supervision.

Informal organization can have either a constructive or destructive influence on the formal organization. To make the best possible use of informal organization, the supervisor must understand its workings and be able to identify its informal leaders. Then the supervisor can work with them in a way that will help accomplish the objectives of the department. For example, the informal group and its leader can be used to break in new employees or transmit messages. Instead of dwelling on the informal organization as a source of conflict, the supervisor should remember that both the formal and the informal organizations are part of a complex system interacting with each other. Instead of viewing it as something antagonistic, it should be approached positively, and its potential for the good of the enterprise should be emphasized. After all, informal groups are similar in many respects to formal committees, and they have many of the same advantages; this can be put to good use by letting the informal groups act as group decision makers.

Part Five

Staffing

16

The Staffing Process

Staffing is the managerial function concerned with the most important asset of an organization, its people. It is the function that supplies the human resources to fulfill the institution's plans and objectives. The staffing process takes place after the managerial functions of planning and organizing. Once goals have been determined, departments set up, and duties and task relationships established, people must be found to give life to what would otherwise be only a theoretical structure. It is the manager's responsibility to vitalize the department by staffing it properly. It must be staffed in such a manner that the capabilities of the employees in the department match their authority and responsibilities. This is important because if an employee's capabilities exceed the challenges and authority of the position, that person is not employed to full capacity and will not derive the necessary satisfaction from the job. On the other hand, if the employee's capability is beneath the demands and authority of the position, he or she will probably not be able to perform the job satisfactorily. The purpose of the staffing function, then, is to achieve the optimal use of human resources, which is only possible when job authority and demands match the employee's capability. And, of course, this balancing of capabilities with job requirements is the essence of the managerial staffing function.

More specifically, the staffing function of the manager includes the selection, placement, development, training, and compensation of the subordinates in the department. It is every manager's and supervisor's job to evaluate and appraise the performance of employees, promote them according to effort and ability, reward them, and, if necessary, discipline or even discharge them. Only if a manager performs all of these duties can it be said that the managerial staffing function has been truly fulfilled. Obviously staffing is a difficult task, and many supervisors depend on the help of specialists to achieve this human resources goal. This is the reason for the availability of a specialized staff department, the personnel department, in almost all organizations.

In checking the above list of activities, many supervisors may be inclined to believe that some of them are more properly the responsibility of the personnel director and the personnel department. It is true that in certain hospitals and related health care facilities some of the above-mentioned activities are performed by the personnel department. In such institutions, the personnel department has very broad jurisdiction. Nevertheless, good management still considers these duties as part of the supervisor's legitimate functions. Although the supervisor may be assisted in the performance of these functions by the personnel staff, they are still primarily the supervisor's responsibility.

The Staffing Function and the Personnel Department

Throughout the following discussion, it will be assumed that within the organizational structure of the institution the personnel department—also known as the department of human resources or similar terms—is considered a staff department as defined in our discussion of line and staff. The usefulness and effectiveness of the personnel department will depend largely on its ability to develop a good working relationship with line supervisors, that is, the quality of the line-staff relationship. This, of course, will be governed in part by how clearly and specifically the administrator has outlined the activities and authority of the department of human resources. In determining its scope and relationship to the staffing function of line supervisors, it is necessary for the administrator to understand the historical place of the personnel department in the institution. Only then will one be able to establish a structure that is meaningful in terms of current needs and patterns.

Historical Patterns

The personnel department started primarily as a record-keeping department. It kept all employment records for the employees and managers, all correspondence pertaining to their hiring, application blanks, background information, various positions held within the enterprise, dates of promotions, salary changes, leaves of absence granted, disciplinary penalties imposed, and other kinds of information that describe the employee's relationship to the enterprise. Of course, proper maintenance of these clerical records is still of great importance today, especially with the growing emphasis on equal opportunity employment, pension and insurance programs, unemployment claims, seniority provisions, and promotional and development programs. By assigning such clerical service activities to the personnel staff, the administrator knows that they will be handled with high technical competence and efficiency because of the specialization of the department. If such a service were not provided by the personnel department, each and every supervisor would have to keep these records for his or her own department. Obviously, this would be a cumbersome and time-consuming task with which to be burdened in addition to the daily chores of getting the job done. Therefore, line supervisors are happy to have the personnel staff perform these complicated clerical services for them. The line supervisors are just not interested in doing the work themselves, and often they may not even have the ability to do so.

As time went on, mainly during the 1920s, many managers in industry believed that the threat of unionization might be thwarted if efforts were made to give employees cafeterias, better rest rooms, bowling teams, company stores, etc. Although most of these benefits have a strong flavor of "paternalism," management thought that they would make the employees happier and less resentful. Since none of these activities fitted into the regular line departments of the enterprise, however, the personnel department took responsibility for an increasing number of them.

During the 1930s, another shift in the emphasis of the personnel department took place. With the increase of union activities, the personnel department was expected to take direct charge of all employee and union relations. It often assumed full responsibility for hiring, firing, handling union grievances, and dealing with general labor problems. In other words, management believed that by having a personnel department, all personnel questions could be handled by them, leaving the line supervisors with practically no staffing function.

This led to serious difficulties, however, because although the duties and power of the personnel department increased significantly, the standing of the supervisor as a manager decreased. The more power the personnel director acquired, the weaker the supervisor's relationship became with his or her own employees. The demoralized supervisor justifiably complained that it was impossible to effectively manage the department without having the power to select, hire, discipline, and reward the employees. The employees no longer regarded the supervisor as their boss. Because someone in the personnel department hired the employees, established their wages, and promoted, disciplined, and fired them, employees looked to someone in the personnel department as their supervisor. Since this obviously led to a bad state of affairs in many organizations, good management now clearly delineates between the functions of the personnel department in a staff capacity and the supervisor's role as a manager of the department.

Current Patterns

During the last decades most organizations have recognized the need for a proper balance of influence and authority between the line managers and the personnel staff. Good management dictates that supervisors and personnel people must work together because their work is intertwined. But their areas of authority and their roles must be clearly stated. Sound management principles advocate that the job of the personnel department is to provide the line supervisor with advice and counsel concerning personnel problems and to help the line supervisors in every possible respect. Going beyond this would lead to a fragmentation of the supervisor's job and make it impossible for the supervisor to be an effective manager within the department. Of course, the supervisor must manage within the framework of the hospital's personnel policies, procedures, and regulations. Naturally, the line supervisor should take full advantage of the expert advice and assistance that is available within the personnel department, but the line supervisor must retain the basic responsibility for managing the department.

Since it is the supervisor's job to get out the work within the department, he or she must make managerial decisions that concern the people who work in the department. Generally, this means that the supervisor defines the specific qualifications expected from an employee who is to fill a specific position. It is the personnel department's function to develop sources of qualified applicants within the local labor market. The personnel department must let the community know what jobs are available and, in general, create an image of the organization as an employer. The personnel department can accomplish this by fostering good community relations and recruiting in high schools, training schools, colleges, and other sources of employees.

The personnel department should conduct preliminary interviews with applicants to determine whether or not their qualifications match the requirements as defined by the supervisor. Necessary reference checks as to previous employment dates and past records should be made by the personnel department, and those applicants who do not meet job requirements should be eliminated from consideration. Those candidates who meet the stated requirements should be referred to the supervisor.

It is up to the supervisor to interview, select, and hire from among the available candidates. It is the supervisor who normally will make the final decision, sometimes in collaboration with the direct line superior. The supervisor assigns the new employee to a specific job, and it is the responsibility of the supervisor to judge how this new employee's skills can best be utilized and developed. It is the personnel department's job to give the new employee a general indoctrination about the hospital, benefits, general rules, shifts, hours, etc. But it is the supervisor's job to introduce the employee to the specific details of the job—wages, departmental rules, hours, rest periods, etc. The supervisor monitors compensation within the pattern of remuneration, instructs and trains the new employee on the job, and assesses the employee's performance to determine, as time goes on, whether or not this person should be promoted into a better job. If the need to take disciplinary measures should arise, it is clearly the supervisor's duty to do so and, if necessary, even to fire the employee; this may be done with higher line management review. During the time an employee is with the organization, the complete employment record is maintained by the personnel department.

In carrying out the staffing function the supervisor will be greatly aided by the department of human resources. They maintain all the clerical services, keep the records, and are there to provide advice, counsel, and guidance whenever personnel problems arise. In making decisions, the supervisor can follow, reject, or alter the personnel department's advice and counsel. In reality, of course, it is often difficult to draw such a fine line of distinction between the advice, counsel, and guidance of the personnel department and the supervisor's decision making.

The following example will illustrate how blurred the distinction can be between providing information and giving advice and, on the other hand, trying to make decisions for the supervisor. When the staff person merely provides information facts are furnished that help the supervisor make a sound decision. For instance, the personnel officer might inform the nursing director that those applying for an open nursing position are expecting a starting salary which is higher than the institution's starting rate. Or the personnel person might advise that if the director of nursing were to hire a nurse at a certain salary, the director may have some dissatisfied older employees in the department. In the latter remark, the staff person is providing not only information but also advice. By selecting the facts and phrasing this advice carefully, the personnel officer may actually sway the line supervisor's decision one way or the other. He or she may even advise paying the new nurse a certain amount per hour. And before anyone realizes it, the information becomes advice and the advice becomes a decision. This may have come about not because of a desire on the personnel officer's part for broader authority or to reduce the supervisor's authority, but rather the line supervisor may have encouraged this growth of staff activity.

Sometimes supervisors will welcome the personnel department's willingness to help them out of a difficult situation. Frequently supervisors ask the personnel department to make a decision for them so that they will not become burdened with so-called personnel problems. They gladly accept the staff person's decision, believing that if the decision is wrong, they can always excuse it by saying it was the personnel department's decision. In other words, the line supervisor is only too ready to capitulate to the personnel person in many instances. In so doing one can "pass the buck" to the personnel department.

Although it is understandable that the supervisor is reluctant to question and disregard the advice of the staff expert, the supervisor must bear in mind that the staff person sees only a small part of the entire picture. The staff officer is not responsible for the performance of the department. There are usually many other factors involved in the overall picture that will affect the department, factors with which staff is not as familiar as the line supervisor. The supervisor cannot separate his or her functions between clear areas of personnel problems and performance problems. Every situation has certain personnel implications, and it is impossible to separate the various components of each problem within the department. Only the supervisor is likely to know what the broad picture is.

If the supervisor capitulates and has the personnel department make decisions, the relationship with the department's employees will sooner or later be damaged. The subordinates will decide that it is the personnel department and not the supervisor who has the real power to influence their jobs within the hospital. The supervisor's leadership position will slowly deteriorate if the employees detect that the personnel staff determines salaries and hiring and firing practices. They will discover that the supervisor does not control rewards and penalties and that, in reality, he or she does not make the decisions in the department.

The supervisor must make it clear that it is he or she who makes the decisions and takes the responsibility for the consequences. Although there are occasions when it may seem convenient to "pass the buck" to the personnel department, such practices sooner or later will backfire. It is not uncommon for supervisors to say that they would gladly give their employees a certain raise but that "they" (the personnel department) will not let them do so. Although this may be expedient for the moment, practices of this type lead eventually to erosion of the supervisor's authority. In this situation the supervisor has to state that *he or she* has explored all possible alternatives and that nothing can be done at this time for the employee, that he or she will keep trying, etc.

At times a supervisor may see the necessity of dismissing an employee, but the personnel department "advises" not to do so. If in the future this particular employee's performance leads to additional difficulties within the department, the supervisor is likely to shrug off responsibility by merely saying that he or she wanted to fire the person a long time ago, but that the personnel officer "advised" not to do so. The supervisor is thus disclaiming all responsibility for this particular employee, and all of this leads to untenable conditions within a department. It is up to the supervisor to make managerial decisions and take the responsibility for them, regardless of the difficulty or risks involved.

Staffing and Legal Implications

During recent years it has become increasingly difficult to carry out the staffing function because of numerous federal, state, and local laws and regulations. Employment practices and policies must comply with these laws which, generally speaking, prohibit discrimination against applicants and employees on the basis of race, sex, color, religion, or national origin. Nor is it proper to use age as a criterion of selection among applicants who are between 40 and 70 years old. There are also laws that might request an organization to hire handicapped persons and veterans. Affirmative-action programs might dictate to the institution to give hiring preferences to minority members who are qualified or have the potential to fill available jobs.

A discussion of equal employment opportunity is beyond the confines of this text; however supervisors must be aware of this concern because it affects their staffing function. Table 16-1 is a partial listing of some of the major laws on equal employment opportunity requirements and the enforcement agencies. It is necessary to mention this important subject, since it clearly affects the staffing function. It will be discussed in more detail in Chapter 17.

Since the problems of equal employment opportunity, discrimination, and similar laws and court decisions are a rapidly growing special area of considerations, it would be impossible for a line supervisor to be aware of all of this or to try to keep up with it. Therefore, members of the personnel department become specialists in these problems and exert a pervasive influence on the staffing function. It is imperative that the organization complies with the multitude of laws and regulations, and in recent years it has become one of the personnel department's obligations to make certain that the institution is in compliance and not in violation.

Figure 16-1. Examples of current laws and regulations affecting employment policies**

Legislation	Concern or content	Administrative agency
Title VII of the Civil Rights Act of 1964*	Sex	EEOC†
Equal Pay Act of 1963		EEOC
Title VII of the Civil Rights Act of 1964*	Color	EEOC
Title VII of the Civil Rights Act of 1964*	Race	EEOC
Title VII of the Civil Rights Act of 1964*	Religion	EEOC
Title VII of the Civil Rights Act of 1964*	National origin	EEOC
Age Discrimination in Employment Act of 1967, as amended in 1978	Age (protection for those 40 to 70 years old)	EEOC
Rehabilitation Act of 1973	Handicapped persons	U.S. Department of Labor
The Vietnam-Era Veteran Readjustment Assistance Act of 1974	Vietnam-era veterans	U.S. Department of Labor
Various executive orders, principally no. 11246 and revised order no. 4	*All* of the above as part of affirmative-action programs	Office of Federal Contract Compliance, U.S. Department of Labor

*As amended by the Equal Employment Opportunity Act of 1972 and the Pregnancy Discrimination Act of 1978.

†Equal Employment Opportunity Commission.

**Effective at the time of publication of this text. The above is a partial—and not exhaustive—list of the framework of laws, regulations, and administrative agencies which govern staffing policies and decisions.

Functional Authority and the Personnel Department

As stated in the beginning of this chapter, all of the above remarks refer to an organizational arrangement in which the personnel director's office is attached to the organization in strictly a staff position. In a number of health care institutions, however, the chief executive officer has decided that all dismissals have to be approved by the director of personnel. The top administrator has the authority to make such a provision, and in this instance functional staff authority as discussed in Chapter 12 has been conferred on the personnel director. In other words, top administration wants the director of human resources to make the final decision as to whether or not an employee who has been working in the hospital longer than the customary probationary period should be dismissed. The administrator is removing this part from the supervisor's authority and conferring it on the director of personnel.

There must be strong reasons behind such a decision, since it clearly runs counter to the principle of unity of command and weakens the authority of the supervisor's position. The chief administrator may have done this to protect the hospital from excessive unemployment compensation claims that result from too many firings. Or the decision may have been based on the administrator's desire to comply with all possible fair and nondiscriminatory employment practices and regulations so as not to expose the hospital to embarrassing situations.

There may be other reasons as to why an administrator may want to delegate this final authority to fire an employee to the director of personnel. In such situations it is desirable for the personnel director to disseminate as much information as possible to all first-line supervisors. For example, the personnel office should familiarize the supervisors with the latest government provisions regarding fair employment practices. Also, the various possibilities of engaging in conscious or unconscious discriminatory practices should be brought to the attention of the supervisors. Supervisors should understand the meaning of affirmative action. Furthermore, first-line managers should be informed as to how unemployment claims by former employees affect the overall wage bill of the hospital.

The chief administrator should explain the importance of documentation, and the line supervisors should be urged to keep meaningful records that they and the hospital can refer to if necessary. If supervisors are familiar with all of these current thoughts and considerations, it is unlikely that they would consider discharging an employee unless all possible ramifications have been considered. Under these circumstances it is likely that the director of personnel will go along with a proposed dismissal, since the supervisor has a well-documented and substantiated case which can become a valid defense. It is desirable, therefore, that the director of personnel who has been given the final authority on discharges will use this authority with much discretion and in a manner of "consultation" with the various supervisors and not use it as if he or she were the "supreme power."

The Supervisor's Staffing Function

The staffing function is a continuous activity for the supervisor. It is not something that is required only when the department is first established. As a matter of fact, it is much more realistic and more typical to think of staffing as a situation in which a supervisor is put in charge of an existing department with a certain number of employees already in it. Although there is a nucleus of employees to start with, it is likely that before too long changes in personnel will take place. Since every supervisor depends on employees for the operating results of the department, it is the supervisor's responsibility to make certain that there is a supply of well-trained employees to fill the various positions.

Determining the Need for Employees

To make certain that the department can perform the jobs required of it, the supervisor must determine both the number and kind of employees

who will be needed for the department. If the supervisor has set up the structure of the department, he or she has designed an organizational structure in
which the functions and jobs are shown in their proper relationships. If the
supervisor takes over an existing department, it is necessary to become
familiar with it by drawing a picture of the existing jobs and functions. For example, the supervisor of the maintenance department may find that there are
groups of painters, electricians, carpenters, and other skilled *persons* within
the department. After taking this inventory of personnel, it should be determined how many skilled *positions* there are or should be within this department, considering budgetary constraints. The working relationships between
these positions should be examined and defined by the supervisor. After
determining the needs of the department, the supervisor may have to adjust
the ideal setup to existing necessities. Or several positions may have to be
combined into one if there is not enough work for one employee. It is only by
studying the organizational setup of the department that the supervisor can
determine what employees are needed to perform what jobs.

Job Description

To fill the various positions with appropriate employees, it is necessary
to match the available jobs in the department with the credentials of prospective employees. This can only be done with the help of job descriptions (Figures 16-2 and 16-3).* The job description tells exactly what duties and responsibilities are contained within a particular job. It describes the content of the
job by listing as completely as possible every duty and responsibility involved. In many instances the supervisor will find a set of job descriptions
available. If none is available, the personnel director can and will be of great
help in establishing a set of job descriptions. But no one is better equipped to
describe the content of a job than the supervisor. It is the supervisor who is
responsible for the accomplishment of the tasks of the department, and he or
she knows or should know the content of each position. Although the final
form of the job description may be prepared in the personnel office, it is the
supervisor who determines its specific content.

Only by describing the job requirements in great detail is it possible to
ascertain the skills necessary to perform the job satisfactorily. Even if the position is one that is already in operation, it is still advisable to follow this procedure of determining the major duties and responsibilities. After this has
been done, it is advisable to compare this list with the current job description
and with what the employee is actually doing. The older job description may
no longer fit the current content of the job, and should be corrected. The
supervisor may find that some of the duties assigned to the job really do not
belong to it. Even if the job in question is a new position, the supervisor should
proceed along similar lines. It should be decided what the duties and responsibilities of the job are, and with the help of the personnel department a job
description should be drawn up. Once the content of the job has been

*See also job descriptions in Appendix B.

Figure 16-2. Position Description

POSITION: _____Nurse Specialist_____ DATE: _____June, 1984_____
DEPARTMENT: ___Nursing Service___ NEXT REVIEW DATE: ___June, 1984___
SECTION: _____3110_____ JOB GRADE: _____20_____
REPORTS TO: ___Clinical Director___ JOB CODE NO.: _____012_____

POSITION PURPOSE: The Nurse Specialist delivers or supervises nursing care, educates patients, families, and staff, serves as a consultant and conducts nursing research.

DIMENSIONS: Indeterminate.

NATURE AND SCOPE: The position reports directly to the Clinical Director of Specialty Nursing along with the head nurses of specialty areas.

A major challenge of this position is to keep current in a specialized field in order to provide effective services throughout the hospital and in the community.

The Nurse Specialist assesses nursing care, collaborates with other disciplines and supports therapeutic medical treatment. Specifically:

The incumbent provides direct/indirect nursing care to a caseload of patients, implements changes based on evaluation of patients and acts as a patient advocate.

Educational functions include education to patients/families and community in prevention, treatment, and rehabilitation of disease and health maintenance. Also, clinical and theoretical health care instruction is provided to nursing personnel, other professionals, and students via workshops, conferences, seminars, and formal courses.

The Clinical Specialist responds to referrals from nursing staff, physicians, social work, and other disciplines and serves as a consultant to assist in identifying clinical problems and planning appropriate intervention. Also consults with health-related organizations/groups for program and curriculum planning, development, and evaluation.

Another important function is to serve as a change agent by influencing attitudes, modifying behavior, and introducing new concepts.

The incumbent uses systematic methods of scientific inquiry to investigate nursing problems related to a specialty area, participates in nursing research projects and in the development of standards of performance and patient care.

Participation in general nursing service endeavors is demonstrated by participation in audit activities, assisting in the development of policies/procedures and membership on committees as appointed.

Problems/decisions referred to the Clinical Director for resolution include those that may involve legal consideration, affect other departments, proposals for special projects, recommendations for change, and requests to attend outside meetings.

Performance is measured by timeliness, completeness, and accuracy of written reports; feedback from involved staffs and observations made by the responsible Clinical Director.

Significant contacts are with Nursing personnel and other disciplines as well as with patients and families. Individual and group meetings will be scheduled with the Clinical Director.

This position requires graduation from an approved school of nursing, current RN licensure in Missouri and a Master's degree in Nursing. Two years clinical practice in the specialty is preferred. Knowledge of teaching-learning theory, utilization of community resources, physical assessment skills, and principles of both change theory and research will enhance the effectiveness of the incumbent.

PRINCIPAL ACCOUNTABILITIES:

1. Provides direct clinical expertise by responding to referrals from medical and nursing staffs.
2. Provides indirect clinical expertise through educational programs for patients/ families, nursing staffs, and other involved disciplines.
3. Remains knowledgeable in field of specialty by attending/participating in formal courses, workshops, and seminars in area of expertise.
4. Ensures current nursing practice and policy making through membership on Standing Nursing Committees and making recommendations for change.

REPLACES JOB DESCRIPTION(S): Nurse Specialist, dated July 1979.

Reprinted with special permission from Barnes Hospital, St. Louis. This description is for illustrative purposes only.

Figure 16-3. Position Description

POSITION: _____Executive Secretary I_____   DATE: _____January 22, 1984_____

DEPARTMENT: _____Nursing Service_____   NEXT REVIEW DATE: __November, 1984__

SECTION: _____3100_____   JOB GRADE: _____10_____

REPORTS TO: ___Director of Nursing___   JOB CODE NO.: _____081_____

JOB DUTIES: Coordinates and performs a variety of secretarial functions in the office of the Director of Nursing:

Receives and transcribes dictation by shorthand or taped dictation.

Types and composes correspondence, drafts, reports, and schedules as assigned or delegated.

Processes Pers-8 forms for nursing administration personnel and maintain files and salary cards for each.

Answers calls and takes messages for nursing administration and refers calls to appropriate nursing service personnel.

Receives and distributes mail.

Orders and maintains adequate supplies and equipment for office of the Director of Nursing.

Plans, coordinates, and schedules meetings. Distributes agenda, takes and distributes minutes of meetings.

Coordinates calendar of Director of Nursing with appointments, meetings, and travel schedules.

Coordinates travel schedules of nursing service personnel and arranges for travel and hotel reservations. Prepares reports on travel expense for Director of Nursing and requisitions approved monies. Reviews expense reports submitted after travel, obtains signatures, and submits to Accounting Department.

Reviews incident reports and assembles information needed by Director of Nursing concerning disposition of report or reimbursements. Initiates correspondence concerning disposition and processes paperwork for approved reimbursements.

TRAINING, EDUCATION, EXPERIENCE, OR OTHER REQUIREMENTS: High school graduate with additional college credits desirable. Types 60 w.p.m. and shorthand 100 w.p.m. Good knowledge of grammar, spelling, and compositional writing. Self-directed with ability to identify problems and subsequent solutions. Ability to communicate courteously and effectively with the general public and all levels of hospital personnel. Must maintain confidentiality of information processed.

PHYSICAL DEMANDS: Sits at desk most of day. Works in clean, air-conditioned environment.

REPLACES JOB DESCRIPTION(S): Secretary-I, Executive, dated January 1983.

Reprinted with special permission from Barnes Hospital, St. Louis. This description is for illustrative purposes only.

---

specified, the supervisor should then specify the knowledge, education, degrees, experience, and skills required of the prospective employee.

In every job there are certain things an employee must know before he or she can perform the job effectively. For example, it may be necessary to be able to read simple blueprints or be familiar with mathematics. To elaborate on this last instance, if a knowledge of mathematics is needed for a certain job, the specific type of mathematics required should be clearly defined. The word "mathematics" could imply knowledge far beyond a working knowledge of simple arithmetic, and a knowledge of simple arithmetic might be all that is required in the job. The more precisely defined the required job knowledge is, the easier it will be to select from among available applicants.

When stipulating the skills needed for a particular job, the supervisor should not ask for a higher degree of skill than is absolutely necessary. One way to avoid this is to check the requirements drawn up with the qualifications of employees who are doing the same or similar kinds of work. Such investigation may quickly reveal that for a certain job, a high school education is not necessary. The supervisor may discover that an older person without a high school diploma can perform this kind of work.

Equal employment opportunity laws and rulings require that job descriptions must not discriminate against certain classes and that they must be job related. Since supervisors could not possibly be aware of all the ramifications in this respect, the personnel department should be consulted. In reality, to comply with these laws and regulations many personnel departments have assumed responsibility for the final draft of the job descriptions.

The supervisor should realize that by setting employment standards unrealistically high, the task of finding the person to meet these specifications will become unnecessarily difficult. There is no need to specify a certain number of years of formal education and experience if all that is required is simple job know-how. This does not mean that the job specifications should ask for less than what is actually needed. It should specify the requirements realistically. If the requirements are set too high, people will be placed on the job who are overqualified. The likely result is that the particular employee may prove to be troublesome because his or her capacities are not completely utilized. By the same token, it is just as disastrous to ask for less than necessary. Once placed on the job, the employee may turn out to be unsatisfactory. Many of these difficulties can be avoided if the supervisor analyzes the job content diligently and specifies the job knowledge and skills required in a realistic manner.

The personnel department will prove to be of great help in drawing up these job descriptions. But the supervisor should be cautioned not to turn over the job of doing this to the personnel person. The content must definitely be specified by the supervisor and by no one else. Once these job descriptions have been drafted, the supervisor should consult with some of the people who are holding these jobs, so as to compare the job descriptions with the actual positions in question. Once all difficulties have been ironed out, these job descriptions are maintained in the personnel department and also in the supervisor's file. Whenever the supervisor needs to fill a certain job, the personnel department is informed that it is open, and the personnel people will try to recruit suitable applicants to fill the job. Personnel can quickly screen out those applicants who are obviously unfit because they do not have the knowledge or necessary skills or cannot fulfill any of the other requirements. But all of those who seem to fulfill the requirements will be referred to the supervisor for his or her acceptance or rejection.

Since job descriptions should be kept up to date, the supervisor must review the contents of the job from time to time. Without regular reviews there is a danger that they may become incorrect because of changing requirements, education, and advances in technology. The supervisor must continually audit the job descriptions in the department. Many activities in the health care field change considerably through new technology, scientific advances, and sometimes because of the creative efforts of the person occupying a position. Ambitious employees may enlarge the scope of their own activities, whereas other employees lose or forego portions of theirs. The extent and character of change must be determined so that accurate information is contained in the job description. This is necessary because the job description is constantly referred to when the personnel department recruits candidates, when the supervisor hires new employees, when their performance is appraised, and when an attempt is made to establish an equitable wage pattern within the department.

If staffing decisions are to possess any validity, they must be based on comprehensive job descriptions that are systematically revised to reflect the current job situation in as accurate a manner as possible. Furthermore, they must reflect the current situation of equal opportunity employment and non-discrimination. The descriptions contained in the Appendix B may well serve as a starting point from which interested persons may prepare descriptions more reflective of their own situation and circumstances.

How Many to Hire

Normally, the supervisor is not confronted with the situation in which a great number of employees have to be hired at the same time. Such a situation could exist when a new department is created and the supervisor has to staff it completely from scratch. It is more typical that the question of hiring an employee will occur only occasionally. Of course, there are some supervisors who continuously ask for additional employees to get a job done. In most of these cases their problems are not solved even if they get more help. As a matter of fact, the situation may become worse; instead of reducing the supervisor's problems, they are actually increased.

Normally, a supervisor will need to hire a new worker when one of the employees leaves the department, either voluntarily quitting or from dismissal or some other reason. In such instances there is little doubt that the job must be filled. Occasionally, changes in the technical nature of the work take place, and manual labor may be replaced by machinery or sophisticated instruments. In such a case a replacement may not be needed. But normally, a new employee has to be hired to replace the one who left.

There are other situations when additional employees have to be added. For example, when departmental activities have been enlarged or when new duties are to be undertaken and no one within the department possesses the required job knowledge and skill, the supervisor has to go out into the open market and recruit employees. Sometimes a supervisor is inclined to ask for additional help if the work load is increased or if the supervisor feels added pressure. But before requesting additional employees under those conditions, the supervisor should make certain that the persons currently within the department are fully utilized and that additional people are absolutely necessary. It is hoped that this can be achieved within the constraints of the budget.

If there are vacancies within the department, the supervisor should inform the personnel department, and the personnel manager in turn should see that a number of suitable candidates for the jobs are made available. The personnel department accomplishes this task by consulting the various job descriptions. Those applicants who are obviously undesirable and unfit for the position in question can quickly be screened out. Those who seem to be generally acceptable and fulfill the required knowledge and skills should be passed on to the supervisor. The actual hiring decision is not to be made in the personnel office; it is to be made by the supervisor in whose department the employee is to work. Although supervisors may believe that this is not necessary in filling an unskilled job, they should not relinquish their prerogative and duty to hire the people who are to work in their department. It does not matter if it is a nonskilled, skilled, or semiskilled job that is to be filled. It is up to the supervisor to hire the employee. Since all applicants are prescreened by the personnel office, the supervisor knows that all of those who are sent to him or her possess the minimum qualifications prescribed for the job. It is the supervisor's job to pick out the one who will probably fill the job best. This is not an easy task, but as time goes on the supervisor will gain more and more experience, and it will become easier to make the right decision. All of this will be discussed in the following chapter.

Summary

Staffing is one of the managerial functions every supervisor has to perform. It means to select, place, train, evaluate, promote, discipline, and appropriately compensate the employees of the department. All of this is the supervisor's line function. In fulfilling this duty the supervisor is significantly aided by the services of the department of human resources. In most enterprises the personnel department is attached to the organization in a staff capacity, and its purpose is to counsel, advise, and service all other departments of the enterprise. In its eagerness to be of service to the line manager, the personnel department may be inclined to take over line functions such as hiring, disciplining, and setting wages. Supervisors must caution themselves not to capitulate any of their line functions to the personnel department, although at times it might seem expedient to let them handle the "dirty" problems. Throughout the staffing function attention must be paid to the many laws and regulations concerning nondiscrimination and equal employment opportunity.

Before the manager can undertake the staffing function, the number and kinds of employees needed in the department must be clarified. The organizational chart combined with job descriptions will specify the kinds of workers necessary to fill the various jobs. In addition, the supervisor must take into consideration the amount of work to be performed and the positions allocated in the budget. In all of these supervisory duties the personnel department is available for assistance and service. But it is the supervisor's function to select, place, develop, evaluate, promote, reward, and discipline *all* the employees within the department.

17

The Employment Interview and Selection Process

Since the selection of the right employee contributes significantly to the supervisor's effectiveness, ultimate responsibility for decision making must reside with the line manager. Personnel specialists can help the supervisor select subordinates by recruiting and screening properly qualified candidates. But the final decision on hiring rests with the manager.

After all of the preliminary work has been performed by the personnel department, such as recruitment, preliminary screening interviews, obtaining biographical data, and formal tests, it is the supervisor's job to see the applicants, talk to them, and select the one who will best fill the vacant job. This is a decisive step for the employee and the supervisor. This is the moment when the supervisor must match the applicant's capability with the demands of the job, authority and responsibility inherent in the position, working conditions, and rewards and satisfactions it offers. The personal interview between the supervisor and applicant is an essential part of the selection process.

The interview is an almost universal selection device. It involves a two-way communication, enabling the interviewer to learn more about the applicant's background, interests, and values, and enabling the applicant to ask questions about the institution and the job. The interview is not a precise technique, and it is difficult to interview skillfully. Since there are no fixed criteria for success or failure, prejudiced interviewers can easily evaluate an applicant's performance according to their own stereotypes. Also job applicants react differently to different interviewers. But as a major means for deciding, interviews are probably more valid for accurately predicting employee behavior than decisions made on tests alone. Generally, structured interviews are more valid than unstructured interviews. It is not an easy task to make an appropriate appraisal of someone's potential during a brief interview. Interviewing is much more than a technique, it is an art that can and must be developed by every supervisor. It can be acquired better by practice than merely by reading articles on it.

Interviews

Over a period of years the supervisor will learn that there are several kinds of interviews. There are preemployment, or selection, interviews between the supervisor and prospective employees, there are discussions when employees are fired, and there are counseling sessions during which the abilities and deficiencies of an employee are discussed. In addition, there are interviews when an employee voluntarily leaves the job, as well as when employees want to discuss complaints, grievances, and any other problem situations. Generally, all of these can be grouped into two kinds of interviews, directive (structured) and nondirective (counseling). Throughout our discussion we will separate these two approaches, but some interviews have aspects of both categories. For example, the appraisal interview (Chapter 18) is, to a large extent, a directive interview. But the discussion may take on some aspects of a nondirective counseling interview.

Directive Interviews

Normally, a directive interview is a discussion in which the interviewer knows beforehand what particular facts will be discussed and what the goals, objectives, and area of the discussion are. The directive interview is structured; the interviewer will ask direct questions and tries to keep the discussion within predetermined limits. The interviewer will try to get the necessary information by encouraging the interviewee to volunteer as much as possible, and, if need be, by asking the interviewee additional questions. The employment interview in which the supervisor selects one applicant over another is an example of directive interview.

Nondirective Interviews

Although we will be primarily concerned with the directive interview in this chapter, it is advisable to call the supervisor's attention to what it means to conduct a nondirective, or counseling, interview. In a nondirective interview the interviewer encourages the interviewee to freely express his or her thoughts and feelings. This kind of interview is usually applied to problem situations in which the supervisor is eager to learn what the interviewee thinks and feels. The nondirective interview is employed in problem situations, such as complaints and grievances or off-the-job problems, or it may take the form of an exit interview when the employee voluntarily leaves the job. Affording your subordinates the opportunity of counseling interviews is a vital aspect of good supervision.

Supervisors must encourage subordinates to come to them with their problems. They must show that they are willing to hear them out. Otherwise minor irritations may turn out to become major problems. The supervisor must realize that there is an invisible barrier between the supervisor and the subordinates inherent in the managerial position. Some employees will have little difficulty speaking to their supervisors; but many are more timid. Therefore, the supervisor must make an effort for those who are reluctant to reveal what is on their mind. The supervisor should see that time is always available to listen to the subordinates and hear them out. If time is not available at the moment, then the interview, if possible, should be postponed for a few hours; the supervisor must allow enough time and not rush through the discussion.

The principal function of the nondirective interview is to give the supervisor a clue as to what the interviewee really thinks and feels and what lies at the root of a particular problem. In addition, it gives the interviewee a feeling of relief, and it helps the subordinate develop greater insight into his or her own problems, often finding solutions while "thinking out loud." There are many sources of frustration within and without the working environment, and, unless frustration is relieved, it may lead to all kinds of undesirable responses.

The ground rule is to let the interviewee say whatever he or she wants to say and to encourage free expression of feelings and attitudes. Conducting a nondirective interview is more difficult than conducting a directive interview. It demands the concentrated and continuous attention of the supervisor. The supervisor must exert self-control and hide his or her own ideas and emotions during the interview. The supervisor should not express approval or disapproval even though the employee may request it. This may prove exasperating, but it is essential.

In such a counseling interview the employee must feel free, perhaps for the first time in his or her life, to express feelings about everything. The fact that the troubled employee can pour out his or her troubles has therapeutic value. In all likelihood, as soon as all of the negative feelings have been expressed, the employee may start to find some favorable aspects of the very same things that he or she had criticized earlier. When the employee is encouraged to verbalize problems, he or she may gain a greater insight into them or possibly may arrive at an answer or course of action that will help solve the difficulties. It is essential that the employee be permitted to work through difficulties alone, without being interrupted and advised by the counselor regarding the best course of action. If the problem concerns the job, work, and organization, however, the supervisor may have to be directive so that the solution is consistent with the needs of the institution.

The supervisor should normally exercise great care not to give advice or become burdened with the task of running the subordinate's personal life. Most of the time the interviewee wants a sympathetic and empathic listener and not an advisor. The average supervisor is not equipped to do counseling, and it is not part of the supervisor's job. If need be, the subordinate should be helped by referral to trained specialists. This may be necessary when sensitive areas and deep-seated personality problems are involved. The patient-psychiatrist relationship is not applicable to that of subordinate and boss.

Frequently, subordinates bring to the supervisor personal off-the-job problems, which even the most stable individuals experience. Again, the supervisor should listen, but should be careful not to give advice or try to run the subordinate's personal affairs. They may ask for advice, but truly want a chance to talk. This is so much more important when deep-seated personality problems are involved. In this situation the supervisor should refer the person to a professional trained specialist.

At first the nondirective interview is difficult to conduct, but as time goes on, a good supervisor will learn to exercise self-control and, by concentrated listening, grasp the feelings of the employee. The counseling interviews can often be very time consuming. Although the supervisor is under many pressures and may not have much time for listening, time for such interviews must be made. The supervisor will find out that by listening, relationships with subordinates will be better, and probably fewer personnel problems will have to be coped with. The supervisor must encourage subordinates to come to him or her and show that he or she is always willing to hear them out.

Skillful listening is an art that can be learned with training and experience. It can be learned better by practice than by reading books on the subject. The supervisor can gain this practice almost every day on the job. Eventually the supervisor will develop a system of listening that is comfortable and fits the supervisor's personality and at the same time puts the employee at ease.

A common purpose of both directive and nondirective interviews is to promote mutual understanding and confidence. It is an experience in human relations that will permit the interviewer and the interviewee to obtain greater understanding. The nondirective approach is not a cure for all human relations problems. Occasionally, as stated before, the supervisor has to be directive in the solution stage of the discussion. After fully listening to the subordinate, the supervisor may still have to overrule the employee so that the solution is in accordance with the needs and within the limits of the organization.

The Employment Interview

The employment interview, also known as the preemployment, or selection, interview, will be discussed as an example of the directive, or structured, interview. The interviewer knows ahead of time what facts will be discussed, what the objectives are, and what area the discussion will cover. The structured interview is conducted using a set of standardized questions that are asked of all applicants; this produces data on applicants that can be compared and provides a basis for evaluating the applicants. The interviewer should prepare the questions in advance. This does not mean that the structured interview must be rigid. Although the questions preferably should be asked in a logical sequence, the applicant should have ample opportunity to explain the answers. At times, the interviewer has to probe until a full understanding has been reached. The supervisor wants to learn as much as possible by first letting the interviewee volunteer information and then by asking direct questions.

Preparing for the Employment Interview

Since the purpose of the directive employment interview is to collect facts and reach a decision, the supervisor should prepare for it as thoroughly as possible. First, it is essential that the supervisor become acquainted with the available background information. By studying all the information assembled by the personnel director, the supervisor can sketch a general impression of the interviewee in advance.

The application blank supplies a number of facts, such as the applicant's schooling and degrees; training; previous work experience, including nature of duties, length of stay, and salary; and other relevant data.

The information contained in a completed application is limited because of laws, regulations, and court decisions regarding equal employment opportunites and discrimination. Generally, federal regulations and guidelines prohibit requiring applicants to state religion, sex, ancestry, marital status, age (except under certain circumstances), birthplace of the applicant or parents, and other data. More details will be discussed later in connection with what questions an interviewer can properly ask of the interviewee. Application blanks may sample the candidates' abilities to write, organize thinking, and present facts clearly. The application blank indicates whether the applicant's education has been logically patterned and whether there has been a route of progression to better jobs. Also, it gives the interviewer points of departure for the formal interview.

While studying the application blank, the supervisor should keep in mind the job for which the applicant will be interviewed. If some questions arise while studying the application blank, the supervisor should write them down so that they will not be forgotten and will be asked. For instance, all previous jobs are stated in chronological sequence; however, these data reveal a gap of six months, during which the applicant did not work or go to school. Careful questions about this will reveal that the candidate spent the time traveling abroad or that a car accident required a lengthy stay at a hospital. There may be some questions concerning results of previous tests given by the personnel department, and any questions in this area should be clarified by the supervisor before the interview takes place.*

Since the purpose of the employment interview is to gather information to make a hiring decision, the supervisor should prepare a schedule or plan for the interview. The interviewer should jot down all the important items about which no information is available. The interviewer should also write down all those points about which further clarification is needed. Once all of these key points have been written down, one is not likely to forget to ask the interviewee about them. It is conceivable that during the interview the supervisor may be interrupted, and the applicant might be dismissed before the supervisor has had a chance to ask about certain points on which still some

---

*The discussion of formal tests as a selection method goes beyond the confines of this text. More information on tests is provided in texts on personnel, personnel management, and human resources management.

information is lacking. Writing them down beforehand will prevent such an occurrence. Having thought out the various questions in advance, the supervisor can devote much of the attention to listening and observing the applicant. A well-prepared plan for the employment interview is well worth the time spent on it.

In addition to getting background information and making out a plan for the interview, the supervisor should be concerned with the proper setting for conducting the interview. Privacy and some degree of comfort are normal requirements for a good conversation. If a private room is not available, the supervisor should create an aura of semiprivacy by speaking to the applicants in a corner or in a place where other employees are not within hearing distance. That much privacy is a necessity. If it can be arranged, precautions should be taken to avoid any interruptions during the interview by phone calls or other matters. This gives the interviewee additional assurance of how much importance the interviewer places on this interview.

Conducting the Interview

After having made preparations, the supervisor is ready to conduct the employment interview. The supervisor should make certain that a leisurely atmosphere is created and that the applicant is put at ease. The wise supervisor will think back about when he or she applied for a job and recall the stress and tension connected with it. After all, the applicant is meeting strange people who ask searching questions and is likely to be under considerable strain. It is the supervisor's duty to relieve this tension, which is certain to be present in the applicant, and possibly in the supervisor also. The applicant might be put at ease by opening the interview with brief general conversation, possibly about the weather, heavy traffic, World Series, or some other topic of broad interest. Any topic that does not refer to the eligibility for the job will be relaxing. The interviewer may offer a cup of coffee or may employ any other social gesture that will put the applicant at ease.

This informal ''warming-up'' approach should be brief, and the interviewer should move the discussion quickly to job-related matters. Excessive non–job-related informal conversation should be avoided. Studies have shown that sometimes the interviewer makes a selection decision in the first minutes of the interview, and it would be wrong to do this without having discussed job-related matters. A good opening question would be to ask how the applicant learned about this job opening.

In addition to getting information from the applicant, the interviewer should see to it that the job seeker learns enough about the job to help the applicant decide whether he or she is the right person for the position. The supervisor, therefore, should discuss the details of the job, such as working conditions, wages, hours, vacations, who the immediate supervisor would be, and how the job in question relates to other jobs in the department. The supervisor must describe the situation completely and honestly. The supervisor must be careful not to oversell the job by telling the applicant what is available for exceptional employees. If the applicant turns out to be an average worker this will lead to disappointments. In his or her eagerness to make the job look as attractive as possible, especially to professionals who are in short supply, it is conceivable that the supervisor may state everything in terms better than they actually are.

After having outlined the job's details, the supervisor should ask the applicant what else he or she would like to know about the job. If the interviewee has no further questions at this time, the supervisor should proceed with questioning to find out how well qualified the applicant is. The supervisor will have some knowledge about the background from the application blank; there is no need to ask the applicant to restate information already given. But the interviewer will need to know exactly how qualified the interviewee is in relation to the job in question. By this time the applicant has probably gotten over much of the tension and nervousness and will be ready to answer questions freely. Most of this information will be obtained by the supervisor's direct questions. The interviewer should be careful to phrase these questions clearly for the applicant. In other words, only terms that conform with the applicant's language, background, and experience should be used. Questions should be asked in a slow and deliberate form, one at a time, to not confuse the applicant. The interviewer should take care not to ask "leading" questions that would suggest a specific answer. For example, the supervisor should refrain from questions such as, "Do you have difficulty adjusting to authority?" or "Do you daydream frequently?" This kind of questioning can only lead to antagonism.

All questions the supervisor asks should be pertinent and job related. This brings up the area of those questions which, although not directly related to the job itself, can become relevant to the work situation. It is helpful to know whether a woman has young children and what arrangements she can make for them to be cared for. Problems of this nature, although only indirectly connected with the job, are relevant to the work situation. A supervisor will have to use good judgment and tact in this respect, since the applicant may be sensitive about some of the points to be discussed. By no means should the supervisor pry into personal affairs that are irrelevant and removed from the work situation merely to satisfy his or her own curiosity.

Equal Employment Opportunity Laws

Before the 1960s the interviewer could ask almost any question that was job related in some way. Today interviewing has become far more complicated and sophisticated because of the many laws, regulations, and decisions affecting equal employment opportunities, discrimination, affirmative action, and so on. A number of questions are still perfectly lawful; for example, the interviewer can ask for the applicant's first and last names, current address, previous employment, educational background, etc. Questions that are clearly unlawful include those about race or color, sex, religion, birthplace, and arrest record. A number of questions are potentially unlawful to ask. For instance, it is certainly lawful to ask the applicant what other languages he or she speaks. In certain areas it is desirable, even sometimes necessary, to also speak Spanish, for instance. But this question should not lead to asking the applicant's native language and the one used at home. It would be inaccurate and presumptuous to provide a "Do and Don't Ask List," since each situation has to be judged in the local context, relatedness to the job, and the particular circumstances. It is far better for supervisors to consult with the personnel department periodically to learn what can be asked and in which way and what should not be asked. The laws and regulations are numerous and ever changing. Almost daily new decisions are made by the courts and administrative agencies so that it is a full-time job to be aware and stay abreast of them. The staff in the personnel division are usually familiar with the most recent developments and proper current practices. The interviewer should consult with them frequently to learn which questions are appropriate, lawful if properly worded, and clearly unlawful. The interviewer may also receive some suggestions as to how to obtain information that is necessary but cannot be asked directly. For instance, the supervisor may have to resort to questions such as, "Can you be away from home overnight if the job requires it?" or "Will your home responsibilities permit you to work around the clock?"

Evaluating the Applicant

The chief problem in employment interviews is how to interpret the candidate's employment and personal history and other pertinent information. It is impossible for supervisors to eliminate completely all their personal preferences and prejudices. Interviewers should face up to personal biases and make efforts to control them. It is not sufficient to claim that he or she has no biases; the supervisor should be able to clearly write down the reasons why one applicant has been selected in preference to another. It might also be helpful if the interviewer has made some notes during the interview or immediately thereafter; this will help in making the final decision. It is essential that the interviewers take great care to avoid some of the more common pitfalls while sizing up a job applicant.

First, it is necessary not to make snap judgments. It is difficult not to form an early impression and look for evidence during the rest of the interview to substantiate this first impression. The interviewer should collect all the information on the applicant before making a judgment. This will help the interviewer not to become a victim of the halo effect.

The *halo effect* occurs when an interviewer lets some prominent characteristic overshadow other evidence. It means basing the overall impression of the applicant on only part of the total information and using this impression as a guide in rating all the other factors. This may work either favorably or unfavorably for the job seeker. In any event, it would be wrong for the supervisor to form an overall opinion of the applicant on a single factor, for instance, the ability to express himself or herself fluently. If an applicant is articulate, there is no reason to automatically project a high rating for all other qualifications. A glance at the employees in the department will remind the supervisor that there are some very successful employees whose verbal communications are rather poor. Another common pitfall is that of overgeneralization. The interviewer must not assume that because an applicant behaves in a certain manner in one situation that he or she will automatically behave the same way in all other situations. There may be a special reason as to why the applicant may answer a question in a rather evasive manner. It would be wrong to conclude from this evasiveness in answering one question that the applicant is underhanded and probably not trustworthy. The halo effect would be there if the interviewer lets an applicant's alma mater overshadow other aspects. People are prone to generalize quickly.

Another pitfall is that the supervisor will tend to judge the applicant by comparisons with current employees in the department. The supervisor may wonder how this applicant will get along with the other employees and with the supervisor. The interviewer may believe that any applicant who is considerably different from current employees is undesirable. In fact, this kind of thinking may do great harm to the organization because it will only lead to uniformity, conformity, and thereafter to mediocrity. This should not be interpreted to mean that the interviewer should make it a point to look for "odd-balls" who obviously would not fit within the department. But just because a job applicant does not resemble exactly the other employees is no reason to conclude that the person will not make a suitable employee.

The interviewer should realize that the applicant may often give responses which are socially acceptable, but not very revealing. The job seeker knows that the answer should be what the interviewer wants to hear. For example, if the interviewer asks a nurse what his or her aspirations are, the reply probably will be to be a head nurse one day. He or she settles for the head nurse's job rather than that of the the director of nursing to avoid appearing conceited or presumptuous; but the nurse knows that a certain amount of ambition is socially acceptable.

Another hazard for the interviewer to avoid is excessive qualifications. Eager to get the best person for the job, the supervisor may look for qualifications that exceed the requirements of the job. Although the applicant should be qualified, there is no need to look for qualifications in excess of those actually required. An overqualified applicant would probably make a poor and frustrated employee for a job.

The above are some of the more commonly known pitfalls in interpreting the facts brought out during an interview. Supervisors should make an all-out effort not to fall into these traps when evaluating applicants.

Concluding the Interview and Making the Decision

The decision whether or not to consider the applicant is made during or immediately after the interview. The supervisor should have made some notes either during or after the interview so that the information can be reviewed and reevaluated. At the conclusion of the employment interview the supervisor is likely to have the choice of three possible actions: hire the applicant, defer the decision, or reject the applicant. We assume that it is within the supervisor's authority alone to decide. The applicant is eager to know which of these actions the supervisor is going to take and is entitled to an answer. There is no particular problem if the supervisor decides to hire this applicant; the person will be told when to report for work, and additional instructions may be given.

It is conceivable that the supervisor may consider it best to defer a decision until several other applicants for the same job have been interviewed. If this choice is made, it is necessary and appropriate for the supervisor to tell the interviewee this and to inform this person that he or she will be notified later. Preferably the supervisor will set a time limit within which the decision will be made.

Such a situation occurs frequently, but it is not fair to use this tactic to avoid the unpleasant task of telling the applicant that he or she is not acceptable. Under such circumstances telling the applicant that the supervisor is deferring action raises false hopes. While waiting for an answer the applicant may not look for another job and, consequently, may let some other opportunities slip by. Of course it is unpleasant to tell an applicant that he or she is not suitable for the job. But if the supervisor has decided that an applicant will not be hired, the applicant should be told by the supervisor in a clear but tactful way. Although it is much simpler to let the rejected applicant wait for a letter that never arrives, the applicant is entitled to an honest answer. If the job seeker does not fulfill the requirements of the job, it is preferable to say so.

It is better not to state the specific reasons beyond a general turndown phrase. Supervisors may have experienced that stating reasons for not hiring someone encourages arguments and comparisons and can lead to many other problems, especially since the chances for being misquoted and misunderstood are great. It is best to turn the applicant down by stating, in a general way, that there is not sufficient match between the applicant's qualifications and the needs of the job. It is also not fair to hold out hope by telling the applicant that he or she will be called if something suitable opens up, when the interviewer knows fully that no hope exists.

The supervisor should always bear in mind that the employment interview is an excellent opportunity to build a good reputation for the institution. The applicant knows that he or she is one of several candidates and that only one person can be selected. A large percentage of applicants are not hired. But the manner in which they are turned down can have an effect on the applicant's impression of the institution and on the job seeker. The only contact the applicant has with the organization is through the supervisor during the employment interview. Therefore, the supervisor should remember that the interview will leave either a good or a bad impression of the institution with the applicant. It is necessary, therefore, that an applicant leave the interview, regardless of its outcome, at least with the feeling that he or she has been courteously treated and had a fair deal. Every supervisor should bear in mind that it is a managerial duty to build as much goodwill for the organization as possible and that the employment interview presents one of the rare opportunities to do so.

Documentation

It is advisable that the interviewer put down in writing the reasons for not hiring a certain applicant, and/or why the one was hired in preference to the others. It is essential to have documentation of this sort because the supervisor could not possibly remember the various reasons, and he or she may be asked to justify the decision at some later time. Such documentation is even more important now because the decision to hire or reject an applicant should be based on job-related factors and should not be discriminatory. Sometimes supervisors might be pressured by the personnel department and/or higher management to give preferential hiring considerations to minorities or women. Supervisors should realize that the organization may have to meet certain affirmative-action goals. Only by careful documentation will supervisors be able to justify their decisions. Notes on a separate piece of paper to be attached to the application, not on the back of the application, will serve the purpose.

Temporary Placement

It may sometimes happen that although the applicant is not the right person for a particular job, he or she would be suitable for another position for which there is no current opening. The supervisor might be tempted to hold this desirable employee by offering temporary placement in any job that is available. The applicant should be informed about this prospect by the supervisor. Sometimes, however, temporary placement in an unsuitable job causes misunderstanding and disturbance within the department. It is usually strenuous for an employee to mark time on a job that he or she does not care to perform, while hoping for the proper job to open up. Normally, such strain causes dissatisfaction after a certain length of time, and this dissatisfaction is usually communicated to other employees within the work group. And sometimes the expected suitable job does not open up. Therefore, interim placements are ill-advised and unsound.

Summary

There are two ways of filling available job openings: to hire someone from the outside or promote someone from within the organization. In hiring from outside the organization the supervisor is aided by the personnel department, since it performs the services of recruiting and preselecting the most likely applicants. It is the supervisor's function and duty, however, to appropriately interview the various candidates and to hire those who promise to be the best ones for the jobs open. To accomplish this, it is necessary for the supervisor to acquire the skills needed to conduct an effective interview. The employment interview is primarily a directive, or structured, interview in contrast to the nondirective interview often encountered in the supervisor's daily work.

During the employment interview the supervisor tries to find out whether the applicant's capability matches the demands of the job. The purpose is to hire the person most suitable for the position open. To carry out a successful employment interview, the supervisor should become familiar with background information, list points to be covered and questions to be asked, be prepared in advance, and have the proper setting. In addition to securing information from the applicant, the interviewer should discuss with the interviewee as many aspects of the job as possible. There will be a number of additional questions and answers before the interviewer is ready to conclude the employment interview, size up the situation, and make a decision. All of this must be accomplished while giving proper attention to the many considerations of equal and fair employment practices.

In addition to conducting directive interviews, the supervisor is often called on to carry on nondirective interviews. This kind of interview usually covers problem situations and gives the employees the opportunity to freely express their feelings, sentiments, and anything else on their mind. There are many sources of frustration within and without the working environment that can easily lead to a variety of undesirable responses. To give subordinates the opportunity of a counseling interview is another vital duty of the supervisory position.

18

Performance Appraisals, Promotions, and Transfers

In the typical organization every employee is subject to a periodic performance appraisal. Performance appraisals are formal evaluations of employee's job-related activities. Every organization needs valid information that enhances management's effectiveness in making decisions which influence the directing of human resources. The performance appraisal system is the continuous process for gathering, analyzing, and disseminating information about the performance of its members. Performance appraisals not only guide management in selecting certain individuals for promotion and salary increases, but they are also useful for coaching employees to improve their performance. Performance appraisals are an important part of long-range personnel planning and the supervisor's staffing function. In addition, well-identified and described appraisal methods and procedures will contribute to a healthy organizational environment of mutual trust and understanding. This kind of atmosphere is necessary if the health care center wants to bring about increased productivity and better patient care. A performance appraisal system helps to identify work requirements, performance standards, analysis and appraisal of job-related behaviors, and recognition of such behaviors.

The Performance Appraisal System

The appraisal of an employee's performance holds a key position in the supervisor's staffing function. It helps management identify those employees who have the potential to be promoted into better positions, points to the need for further development, and shows how effectively various subordinates contribute to departmental goals. Obviously, it is important for a supervisor to be in a position to objectively assess the quality of the performance of the employees in the department. Therefore, most organizations request that their supervisors periodically appraise and rate their employees through a formal appraisal system, also known as *performance appraisal, employee evaluation, employee rating,* or *merit rating.*

Purposes of the Performance Appraisal System

The performance appraisal system serves many purposes. It is a guide for possible promotion and further development, and it provides a basis for merit increases. One purpose of such a formal rating system is to translate into objective terms the performance, experience, and qualities of an employee and to compare these items with the requirements of the job. The appraisal system is designed to take into consideration such criteria as job knowledge, ability to carry through on assignments, judgment, attitude, cooperation, dependability, output, housekeeping, safety, and so on. Such a system of evaluation helps the supervisor to take all factors into account when considering merit increases or a promotion. It also provides a rational basis for decision, since it reduces the chances for personal bias. Such a formal appraisal system forces the supervisor to observe and scrutinize the work of the subordinates not only from the point of view of how well the employee is performing the job, but also from the standpoint of what can be done to improve the employee's performance. It is difficult to make such judgments because in most health care situations we are not dealing with concrete performance measures, such as the number of units produced, but with concepts such as leadership, teamwork, cooperation, etc.

Since an employee's poor performance and failure to improve may be due to inadequate supervision, a formal appraisal system is bound to improve supervisory qualities.

In addition to these reasons, a formal evaluation system serves another purpose. Employees have always expected security from the work they do. In addition to security, they also seek satisfying and interesting work that enables them to grow. A well-designed appraisal system reduces ambiguity concerning job requirements and uncertainty by providing employees with information about what is expected from them and feedback on how they have performed. Every employee has the right to know how well he or she is doing and what can be done to improve the work performance. It can be assumed that most employees are eager to know what their supervisors think of their work. In some instances the employee's desire to know how he or she stands with the boss can be interpreted as asking for reassurance about the employee's future in the organization. In other instances this expressed desire has different interpretations. For example, a subordinate may realize that he or she is doing a relatively poor job but hopes that the boss is not aware of it; the subordinate is anxious to be assured in this direction. On the other hand, another subordinate who knows that he or she is doing an outstanding job may wish to make certain that the boss is aware of it, and this subordinate will want to receive more recognition.

The mere existence of regular appraisals is an important incentive to the employees of an organization. It is only too easy in a large complex organization for employees to feel like they and their contributions are forgotten and lost. Regular appraisals provide the assurance that there is the potential for improving oneself in the position and that one is not lost within the enterprise. It gives employees the assurance that supervisors and the entire organization care about them.

The appraisal program is a critical tool at the disposal of the supervisor, since it influences all human resource functions. It is a determinant in the planning, development, and recognition of the human resources of the organization. The performance appraisal system serves all of these purposes. Another result of good implementation of performance appraisals is to direct employee behavior so that it benefits the employees and the organization. The supervisor will have ample opportunity to include the topics of motivation, such as Theories X and Y and hierarchy of needs,* in the appraisal procedure, particularly during the postappraisal interview. These motivational theories can be incorporated into the performance appraisal, thus leading to an environment of trust.

In addition to creating a healthy organizational climate of trust, performance appraisals are beneficial in the following ways. They help management in decisions about compensation. They help in the area of the training and developmental needs of the employees. They provide an inventory of human resources suitable for promotions. They aid the supervisor, since they show whether an employee is in the right job or not. They identify for the boss those employees who are going ahead and those who are not progressing satisfactorily. They show whether or not the supervisor is succeeding in the job as a coach and teacher. As far as the employees are concerned, an appraisal program has many advantages. It reflects the quality of their work and gives them a sense of being treated fairly and of not being overlooked. The employee knows what he or she can do to be promoted to a better job. It gives the subordinate an opportunity to complain and criticize and express personal goals and ambitions. In this respect appraisals are motivational because they create a learning experience for subordinates that inspires them to improve.

Timing of Appraisals

Appraisals must be conducted on a regular basis to be significant to the employee and the organization. A one-time performance measure is of little importance. Therefore, the supervisor should appraise all the employees within the department at regular intervals—at least once a year formally. This formal appraisal means the completion of special forms and a follow-up evaluation interview. One year is normally considered a sufficient period of time. If held more frequently, formal appraisals are likely to become mechanical and meaningless. If an employee has just started in a new or more responsible position, however, it is advisable to make an appraisal within six

---

*These topics are discussed in Chapter 20.

months or so. These periodic annual appraisals will assure the employee that whatever improvement was made will be noticed and that he or she will be rewarded for this progress. As time goes on, periodic ratings and reviews will become an important determinant of an employee's morale. It reaffirms the supervisor's interest in the employees and in their continuous development and improvement.

Annual formal appraisals and their review do not exclude the feedback on performance that is part of the day-to-day coaching responsibilities of the supervisor. It is a well-known fact that performance feedback is most effective when it takes place immediately after the behavior to which it relates. This applies equally for feedback on below-par performance, as well as for recognition of above-standard performance.

Who Is the Appraiser?

A major difficulty in effective performance appraisal is human nature because the measurement and appraisal depend on the eye and brain of the appraiser. This creates *intellectual* and *perceptional* problems, leading to the rater's own interpretation of reality and not necessarily absolute reality. To minimize these shortcomings some organizations devise an appraisal system in which the employee is appraised by various appraisers and these appraisals are subject to reviews by those higher up in the administrative hierarchy. A few organizations have assessment centers for evaluating employees for their future potential as managers.*

Most organizations, however, have come to the conclusion that immediate supervisors are best able to appraise subordinates. Among all other appraisers, the immediate supervisor is the one person who should know the duties of the jobs within the department better than anyone else. The immediate supervisor has the best opportunity to observe the appraisee on the job and provide feedback. Furthermore, most subordinates want to receive performance-related feedback from their immediate supervisor and feel more comfortable in discussing the appraisal with him or her.

Therefore, it is best for the immediate line-supervisor to make the evaluation. In some instances it may be necessary for the first-line boss to call on the help of the next higher supervisor. Some organizations require that managers or administrators at levels higher than the immediate supervisor review performance ratings. In some institutions the appraisal is made by a committee made up of the first-line supervisor, his or her boss, and possibly one or two other supervisors, as long as the appraisers have adequate knowledge of the performance of the employee being rated. This has the advantage of reducing some of the immediate supervisor's personal prejudices. Some health care organizations advocate self-ratings and peer evaluations in addition to the immediate supervisors and higher level administrators.

Since some organizations have become involved in participative goal setting, *self-appraisal*, or *self-rating*, has become one more input. Setting goals and then analyzing success and failure gives the employee a good opportunity

*This concept is discussed more fully toward the end of this chapter.

for self-appraisal. This can often lead to a conflicting situation when the supervisor's appraisal differs significantly from that of the employee. This gives the employees the opportunity to express their discontent with the rating, bringing into the open differences in appraisee and appraiser perception.

At times *peers* are used as appraisers. Of course, they can provide some valuable information about their colleagues. Some powerful influences in organizational life may distort or cloud a peer's perception. For all practical purposes, most employees have a strong need for security and work for present and future rewards from the employer. If someone else receives additional rewards, the chances for additional rewards become smaller for everyone else, since the resources are limited. This competition for current or future employer rewards—whether readily apparent or not—is likely to cloud or distort a peer's perception of a colleague's performance and potential. In addition, friendships and stereotyping may bias the rating. Friendship does not relate only to individuals, but also to groups. For instance, the appraiser is evaluating some peer in a group of which he or she was once a member. The appraiser may be tempted to rate members of that particular group higher than individuals in another group.

For all practical purposes, appraisal done by the immediate supervisor should suffice, and in most organizations the immediate supervisor is the one, if not the only, appraiser of employee performance. Performance appraisal consists of two distinct steps: the performance rating and the evaluation interview that follows.

Performance Rating

To minimize and overcome the difficulties in appraising an employee, most enterprises find it advisable to use some kind of appraisal form. These appraisal forms are prepared by the personnel department, often in conjunction with outside consultants and the supervisors' suggestions. Although innumerable types of appraisal forms are available, most of them include criteria for objectively measuring job performance, intelligence, and personality traits. The instrument most used in the appraisal process will be both behavior and trait based. The following are a number of qualities and characteristics most frequently to be rated. For nonsupervisory personnel typical qualities rated are quantity and quality of work, job knowledge, dependability, cooperative attitude, supervision required, housekeeping, unauthorized absenteeism, tardiness, safety, personal appearance, and so on. For managerial and professional employees typical factors are analytical ability, judgment, initiative, leadership, quality and quantity of work, knowledge of work, attitude, dependability, emotional stability, and so on. For each of these factors the supervisor is supposed to select the degree of achievement attained by the employee. In some instances a point system is provided to arrive at a numerical scoring. The form is usually of a "check the box" type and reasonably simple to fill out (Figures 18-1 and 18-2).

Figure 18-1. Example of a performance appraisal form.

PERS 22
Barnes Hospital
l4067-3

JOB PERFORMANCE EVALUATION (Management and Professional Employees)

NAME   EMPLOYEE NUMBER   ACCOUNT NUMBER

A. Complete in triplicate and attach the original and one copy to a Pers-8 at the time of Periodic Review, Promotion, Demotion, or Interdepartmental Transfer. Third copy may be given to the employee.

B. Evaluate individual's performance since employment, last performance evaluation, promotion, or transfer.

C. Check the block after each factor that best describes this employee. Use supportable, careful judgment.

D. Use "Comment" section to describe employee's strengths and weaknesses. State suggestions for improvement.

E. Use first 7 factors to evaluate employee other than department heads and supervisors.

F. Complete all 10 factors to evaluate department heads and supervisors.

Exceeds Requirements
Meets Requirements
Improvement Needed   COMMENTS

1. QUALITY: Meets expectations for thoroughness and accuracy. Decisions are sound and based on all available facts. Work is performed within the framework of hospital policies, procedures, and supervisor's instructions. ☐ ☐ ☐

2. QUANTITY: Meets established standards for rate of progress on assignments. Makes efficient use of working time. ☐ ☐ ☐

3. KNOWLEDGE: Understands all aspects of position and its proper relationship to other operations. Actively keeps informed of current developments in own and related fields. ☐ ☐ ☐

4. INITIATIVE: Requires minimum supervision in completing routine duties of special assignments. A self-starter. Assumes responsibility when orders are lacking. Sees problems and recommends solutions. ☐ ☐ ☐

5. ABILITY TO WORK WITH OTHERS: Maintains effective yet courteous relationships with all levels of personnel without compromising the responsibilities of the job. Promotes a cooperative attitude toward the hospital, patients, and visitors. ☐ ☐ ☐

6. ATTENDANCE: Works scheduled days. ☐ ☐

7. PUNCTUALITY: Reports on and off duty as expected. Adheres to schedules for meetings and assignments. ☐ ☐

Reproduced with special permission from Barnes Hospital, St. Louis, Mo.

Complete remaining items in case of Supervisors, Department Heads and other Management Employees only

8. LEADERSHIP: Motivates employees to ☐ ☐ ☐
   work to the maximum of their abilities. Encourages them in self development. _____
   Delegates work effectively. Communicates
   adequately with all levels of personnel. _____

9. PRODUCTIVITY OF EMPLOYEE/ ☐ ☐ ☐
   EMPLOYEES SUPERVISED: Meets
   established quantity, quality, and cost _____
   standards for performance during the
   review period. _____

10. APPRAISAL: Rates employees' perform- ☐ ☐ ☐
    ance objectively and thoroughly in relation
    to contributions and progress. Conducts
    job performance evaluations and appraisal _____
    interviews within established time limits
    and in a way which has a constructive in- _____
    fluence on employees' desire to improve
    performance. _____

REMARKS _____

_____

_____

_____

_____

_____

_____

_____

_____

(Check one block only)

☐ This employee is being recommended for a pay increase on the basis of this evaluation and such increase is reflected on the attached Pers-8 form.

☐ This employee is NOT being recommended for a pay increase because _____
  _____. Please change periodic

  review date to_____ and resubmit for

  reevaluation on (date)_____

☐ Employee's address as showing under Section II of attached Pers-8 form is correct;
  otherwise, it has been corrected under SECTION III of the attached Pers-8 form.

After comparing this employee's performance with that of others in similar or like positions of responsibility, I feel this to be an impartial evaluation of his/her performance.		I have read this evaluation of my job performance. Should I not agree with this appraisal, I understand that I may make my own explanation on a separate sheet and it will become a part of this evaluation.
_____ _____	_____ _____	_____ _____
Signature of Evaluator Date	Signature of Dept. Head Date	Signature of Employee Date

Figure 18-2. Example of a performance appraisal and status change form.

V – EMPLOYEE PERFORMANCE EVALUATION (NONEXEMPT PERSONNEL)

REASON FOR EVALUATION: ☐ Periodic Review ☐ Promotion ☐ Transfer
☐ Other (Specify)_____

INSTRUCTIONS

A. Use this form to evaluate personnel who ARE NOT or CANNOT be exempted from overtime as Professional, Executive, or Administrative employees under the FLSA.

B. Complete Section 1 – EMPLOYE IDENTIFICATION, other side.

C. Evaluate employee's performance since hire, last pay increase, or promotion, etc., as applicable.

D. Disregard your own personal stereotyped feelings, judge this employee on the factors listed below.

E. Try to remember specific instances that are typical of employee's work and behavior.

F. Level of rating is to be based on performance of employee as compared with that of other employees in same or similar job, or is to be based on job standards, if any.

G. Using supportable, careful judgment, check the appropriate BLOCK after each factor that best describes this employee.

Exceeds Requirements _____
Meets Requirements _____
Improvement Needed _____

COMMENTS

1. QUALITY OF WORK ☐ ☐ ☐
   Consider neatness, accuracy, dependability of results, as compared with others in like or similar job or based on job standards, if any.

2. QUANTITY OF WORK ☐ ☐ ☐
   Consider amount of work turned out, as compared with others in same or similar job or based on work standards, if any.

3. WORK HABITS ☐ ☐ ☐
   Consider organization of work, compliance with procedure, ability to follow through on instructions, observance of safety regulations, industriousness, initiative, care of equipment and work area.

4. ABILITY TO WORK WITH OTHERS ☐ ☐ ☐
   Consider courtesy, concern with patients and other workers, cooperative attitude.

5. ATTENDANCE ☐ ☐ ☐
   Degree to which employee works scheduled days.

6. PUNCTUALITY ☐ ☐ ☐
   Consider degree to which employee reports on and off duty daily as scheduled and adheres to meal and break schedule.

Reproduced with special permission from Barnes Hospital, St. Louis, Mo.

7. PERSONAL APPEARANCE ☐ ☐
   Consider suitability of dress
   and personal neatness as applicable to hospital environment
   and the job.

SUGGESTIONS FOR IMPROVEMENT (refer to each factor, by number, listed above):

☐ Employee states address showing on other side is correct; otherwise, latest
  address is recorded under Section III, other side.

☐ Pay increase is recommended.

☐ Pay increase is not recommended due to _____

_____ Please change review date to (date) _____

| After careful consideration and comparing this employee's performance with that of other employees in similar or like jobs, I feel the above to be a fair and impartial evaluation of his/her performance. | I have reviewed my perform-ance evaluation above and have been advised by my evaluator of areas where im-provement may be needed and how to go about making such improvements. |

_____ _____ _____
Signature of Evaluator   Date   Signature of Dept. Head   Signature of Employee

(Submit in triplicate)   **EMPLOYEE STATUS CHANGE**   PERS 8

Barnes Hospital   Rev. 1/81

13064—1

INSTRUCTIONS: All information on this form must be typewritten or plainly printed. Section I is to be completed in all cases. Show base rate of pay, not including any differential, under appropriate headings labeled "Hourly Rate." Under headings "Differential Pay," show only cents per hour actually given as differential pay. Administrative approval required for all changes occurring in Section III and for employee DISMISSALS. Other approvals are at the discretion of the individual administrator. For interdepartmental transfers, both concerned administrators must approve before submission to Personnel. EFFECTIVE DATE ON STATUS CHANGES (Section III): Pay increases are to be dated on a Sunday, the first day of a pay period, and are to reach Personnel Administration no later than 9:00 a.m. on the first Monday after the start of the pay period in which the pay change is effective. All other changes are to be submitted promptly as they actually occur.

SALARY BASE CODE		SICK LEAVE CODE	VACATION CODE
1 Full-Time Salaried 2 House Staff 3 Permanent F-T hrly. 4 Temp. F-T hrly. 5 Permanent P-T hrly.	6 Temporary P-T hrly. 7 Fixed Fee or % Basis 8 Part-Time Salaried (M.D.'s only) 9 Non Pay Status	0 None 3 Permanent Part-Time (SBC 5 or 8) (22 hours paid equals one hour accrual). 4 Permanent Full-Time (3.7 hours per pay period accrual).	1 Permanent part-time (SBC 5 or 8) (26 hours paid equals one hour accrual). 2 Two Weeks (3.0770 hours per pay period). 3 Three Weeks (4.6154 hours per pay period). 4 Four Weeks (6.1539 hours per pay period).

I. EMPLOYEE IDENTIFICATION

Name in full, last name first		Employee No.	Account No.
Job Title *(as listed on Departmental Job Listing)*	Grade	Job Code No.	Department

II. ☐ EMPLOYMENT   ☐ RE-EMPLOYMENT

FOR PERSONNEL AND DATA PROCESSING USE ONLY

Starting Date	Hourly Rate (not incl. diff.)	Diff. Pay (cents per hour)	Address (Street No., Street, City, State)						
Salary Base Code	Sick Leave Code	Vacation Code	Sex	M.S.	F.T.C.	Dollars	S.T.C.	Periodic Review Date	Zip Code
If Temporary, how long _____			Social Security Number			Date of Birth			Qual. Code
If Part-Time, hours per pay period _____									

III. INTERIM STATUS CHANGE

FOR PERSONNEL AND DATA PROCESSING USE ONLY

Effective Date	New Hrly. Rate (not incl. diff.)	Diff. Pay (cents per hour)	New Name				
Old Pay Rate	Effective Date of Old Pay Rate	Increase Budgeted? ☐ YES ☐ NO	Social Security Number	M.S. F.T.C. Dollars S.T.C.			New P.R. Date

New SBC	New SLC	New VC	New Address (Street No., Street, City, State and Zip Code)	Telephone No.

New Job Title	Grade	New JCN	New Account Number	New Department

REASON: ☐ Merit Pay Increase; ☐ Promotion; ☐ Assign Diff., ☐ Drop Diff.; ☐ Transferred to another Account Number;

☐ Transferred to Part-Time; ☐ Transferred to Full-Time; ☐ Other (Specify)

LEAVE OF ABSENCE GRANTED From: To: Reason:	Date Returned from L.O.A.

IV. TERMINATION OF EMPLOYMENT

Date Terminated	TOTAL NUMBER OF VACATION HOURS PAID UPON TERMINATION (if none, so state): _____ *(place X in applicable box)* A. Outstanding B. Good C. Fair D. Unsatisfactory

Evaluation of Employee:	A	B	C	D
Quality of Work				
Quantity of Work				
Reliability				
Cooperative Attitude				
Personal Appearance				
Recommended for Rehire? ☐ yes ☐ no				

TERMINATION ACTION DUE TO:
(CIRCLE ONE ONLY - USE NO OTHER TERM.)

1. Resignation with Notice   2. Retirement   3. Disability
4. Dismissal   5. Death   6. Resignation without proper notice
7. Successfully Completed Training
8. Unauthorized absence for three scheduled work days

REASON FOR ABOVE ACTION: _____

SUBMITTED: APPROVED: ☐ Recommended   ☐ Not Recommended

_____   _____   _____   _____

(Department Head Signature)   *(Date)*   Associate Director or equivalent   *(Personnel Officer)*   *(Date)*

_____   _____   _____   _____

(Department Head Signature)   *(Date)*   Associate Director or equivalent   Director (or representative) when required

Despite the outward simplicity of these rating blanks, the supervisor will probably run into a number of difficulties. First, not all supervisors agree on what is meant by a simple adjective rating scale, such as unsatisfactory, marginal, satisfactory, above average, and superior. It is advisable, therefore, that the form contain a descriptive sentence in addition to each of these adjectives: for unsatisfactory, "performance clearly fails to meet minimum requirement"; for marginal, "performance occasionally fails to meet minimum requirements"; for satisfactory, "performance meeting or exceeding minimum requirements"; for above average, "performance consistently exceeds minimum requirements"; and for superior, "performance clearly exceeds all job requirements." Or in place of the adjective, the supervisor can choose from descriptive sentences the one that most adequately describes the employee. For example, in rating the degree of emotional stability of a nurse, the appraiser may have the following choices: first, "unreliable in crises, goes to pieces easily, and cannot take criticism"; second, "unrealistic, emotions and moodiness periodically handicap her or his dealings, she or he personalizes issues"; third, "usually on an even keel, has mature approach to most situations"; fourth, "is realistic, generally maintains good behavior balance in handling situations"; fifth, "self-possessed in high degree, has outstanding ability to adjust to circumstances, no matter how difficult"; and so on.

Performance rating is frequently subject to a number of errors and weaknesses because subjectivity is a part of the entire process. Appraisers are human and are subject to the same forces that influence all human behavior. Some of these errors are more common than others. The supervisor should be aware of these pitfalls in order to minimize the human weaknesses in processing, storing, and recalling observed behavior.

Problems in Performance Rating

Some supervisors have a tendency to be overly *lenient* in their ratings, rating appraisees higher than normal. Some supervisors are afraid that they might antagonize their subordinates if they rate them low, thus making them less cooperative.

Other supervisors are overly *harsh* in rating their employees and appraise them lower than the average appraiser. This tendency of some supervisors to give consistently low ratings is equally damaging. A low rating for a subordinate may also reflect on the supervisor's own ability to encourage subordinates to improve themselves.

If, for example, the nursing personnel on one station are consistently appraised higher than those on the next station, it is difficult to determine whether this is because of the strictness of one head nurse or leniency of the other or whether this reflects real differences in the employees' abilities and performance.

Another subjective error of the appraiser is to be influenced by the *halo effect*. The halo effect is the tendency of most raters to let the rating they assign to one characteristic influence their rating on all subsequent ratings.

This works in two directions. Rating the appraisee excellent on one factor influences the rater to give the employee a similar high rating or higher rating on other qualities than actually deserved. Or rating the employee unsatisfactory in one factor influences the appraiser to give the appraisee a similar low rating or lower than deserved rating in other qualities. One way to minimize the halo effect is to rate all employees on a single factor or trait before going on to the next factor. In other words, the supervisor only rates one factor of each employee at a time and then goes on to the next employee for the same factor and so on. This enables the supervisor to consider all appraisees relative to a standard or to each other on each factor.

Another common error is *central tendency*; the appraiser rates the employees average or around the midpoint. The supervisor often is reluctant to rate employees at the edges of the scale. This may be caused by a lack of knowledge on the appraiser's part and permits an easy escape from making a valid decision by neither praising nor condemning.

A further distortion is due to interpersonal relations and *bias*. The ratings will be influenced by the supervisor's likes and dislikes about each individual working in the department. This is especially apparent when objective standards of performance are difficult to determine or not available. Another source of difficulty arises from *organizational influences*, namely, the way administration uses the ratings. Often raters are lenient when they know that pay raises and promotions depend on the appraisals. If the organizational emphasis is on further employee development, appraisers are inclined to emphasize weaknesses and are harsher on the rating.

The supervisor's judgment must be based on the total performance of the employee. It would be unfair to appraise a subordinate based on only one assignment on which he or she had done particularly well or poorly. Instead of recognizing performance during the entire appraisal period, the supervisor merely rates the appraisee's most recent behavior. Supervisors must caution themselves not to let random or first impressions of an employee influence judgment that should be based on the employee's total record of performance, reliability, initiative, skills, resourcefulness, and capability. Nor should supervisors allow past performance appraisal ratings to unjustly influence current ratings either way. Another aid to minimize these errors and biases is to document employee behaviors as soon as possible after the occurrence. When the formal appraisal takes place, supervisors can refer back to the documentation, thus minimizing biases and other pitfalls in rating.

Observing all of these problems in rating will aid supervisors to overcome human weaknesses in processing, storing, and recalling observed behavior when evaluations are made. Although the results are by no means perfect, many human errors can be avoided and counteracted by top administration's continuous emphasis on training for those who do the appraising. The necessity for training supervisors in observing behavior never ends. The success of the performance appraisal depends to a large degree on the supervisor's ability to obtain accurate information and then to discuss it with the appraisee in a nonthreatening and constructive, growth-producing manner. The evaluation interview that follows the appraisal fulfills this function.

The Postappraisal Interview

The second step in the appraisal procedure, the postappraisal interview, takes place when the immediate superior who has performed the evaluation sits down with the subordinate to discuss the appraisee's performance. Some supervisors would like to shy away from the idea of having to tell their subordinates how they stand in the department and what they should do to improve. They are reluctant because, unless it is done with great sensitivity, this type of interview can lead to hostility and even greater misunderstanding. Many employees distrust anything that relates to their review and are often reluctant to discuss their workplace behavior.

The supervisor must be well prepared for this review session. The appraiser must know what should be covered and achieved in this meeting and gather all the information that has any meaning for the discussion. The various events that occurred during the entire evaluation period must be clear in the interviewer's mind. It may be advisable to prepare an agenda for this meeting. Thorough preparation enables the appraiser to be ready for any direction the discussions will take. It is difficult to predict what will happen in this review session. It may be an exceedingly dull meeting and the appraisee's responses can be minimal, for instance, an occasional yes or no or nod of the head. Another meeting, however, may end up as a major bitter confrontation.

Because of the importance and sensitivity of the performance review, the appraiser must not only be well prepared for this session, but also be skilled in interviewing and counseling; the reviewer must ask the right question at the right time and be a constructive listener. In the review session information must be shared. The appraisee must feel that his or her concerns are of utmost importance. Success of this review session can be improved if the appraiser has empathy, listens constructively, asks the right questions at the proper time, and observes keenly. Last, the appraiser must allow enough time to conduct the interview.

It is essential for top administration to spend a great deal of effort in teaching supervisors how to carry on the postappraisal interview, impart to supervisors the necessary skills of directive and nondirective interviews, and show that in the final analysis this is a part of every supervisor's coaching function. Although it would be better not to follow a formalized system, administration often suggests that supervisors follow a standardized outline. According to this outline, the supervisor should first state the purpose of the evaluation procedure and the interview. The supervisor should go on to a discussion of the evaluation itself, first stating the subordinate's strong points and then the weak points. Next, there should be a general discussion giving the employee an opportunity to state his or her feelings. Another possible procedure is to let subordinates appraise themselves first. This gives the appraisees the opportunity to state their side of the story first; it is easier for many subordinates to criticize themselves than to take criticism from the supervisor. Hopefully the interview will end with a discussion of what the subordinate can and wants to do about the deficiencies and what the supervisor will do for the employee in this connection. Although such suggested schemes will help some supervisors, it is better not to formalize this process. As supervisors gain experience they will devise their own plan, and it is likely that each subordinate will be treated in an individual manner.

Everything regarding general techniques of interviewing is applicable to the postappraisal interview. But additional skills are necessary, since the direction of evaluation interviews cannot be predicted. At times it may be very difficult for the supervisor to carry on this interview, especially if the subordinate shows hostility when the supervisor discusses some negative evaluations. Positive judgment can be communicated effectively, but it is difficult to communicate criticisms without generating resentment and defensiveness. It will take much practice and insight to acquire skills in handling this evaluation interview. Therefore, many administrators provide practice sessions and role-playing experiences for supervisors to aid them in effectively carrying out appraisal interviews.

Some supervisors believe that there is no need for an evaluation interview because they are in daily contact with their employees, and these supervisors claim that their door is open at all times. This, however, is not enough. The employee knows that he or she has been formally appraised, and it is understandable that the subordinate might be eager to have a first-hand report on how he or she made out. Also, employees may have some things on their mind that they do not want to discuss in the everyday contacts with the supervisor.

The appraisal interview should be held shortly after the appraisal has been performed, and, as stated before, supervisors should refresh their memory regarding the reasons for the opinions expressed in the appraisal. Appraisees should be given enough notice so that they can prepare themselves also for the interview. At the outset the supervisor should state that the main purpose of the interview is to be a constructive and positive experience for both the appraisee and the appraiser, for the benefit of the employee, the supervisor, and the hospital. It is sometimes suggested that the supervisor ask the employee to appraise his or her own performance. This will give the supervisor a chance to refer to the progress the worker has made since the preceding counseling interview, compliment the subordinate on achievements, and then discuss areas that need improvement. The formula of starting with praise, following it up with criticism, and ending the interview with another compliment is not necessarily the best method. As a matter of fact, good and bad may cancel each other out and the worker may forget about the criticism. A mature employee is able to take deserved criticism when it is called for. By the same token, when praise is merited it should be expressed. It is not always possible to mix the two together effectively. Since the idea of being rated imposes some extra tensions and strains, a feeling of friendliness and privacy in the interview are more important than probably at any other time.

Since it is likely that personal feelings and points of view will be brought out in the discussion, the appraisee must be assured of privacy and confidentiality. There should not be any distractions or interruptions. If possible, coffee and ashtrays should be available.

The supervisor should stress the fact that everybody in the same job in the department is rated according to the same standards and that the

employee has not been singled out for special scrutiny. The supervisor should
be in a position to document the rating by citing specific illustrations and actual instances of good and poor performance. The supervisor should be
careful to relate the measured factors to the actual demands of the job. The
rating must be geared to the present qualities of the employee's performance.
This is particularly important if an employee is already doing good work and
the supervisor is tempted to leave well enough alone. These are probably the
very employees who are likely to make further progress, and to simply tell
them to keep up the good work is not sufficient. These employees may not
have major problems, but nevertheless they deserve thoughtful counseling.
Such an employee is likely to continue to develop, and the supervisor should
be specific as far as future development plans are concerned. The appraiser
must be familiar, therefore, with the opportunities available to the employee,
requirements of the job, and the employee's qualifications. Whenever discussing a subordinate's future, however, the supervisor should not make promises for promotion that may not be possible to keep.

The interview should also give the employee an opportunity to ask
questions so that the supervisor can answer them fully. Any misunderstanding cleared up at this time may avoid future difficulty. The appraiser should
also make it clear that further performance ratings and interviews are regular
procedure with the enterprise. The supervisor should always bear in mind
that the purpose of the appraisal interview is to help employees to see their
shortcomings and aid them in finding solutions. The real success of the interview lies in the employees' ability to see the need for their own improvement
and stimulate in them a desire to improve.

Since the postappraisal interview is the most important part of the
evaluation procedure, supervisors should do all in their power to make certain that at its termination, the employees have a good objective view of their
performance, the ways in which they can improve, and a desire to improve.
Hopefully employees will establish goals that are mutually satisfying to both
the supervisors and themselves. A commitment on the part of the employee
will provide some quantitative measurable goals against which future performance can be judged. At the end of the next period, both supervisor and subordinate will meet to evaluate how well the goals have been achieved and
what the next objectives will be. This will give the subordinate a custom-
made standard of evaluation. It provides him or her with a specified goal
within a specified period. The employee will be so much more motivated,
since the goal was a commitment on his or her part.

Management by objectives (MBO) has been discussed on several occasions in this text. The underlying concept of MBO is that identified, measurable, and workable objectives are agreed on by the supervisor and the
employee; this leads to improved performance and a motivating environment. It creates a participative climate because it involves the subordinates in
the identification of required performance. Although MBO is primarily a
planning tool and a process that goes beyond performance appraisals, it can
be logically and conveniently linked together with performance evaluation
and postappraisal interviews. The review lends itself very well to measuring
the quality of an employee's on-the-job performance and achievements and

participation in setting new objectives; these new goals are to be achieved during the next period and appraised and reviewed in a year. Thus the subordinate is judged by standards he or she helped determine.

Some experts strongly advocate that the annual performance appraisal review should be separated from salary review. They suggest that discussions of the past, future potential, coaching inputs, counseling inputs regarding desired behavior changes, further education, and development should not be tainted by discussions of pay and compensation. In all likelihood, however, the appraisee listens to everything that is said, figuring out what all of this means in terms of future reward opportunities, possible promotions, and so on. A proposed solution is to have two separate review sessions. The first would be concerned with the review and employee development, and the second session, coming any time 4 to 8 weeks later, would cover the compensation issue.

It is customary that appraisal forms require the appraisee to sign the evaluation form on completion of the review. There usually is a statement above the signature line stating that the employee's signature confirms merely that the interview has taken place and that the appraisee in no way approves or disapproves of the statements contained in the evaluation. With this understanding the subordinate will probably sign. If, however, the appraisee would like to state his or her views, no harm is done in letting him or her do so. Many employees will not verbalize their disagreement with the rating; signing the forms with such feelings can create resentment against the organization. The real purpose of the signature is that the supervisor's own boss can be certain that the evaluation interview has taken place. As stated above, many supervisors have mixed reactions about the postappraisal interview. Since it is essential as feedback in the entire evaluation procedure, administration must make certain that it takes place and the signature is the simplest way to ascertain this.

Proper Wages and Salaries

Although people want more from their jobs than just a wage or salary, these are a basic necessity. Pay provides more than the means of satisfying physical needs; it provides a sense of accomplishment and recognition. Most people at work consider relative pay as very important, and real or imagined wage and salary inequities are frequent causes for dissatisfaction, friction, and low morale. It is top management's duty* to pursue a sound policy of wage and salary administration throughout the entire organization; the goal is to have a sound and nondiscriminatory compensation structure. By setting wages high enough, the health care center will be able to recruit satisfactory

---

*The personnel department or a special division within it is concerned with the administration of the wage and salary program; but top administration has the continuing responsibility and overall authority regarding wage and salary policies. Managers at all levels often become involved in these problems.

employees and motivate their present employees to work toward pay increases and promotions. Reducing inequities among employee's earnings will raise morale and reduce friction.

There is no doubt that in most health care centers wage rates and schedules are set by top administration, and the supervisor's authority in this respect is severely limited and handicapped. Still it is a part of the supervisor's staffing function to make certain that the employees of the department are properly and equitably compensated. It is every manager's job to offer the kind of compensation that will retain competent employees in the department, and, if necessary, attract good workers from the outside. Monetary rewards are an exceedingly important factor for all employees. Many employees are much more concerned about how their salaries compare to the earnings of others than they are about their absolute earnings. No doubt many of the wage rates and schedules have followed historical patterns and others are often accidental. For instance, the problem of personalities has frequently distorted certain wage rates. In the long run such a situation cannot be tolerated. It is the supervisor's duty to see that the wages paid within the department are properly aligned *internally* and *externally*. *Internal alignment* means that the jobs within the department are paid according to what they are worth. *External alignment* means that the wages offered for the work to be performed in the department compare favorably with the going rate in the community and area. If they do not, the supervisor knows that some of the most experienced workers will leave and that it will be difficult to attract new ones from the outside.

Job Evaluation: Internal Alignment

To pay the various jobs within the department according to what they are worth, the supervisor should call on the help of the personnel department to conduct a job evaluation. Job evaluation is a method of determining the relationships between pay rates; it is a system for determining the relative money value of jobs within a department. In such a procedure the jobs are evaluated according to various factors, and an appropriate wage rate can be devised based on the worth of each job. Based on the results of what the jobs are worth, an appropriate wage schedule can be instituted. Of course, there will be some questions about what to do with exceptional cases, namely, those employees who are receiving either excessively high or exceedingly low salaries in relation to others. But once a plan has been designed, it is necessary to maintain it properly, so that no new inequities arise.

The job evaluation program is usually administered by a committee under the general guidance of the personnel department. It is a procedure with which the personnel department is acquainted, and if it has not been performed at a recent date, the supervisor might request a job evaluation for his or her department. Sometimes the help of an outside consultant is used. There are several methods of job evaluation. Although they are systematic, they are not totally precise because they involve questions of human judgment. In addition to the most widely used point system, other methods such as ranking, factor comparison, and job classification methods are common.*

Wage and Salary Survey: External Alignment

If the wage and salary policy of the institution is to be competitive in the labor market, that means to pay rates that are approximately the same as those prevailing in the community, accurate wage and salary data must be collected. This is achieved by wage and salary surveys. Job evaluations establish differentials between jobs based on different job content; wage surveys provide management with information on whether the organization's wage level is competitive and properly externally aligned. A wage survey involves collecting data on wages paid in the community for similar key jobs in similar or related enterprises. Without proper external alignment the supervisor cannot recruit competent employees or prevent present employees from leaving for better paying jobs.

To conduct such a survey is a rather costly and sophisticated procedure; conducting one's own survey will probably produce the most meaningful results. Many other sources publish reliable surveys; some are done by government agencies, such as the Bureau of Labor Statistics, and by many professional associations in the health care field, metropolitan hospital associations, and so on. The area normally to be considered is the geographical area within which workers seek employment and employers recruit workers without necessitating a change of residence.

Most enterprises also provide fringe benefits for employees, such as vacations with pay, retirement plans, insurance and health services, low-cost meals, etc. In general, they are incentives to do a better job. Most of these additional benefits are established by the administrator as institution-wide measures; the supervisor has little to do with them other than to make sure that the subordinates understand how they operate and to be sure that each subordinate receives his or her fair share of these benefits. It is advisable to include information along these lines in any wage survey.

To determine whether or not the rates offered by the department are competitive, it is advisable to request the personnel department to undertake such a wage and salary survey unless recent reliable information is available. Then by comparing this information with the wage patterns, the supervisor can determine whether or not wages are properly aligned externally. A sound wage and salary pattern should always be of great concern to the administrator; it is a subject in which the supervisor has very little direct authority. The supervisor's awareness of inadequacies and inconsistencies will often cause the administrator to investigate.

*For more information on how to conduct a job evaluation, see Herbert J. Chruden and Arthur W. Sherman, Jr., *Personnel Management—The Utilization of Human Resources*, 6th ed. (Cincinnati: South-Western Publishing Co., 1980); or George Strauss and Leonard R. Sayles, *Personnel —The Human Problems of Management*, 4th ed. (Englewood Cliffs, N.J.: Prentice-Hall, Inc., 1980), 565-581.

In most instances supervisors will not have enough authority to make wage and salary adjustments except within the framework of the departmental wage scale. But they should definitely plead their case with top administration. To make an intelligent presentation, however, it is necessary for the supervisor to know the value of the various jobs within the department and also the going rates within the community. As every supervisor knows, proper compensation of employees is a significant aspect of the employee's continuing satisfaction and motivation. Without a sound wage and salary pattern, it is almost impossible for a supervisor to recruit competent employees or keep the subordinates motivated.

Promotions

A promotion is a transfer involving the reassignment of an individual to a position of higher rank. This higher level job will entail more demands on the individual but also brings with it higher pay, more authority and responsibility, more privileges, higher status, increased benefits, greater potential, and so on. Along with this go symbols of higher status, such as a more important job title, a larger office, a bigger desk, secretary, etc. Although some people do not want to get ahead, promotions are sought by most people who have a high level of aspirations. It is part of our culture to start at the bottom of the ladder and rise in status and income as one grows older. Since the majority of our society looks on promotions in this way, it is essential that organizations develop and pursue sound promotion policies.

Promotion From Within

Organizations depend heavily on promoting their own employees into better and more promising positions. The policy of promoting from within the organization is one of the most widely practiced personnel policies today. It is a policy that will help to achieve the organizational objective of being a good employer and a good place to work. The latter is undoubtedly one of the many goals of all health care centers. No organization should rely completely on recruiting employees from the outside, however.

The policy of promotion from within vs. recruitment from without is of considerable significance to the enterprise and the individual employee. For the enterprise it ensures a constant source of trained people for the better positions; for the employees it provides a powerful incentive to perform better. After an employee has worked for an enterprise for a period of time, much more is known about that person than even the best potential candidate from outside the organization. Additional job satisfaction will result when employees know that with proper efforts they can work up to more interesting and more challenging work, higher pay, and more desirable working conditions. Most employees like to know that they can get ahead in the enterprise in which they are working. All of this provides strong motivation. There is little motivation for employees to do a better job if they know that the better and higher paying jobs are always reserved for outsiders.

The internal promotion policy should be applied whenever possible and feasible. Most organizations are aware that under special circumstances outside people must be hired; there will be some occasions when strict adherence to internal promotion would do harm to the organization. For instance, if there are no qualified candidates for the job, the internal promotion policy cannot be followed. If no one with the necessary skill is available, them someone from the outside has to be recruited for the position. It could also happen that an organization is forced to go outside because employees with inadequate potential for promotion have been hired in the past.

At times the injection of ''new blood'' into an organization may be very important because it will keep the members of the enterprise from becoming conformist and repetitious. Such a threat is important primarily in managerial jobs and less important in hourly paid jobs. Another reason the enterprise may have to recruit employees from the outside is that the organization cannot afford the expense of training and schooling current employees. A particular position may require a long period of expensive and sophisticated training and the hospital simply cannot afford this kind of upgrading program. Only large organizations can afford such expenses. Another problem with promotion from within is that the organization must continue to live amicably with those who were bypassed. Such a problem does not exist with an applicant from the outside who was rejected.

On the other hand, the supervisor should remember that not every employee wants advancement; many people know their limitations. Some employees are quite content with what they are doing and where they are within the enterprise. They prefer to remain with employees whom they know and responsibilities with which they are familiar. These employees should not be coerced into better positions by the supervisor. The supervisor should also bear in mind that what he or she may consider a promotion may not seem like a promotion to the employee. A nurse may feel that a ''promotion'' to administrative work is a hardship and not an advancement. She may find the administrative activities less interesting than the professional duties, and she may be concerned about her professional future. The supervisor will have to provide promotional opportunities that do not entail compromises of professional feelings.

Sometimes a supervisor does not want to release an employee because this employee is viewed as indispensable and the supervisor does not want to release him or her to take a better job in another department. This could be due to the fact that the supervisor is extremely good in developing subordinates; for example, as soon as a head nurse has developed a number of outstanding nurses, they are promoted out of that unit. The head nurse may believe that the unit suffers because of it. In such a situation administration should give credit to this head nurse for developing promotable employees and show him or her that there will also be a number of good employees entering the unit from other head nurses' units.

At times, the supervisor may be inclined to bypass someone for promotion because the promotion would cause the supervisor some extra work in replacing the promoted employee and training a new employee. The supervisor may fear that the productivity of the department will suffer. This, of course, is shortsighted, since promotion from within is one of the prime motivators. Supervisors who are tempted to think this way should ask themselves where they would be today if their former superiors had had this attitude.

Basis of Promotion

Despite the objections stated above, there are usually more applicants for promotions than there are openings within the organization. Because of this it is important for the organization and supervisors to formulate a sound basis on which employees are chosen for promotion. Since promotions are considered an incentive for employees to do a better job, it would follow that the employee should be promoted who has the best record of quality, productivity, and skill. But in many situations it is difficult to objectively measure some employees' productivity, although a continuous effort in this respect is made by supervisors in the form of merit ratings and performance appraisals. The most important criteria for choice are *merit* (current performance), *ability* (potential future performance), and *seniority* (experience).

Merit and Ability

Since promotion is an incentive for good performance, the best-performing employees should be promoted. In our discussion of performance appraisals the difficulty in measuring performance was emphasized. The differences in *merit* between different employees in health care jobs are often difficult to measure precisely. The person who was not promoted may feel that bias and favoritism were involved. Nevertheless, performance in one's present job is one of the criteria.

Ability and *potential* to assume the responsibilities of a higher level position are another input. The performance appraisal process is a major source of information regarding employee potential. Some of the factors of evaluation, such as oral and written communication, flexibility, decision making, leadership, and planning, are dimensions for appraising potential and future performance.

Since it has been recognized that traditional methods of selecting managers are fraught with many shortcomings and subjectivity, a number of industrial and utility organizations have adopted an *assessment center* approach for evaluating and selecting managers. An assessment center is a place where a number of individual and group exercises are administered to a group of candidates who are seeking promotions to managerial jobs. The candidates are evaluated for their potential for success in management. The exercises and activities include job-related simulations that are designed to bring forth skills the organization considers critical to success. After the session the candidates are evaluated by assessors and observers.

Seniority

But the exclusive use of merit and ability, which are to a great degree subjective criteria, often gives employees the feeling that promotions are not made fairly. Also, since many factors beyond the control of an employee may affect productivity and performance, it would be unfair to base a promotion solely on these factors. Frequent charges of favoritism and bias caused managers to search for more automatic decision criteria that would not create morale problems. Since it is difficult to find objective criteria that eliminate favoritism and possible discrimination, it has been stated that the only objective criterion is length of service. Supervisors generally believe that their relations with their employees will be easier if they promote on the basis of seniority. Therefore, all organizations give some weight to seniority, whether they have a union or not. Unions have put the greatest stress on seniority; and this sort of thinking is now regularly accepted even by those enterprises which do not deal with unions or for those jobs which are not covered by union agreements. Regardless of unions, managers have come to depend heavily on this concept of seniority as a basis for promotion.

Basing promotion on the length of service assumes that the employee's ability increases with service. Although this may be questionable, it is likely that with continued service the ability to perform and knowledge about the organization are increasing. If management is committed to promotion based on length of service, it is likely that the initial selection procedure of a new employee will be a more careful one and that the employee will get as much training as possible in the various positions. Most managers believe that an employee's loyalty is expressed by the length of service and, consequently, this loyalty deserves the reward of promotion. On the other hand, some good employees may become discouraged and leave the organization, realizing that their chances for promotion are slim because of many long-service employees ahead of them.

Balancing the Criteria

Good supervisory practice will attempt to draw a happy medium between the criteria of merit and ability on the one hand and length of service on the other. When the supervisor selects from among almost equally capable subordinates the one with the longest service will no doubt be chosen. Then again, the supervisor may decide to promote an employee who is more capable but has less seniority than another employee because the first stands "head and shoulders" above the one with longer service. If this is not the case, then the one with more seniority will be promoted. Obviously, these decisions become increasingly difficult, and it is easy to see why some supervisors have finally resolved the matter by making length of service the sole determinant of selection for promotion. The ideal solution, of course, is to combine both factors. It is rare that a supervisor will choose a person with the greatest merit and ability from all eligible candidates without giving any weight to length of service.

Selection for promotion will also depend on the type of work involved, demands of the position to be filled, degree requirements prescribed by accrediting and professional associations, and many other factors. It is likely that increasingly more emphasis will be placed on merit and ability when the position to be filled is a demanding and sophisticated position on a higher level, whereas more weight can be given to seniority for promotion into a lower level position. Every organization must decide on the relative weight of these factors in each case when deciding who is to be promoted.

Transfers

A transfer is a reassignment of an employee to another job of similar pay, status, and responsibility. A transfer is a horizontal move, whereas a promotion is a vertical move in rank and responsibility. Transfers take place either because the organization makes it necessary or because the employee requests a transfer. Employees may want a transfer for all kinds of reasons, for example, to gain broader experience or to avoid some friction in a department. If an employee has problems causing frictions, a transfer is not always the right solution unless these problems are dealt with. Sometimes technological changes in one department free a number of employees for transfer into a unit where needs for employees are expanding.

Transferring an employee from one position to another within the hospital often results in greater job satisfaction. For example, a nurse's aide may consider a job as an aide in the operating room to be more prestigious than being an aide on the nursing floor. In reality the pay is the same and one cannot speak of a promotion. But to the aide such a transfer means greater job satisfaction and constitutes an achievement. It is necessary, therefore, that a health care institution have sound transfer policies and procedures so that those who desire a lateral transfer will be given the possibility of doing so. The personnel director, together with the various line managers, should design these policies and procedures and see to it that employees are prepared to make successful transfers.

It is probably best for the employment office to act as a clearance center for interdepartmental transfers. If the responsibility is given to supervisors, the subordinate may be reluctant to request interdepartmental transfers. Some supervisors may be understanding in these matters, whereas others may be resentful and not give their consent. In whatever procedures are instituted there must be provisions that the employee inform the immediate supervisor of the desire to transfer. It is only fair that the present supervisor should be familiar with what the employee intends to do. In case the immediate supervisor does not recommend the transfer, if this is necessary, the employee should be able to appeal this decision to a higher line officer or possibly to the personnel director.

There must be provisions as to whether transfers are to be made only within departments or between departments. There must be a statement as to whether the employee carries previous seniority credits with him or her and provisions for the transfer decision when two or more persons desire transfer to the same job. For example, should length of service be the sole determinant or should capacity to handle the job be taken into consideration also? Good transfer policies and procedures must cover many additional aspects. But in any event there must be the opportunity for employees to be transferred, since this will provide more job satisfaction and will motivate employees in much the same way as a promotion.

Summary

An important source of employees for job openings is the reservoir of employees who are currently with the institution. Promotion from within whenever possible is one of the most rewarding personnel policies any enterprise can practice. It is of great benefit to the enterprise and to the morale of the employees. Although it is difficult to clearly specify the various criteria for promotion, it is normally acknowledged that a happy balance between merit and ability on the one side and length of service on the other should be used. To be able to assess the ability and merit of the employee, however, it is necessary that supervisors remain continuously aware of the employees' achievements. To do this the supervisor must regularly appraise the performance of the employees of the department.

Performance appraisals are formal evaluations of employees' job-related activities. Such a system not only guides management in the process of gathering and analyzing information but also provides guidance for merit increases, promotions, and coaching employees. An evaluation system consists of the process of rating the employee and the appraisal interview, which regularly takes place thereafter. Although the appraisal interview between the supervisor and the employee may prove to be a difficult situation, the entire performance appraisal system is of no use if this aspect is ignored or not carried out appropriately.

In addition to all these duties, the staffing function includes making certain that the employees of the department are properly compensated. Although much of this is out of the domain of the supervisor, it is a supervisory duty to make certain that within the department there is good internal wage alignment, meaning that each job is paid in accordance with its worth and difficulties. To achieve this, a job evaluation is necessary. In addition to good internal alignment, it is also essential that the enterprise have a sound external alignment. This means that the wages paid must be high enough to attract people from outside the organization if need be and to prevent present employees from leaving for higher wages. To do this, it is essential to be familiar with the going rates being paid in the community in similar occupations. Such information can be obtained by wage and salary surveys conducted by the personnel department.

Part Six

Influencing

19

Giving Directives and Managing Change

Influencing is a human resources function that is particularly concerned with behavioral responses. It is the managerial function by which the supervisor evokes action from others to accomplish organizational objectives. It is the process that management uses to achieve goal-directed action from subordinates and colleagues in the organization.

The influencing function is also known as motivating, directing, leading, and actuating. Regardless of the terminology, however, it is that managerial function which the supervisor exercises to get the best and most out of the subordinates and at the same time create a climate in which the subordinates find as much satisfaction of their needs as possible. In the past, managers depended largely on negative persuasion, disciplinary action, and a few incentive programs to influence their employees. The notion of organizational hierarchy dominated managerial thinking until the behavioral sciences brought about new understanding of human motivation and taught us better methods of influencing. Today every manager must be aware of the human activities of which the supervisor is an essential part and of the potential for influencing them. That is, the manager must understand some of the psychology involved in interpersonal relations.

As stated before, it is the role of every manager, of every supervisor, to influence in order to get the work done through and with the help of employees. Influencing is the managerial function that *initiates* action. Without it, nothing, or at best very little, is likely to be accomplished. Planning, organizing, and staffing can be considered preparatory managerial functions; the purpose of controlling is to find out whether or not the goals are being achieved. But the connecting and actuating link between these functions is the managerial function of influencing. This function includes the issuance of directives, instructions, assignments, and orders, as well as the guidance and overseeing of employees. It also includes the problems of motivation.

Moreover, the manager should consider the influencing function as a means not only for getting the work done and motivating, but also for developing the employees. The most effective way to achieve such development of employees is diligent coaching and teaching by their immediate superior. Thus, influencing is more than just giving orders or supervising the employees to make certain that they follow directives. Influencing means building an effective work force and inspiring members of it to perform their best. Influencing is the function of getting the employees to work in a large enterprise as effectively as possible and with the same amount of enthusiasm that they would display if they were working for themselves, either in their own enterprise or at a hobby. Only by appropriately influencing and supervising the employees will the manager be able to instill in them this motivation to work energetically on the job and at the same time to find personal satisfaction.

Of course, influencing is the job of every manager whether that person is the administrator of a health care facility or the supervisor of one of its departments. Every manager performs the influencing function, regardless of the position held. The amount of time and effort a manager spends in this function will vary, however, depending on the level, number of employees supervised, and other duties. It is a fact that the supervisor of a department will spend most of the time influencing and supervising, more so than the administrator of the hospital. Indeed, influencing is an ever-present continuous function of the supervisor that covers the day-to-day activities within the department.

Naturally, the supervisor's influencing function is interconnected with the other managerial functions. It is obvious that influencing is largely affected by the kind of employee the supervisor has selected while performing the staffing function. Obviously the plans the supervisor made and the organization drawn up also have a bearing on the influencing function. The controlling function is likewise affected by influencing, inasmuch as control often involves human problems.

To get the job done, every supervisor spends a great deal of time and effort in giving directives to subordinates. In this connection, it is advisable to recall the principle of *unity of command* to which reference was made earlier. Unity of command means that in each department only one person has the authority to make decisions appropriate to his or her station. It means that each employee has a single immediate supervisor, who is in turn responsible to his or her immediate supervisor, and so on up and down the chain of command. It also means that a subordinate is responsible to only one supervisor. The principle of unity of command further states that the supervisor is the only one who can give directives to the employees. All directives can come only from the immediate supervisor, and there should be no interference in the guiding and overseeing of the employees by anyone else. In other words, there is a direct line of authority from the supervisor to the subordinate, just as there is one from the administrator to the director of a service and from there to the supervisor of a department. The administrator's line, however, extends only to the director of a service and not to the supervisors and employees

under these supervisors. Thus, all supervision of the employees in a department rests with the supervisor or the head of that department and must not be
exercised by anyone else, emergencies excepted. Otherwise, the principle of
unity of command is violated; no person can serve two bosses.

Characteristics of a Good Directive

Because issuing directives is such a basic and integral part of the supervisor's daily routine, it has often been taken for granted that every supervisor
knows how to give orders. It is frequently assumed that anybody can give
orders. This is probably not true. But even if it were true, there is general
agreement that some ways of issuing directives are much more effective than
others. The experienced supervisor knows that faulty or bad order giving can
easily upset even the best-laid plans, and, instead of coordination of efforts, a
general state of chaos is created.

To the uninitiated outsider, it may seem that some supervisors can get
excellent results even though they appear to break every rule in the book.
Other supervisors may use all the best techniques of order giving and phrase
their requests in the most courteous ways and still only get grudging compliance. The question of what is the most appropriate method of order giving
depends on the employees concerned, work situation, supervisors, the way
they view their job, their attitude toward people, and many other factors.
There are definite techniques for giving orders, however, and since the supervisor's own success depends largely on how the subordinates carry out the
orders, it is essential for the manager to possess the knowledge and skill for
good directing. In other words, since directing is the fundamental tool
employed by supervisors to start, stop, or modify activities, it is necessary for
every supervisor to become familiar with the basic characteristics that
distinguish good and accomplishable directives from those which are not.
These characteristics are fulfilled when directives are reasonable, intelligible,
worded appropriately, compatible with the objectives, and within reasonable
time limits.

Reasonable Directives

The first essential characteristic of a good directive is that it must be
reasonable, that is, compliance can reasonably be expected by the supervisor.
Unreasonable orders will not only undermine morale, but they will also make
controlling impossible. The requirement of reasonableness immediately excludes orders pertaining to activities that physically cannot be done. In judging whether or not a directive can be reasonably accomplished, supervisors
should not only appraise it from their own point of view, but they should also
try to place themselves in the position of the employee. The supervisor should
not issue a directive if the capacity or experience of the employee is not sufficient to comply with the order. This becomes particularly important in the
case of recent graduates who may have had an excellent education in many

areas, but certainly lack experience and even some of the basic knowledge required. Supervisors should not forget the value of their own on-the-job training.

It easily can happen that a supervisor issues unreasonable instructions. For instance, to please the superior, a supervisor promises the completion of a job at a particular time and then issues such an order without considering whether the employee who is to carry out the order can actually do so. In this situation, the supervisor should make it clear that he or she will try to get the job done in time; but unreasonable pressure should not be put on the subordinate. The supervisor should place himself or herself in the position of the subordinate, and ask if compliance reasonably can be expected. The decision will depend on all the conditions prevailing at the time. In some borderline cases the directive may actually be intended to stretch the subordinate's capabilities a bit beyond what had previously been requested. Then the question of reasonableness becomes a question of degree. But generally, a prime requirement of a good directive is that it can be accomplished by the employee to whom it is assigned without undue difficulty.

Intelligibility

Another requirement is that a good directive should be intelligible to the employee, the employee should be able to understand it. The subordinate cannot be expected to carry out an order that he or she does not understand. For example, a directive in a language not intelligible to the subordinate cannot be considered an order. But the same also applies if both speak English, and the supervisor uses words that the employee does not comprehend. This, then, becomes a matter of communication. (See Chapter 5.) The supervisor must make certain that the employee understands, and it is the supervisor's duty to communicate in words and forms that the employee actually understands and not merely should understand. Instructions must be clear but not necessarily lengthy. What is clear and complete to the supervisor, however, is not always clear and complete to the employee. And sometimes the supervisor has not made up his or her mind as to exactly what it is that he or she wants done. Here, too, it is advisable for the supervisor to project himself or herself into the position of the employee. A supervisor simply cannot expect subordinates to carry out directives that have not been made clear and intelligible.

Appropriate Wording

Every good supervisor knows that the tone and words used in issuing directives significantly affect the subordinates' acceptance and performance of them. A considerate tone is likely to stimulate willing and enthusiastic acceptance, which, of course, is preferable to routine or grudging acceptance or outright rejection. Although in the patient care field the word "order" is normally used without unpleasant connotations, most other supervisors should refrain from using the term "order" as much as possible and instead use such terms as directives, assignments, instructions, suggestions, and requests.

Requests

Phrasing orders more as requests does not reduce their character as a directive, but there is a big difference in the reaction a request will inspire as compared to a command. With the majority of subordinates, a request is all that is commonly needed and used. It is a pleasant and easy way of asking an employee to get the job done, particularly with those employees who have been working for the supervisor for some time and who are familiar with the personality of the supervisor and vice versa. A request works best with this kind of employee, and it usually does not rub that person the wrong way.

Suggestions

In other instances, it might be advisable to place the directive in the form of a suggestion, which is a still milder form than a request. For example, the supervisor might say, "Mary, we are supposed to get all of this work done today and we seem to be a bit behind. Do you think we can make up for it?" Suggestions of this type will accomplish a great deal for the supervisor because they will be understood and accepted by responsible and ambitious employees. Such employees like the feeling of not being ordered around and of being on their own to get the job accomplished. This suggestive type of order would not be advisable in dealing with new employees, however. New employees simply do not have the background of the department and have not been around long enough to have received sufficient training and familiarity with its activities. Nor is suggestion the proper way of giving orders to those employees who are less competent and less dependable.

Moreover, some subordinates must be told what to do simply because a request or suggestion might invite an argument as to why they should not do it. Sometimes the command type of order is the only way to get things done. Everyone remembers commands from parents and schoolteachers as part of growing up. Most people, however, feel that once they are adults commands are no longer necessary. Thus, the best rule for a supervisor is to avoid commands whenever possible but to use them when necessary.

Compatibility With Objectives

A good directive must be compatible with the purposes and objectives of the organization. If the instructions do not conform with the objectives of the enterprise, chances are the subordinate may not execute them adequately or may not execute them at all. It is therefore necessary that the supervisor, when issuing directives that appear to conflict with the main organizational objectives, explain to the employee why such action is necessary. Or the supervisor can explain that the directive merely appears to be in conflict, but actually is not contrary to the objectives of the enterprise. Instructions must also be consistent; they must not be in opposition to orders or directives previously given unless there is a good reason for the discrepancy.

Time Allotment

An additional characteristic of a good directive is that it specify the time within which the instructions should be carried out and completed. The supervisor should allow a reasonable amount of time and, if this is not feasible, must realize that the quality of the performance will only be as good as can be produced under the time limit. In many directives, the time factor is not clearly stated, although it is probably implied that the assignment should be carried out within a reasonable length of time. What is a reasonable length of time will, of course, depend on the circumstances of the situation.

• • •

These are some of the major characteristics which should be incorporated in a good directive. Because the performance of the employee depends to a great extent on the quality of directives given, the supervisor should make certain that the directive fulfills these most essential characteristics.

Major Techniques of Directing

On several occasions, we have discussed various theories describing the supervisor's underlying managerial attitudes, such as Theories X and Y,* autocratic and democratic leadership, participation in decision making, and broad or narrow delegation of authority. The following is a more detailed discussion of how these managerial attitudes manifest themselves in the daily working environment, in which the supervisor depends on the subordinates to actually get the job done.

Generally, the supervisor may choose from two basic techniques of direction: *autocratic,* or *close, supervision* on the one hand or *consultative,* or *participative, general supervision* on the other. In our discussion, we can clearly distinguish between these two extremes, but in practice, the supervisor usually combines and blends the techniques. It is conceivable, for example, that the manager might use the autocratic technique for one situation and the democratic technique for another. For some employees the supervisor might consider it more advisable to use one method and for other employees another. No one form of supervision is equally good in all situations. Whether it is better to apply a more autocratic or a more democratic type of supervision will depend on many factors: the kind of work, situation at hand, attitude of

*Douglas McGregor, *The Human Side of Enterprise* (New York: McGraw-Hill Book Co., 1960); Chapters 3 and 4.

the employee toward the supervisor, personality and ability of the employee, and personality, experience, and ability of the supervisor. A good supervisor is sensitive to all of these factors and to the needs of each situation, and the style of supervision will be adjusted accordingly.

Autocratic, Close Supervision

When the autocratic technique of directing—close supervision—is employed, the supervisor gives direct, clear, and precise orders to the subordinates with detailed instructions as to exactly how and in what sequence things are to be done. This, as we know, allows little room for the initiative of the subordinate. The supervisor who normally uses the autocratic technique will delegate as little authority as possible and believes that in all probability he or she can do the job better than any of the subordinates. The supervisor relies on command and detailed instructions, followed by close supervision. An autocratic supervisor believes that subordinates are "not paid to think," they are expected to follow instructions. The boss alone is to do the planning and decision making; this is what he or she is trained and paid for. This kind of supervisor does not necessarily distrust the subordinate, but believes that without detailed instruction the subordinate could not properly carry out the directive. This person believes that only he or she can specify the best method and that there is only one way, namely, the supervisor's way, to get the job done. In other words, Theory X management is practiced.

With most people the consequences of autocratic supervision can be fatal. Employees lose interest and initiative; they stop thinking for themselves because there is no need or occasion for independent thought. They are obedient but silent and lack initiative, sparkle, and ingenuity. It becomes difficult to remain loyal to the organization and to the supervisor; the subordinates secretly rejoice when the boss makes a mistake. This kind of supervision tends to make the employees somewhat like an automaton. Freedom is curtailed, and it is difficult for them to learn even by making mistakes; they justly conclude that they are not expected to do any thinking about their job, and, although they perfunctorily perform their duties, they find little involvement in the work. They are certainly not motivated.

Shortcomings of the autocratic technique of supervision are obvious. Generally, young men and women who have been brought up in a democratic and permissive society from their earliest days resent autocratic order giving. It is contrary to our traditional democratic way of life in America. No ambitious employee will remain in a position where the supervisor is not willing to delegate some degree of freedom and authority. Any subordinate who is eager to learn and progress will resent being constantly given detailed instructions that leave no room for his or her own thinking and initiative. The employee will be stifled, and sooner or later will leave the enterprise if utterly possible. This method of supervision does not produce good employees and will only chase away those who have the potential.

On the other hand, it must not be forgotten that under certain circumstances and with certain people a degree of close supervision may be necessary. But this is the exception, not the rule. Suppose, for example, that the subordinate is the kind of person who does not want to think for himself or herself and prefers to receive clear orders. Firm guidance gives reassurance, whereas loose and general supervision may be frustrating. Some employees lack ambition and imagination and do not want to become at all involved in their daily job. There are also employees who have been brought up in an authoritarian manner by their families here or in a foreign country, and whose previous work experience leads them to believe that general supervision is no supervision at all. Moreover, there are occasions when a work situation is so chaotic that only autocratic techniques can bring order. Aside from these rather unusual situations, however, it can generally be assumed that autocratic, or close, supervision is the least desirable and effective method.

Moreover, the autocratic supervisor usually makes the basic Theory X assumption that the average employee does not want to do the job, that close supervision and threats of loss of the job are needed to get people to work. Such a supervisor believes that if he or she were not on the job and "breathing down their necks," all the subordinates would stop working. And under these conditions, they probably would. On the other hand, the supervisor who follows Theory Y and believes in general supervision assumes that the average employee is eager to do a good job, wants to do the right thing, and must have motivation to perform his or her best. Obviously, autocratic, or close, supervision is not conducive to motivating employees to perform their best; general supervision, however, will.

Consultative, General Supervision

The opposite of autocratic supervision is consultative. Consultative supervision is also known as participative, democratic or permissive supervision. This is similar to the concept of general supervision referred to earlier. Its basic assumption is that employees are eager to do a good job and are capable of doing so. The supervisor behaves toward them with this basic assumption in mind, and the employees in turn tend to react in a manner that justifies the expectations of their supervisors.

This democratic approach to the directing function manifests itself in the practice of general supervision when it comes to routine assignments within the department. When new jobs have to be performed and new assignments made, the democratic method of supervising will manifest itself in the consultative, or participative, technique of directing. Both, of course, have the underlying assumption that employees will be more motivated if they are left to themselves as much as possible. We shall first discuss situations that require consultation and then the meaning of general supervision for routine assignments.

Consultation

The essential characteristic of consultation is that the supervisor consults with employees concerning the extent, nature, and alternative solution to a problem before the supervisor makes a decision and issues a directive. The supervisor who uses the consultative approach before issuing directives is earnestly seeking help and ideas from the employees and approaches the subject with an open mind. More important than the procedure is the attitude of the supervisor. A subordinate will easily sense superficiality and is quick to perceive whether or not the boss genuinely intends to consult on the problem or only intends to give the impression of so doing.

There is a danger that some supervisors are inclined to use such pseudoconsultation merely to give employees the feeling that they have been consulted. In many instances, supervisors ask for participation only after they have already decided on the directive. Here the supervisor is using the consultative technique as a trick, a device for manipulating people to do what he or she wants them to do. The subordinate will quickly realize that he or she is not being taken seriously and that this participation is not real. The results achieved will be much worse than if the superior had used the most autocratic method. To really practice consultative management when issuing new directives and assignments, the supervisor must be ready to take it seriously and be willing to be swayed by the employee's opinion and suggestions. If the manager is not sincere, it would be better not to apply this technique in the first place.

If the subject matter concerns only the supervisor and one employee, the consultative, or participative, method can be carried out informally. There are numerous occasions during the day to hold such private consultations; however, if this approach is used all the time, the subordinates may begin to doubt whether the supervisors have any opinions of their own and are able to make any decisions. Although some supervisors are incapable of making a decision, many just go too far in utilizing this philosophy of direction, and while implementing the technique of participation, they cannot retain the atmosphere of managing.

To reinstate the atmosphere of managing it should be recalled that consultative direction does not lessen or weaken formal authority because the right of decision making still remains with the supervisor. Moreover, the supervisor using this approach is just as much concerned with getting the job done economically and expeditiously as the manager who uses another kind of approach. Although the supervisor must not dominate the situation to the exclusion of any employee participation, this is not to say that the supervisor cannot express an opinion. It must be expressed in a manner which indicates to the employee that even the supervisor's opinions are subject to critical appraisal. Similarly, participative consultation does not mean that the suggestions of the employee cannot also be criticized or even rejected. True consultation implies a sharing of information between the supervisor and employee and a thorough and impartial discussion of alternate solutions, regardless of who originated them. Only then can it be said that the manager really consulted the subordinate.

For such consultative practices to be successful, it is not only necessary that the supervisor be in favor of them, but the employee must also want them. If the employee believes that "the boss knows best" and that making decisions and giving directives is none of his or her concern, then there is little likelihood that the opportunity to participate will induce better motivation or morale. It must also be kept in mind that an employee should be consulted about those areas in which that person is capable of contributing and in which he or she can draw on a certain fund of knowledge. The problems involved must be consistent with the subordinate's ability. Asking participation in areas that are outside their scope of experience will make the employees feel inadequate and frustrated instead of motivating them.

In using consultation there is the danger that at the end of an extended discussion the employee may not have a clear crisp idea of the solution. It is therefore desirable and even necessary for the supervisor or subordinate to summarize the conclusions to avoid such a pitfall. This is even more essential if several employees participated in the consultation.

One of the obvious advantages of summarizing the results of the consultation is that the emerging directive does not appear to the employee as an order, but rather as a solution in which he or she participated. This assures the subordinate's best cooperation and enthusiasm in carrying the directive out. It imparts a feeling of importance, since it is evident that the ideas were desired and valued. Active participation also provides an outlet for reasoning power and imagination and an opportunity for the employee to make a worthwhile contribution to the organization. Since there is a considerable degree of talent among employees, their ideas often prove to be valuable in improving the quality of directives. An additional advantage of this technique is that it will bring the employee closer to the supervisor, which will make for better communication and understanding between them. Looking at these impressive advantages of consultation, it becomes apparent that it is by far the best method to use whenever the supervisor has to issue new assignments, directives, and instructions.

Quality Circles

Quality circles, sometimes called quality control circles, is an application of participative management in the daily work routine. Although the underlying ideas came from the work of Douglas McGregor, Maslow, Herzberg, Deming, Drucker, and others, the first practical applications were made in Japanese industry. This Japanese management technique claims much credit for the high level of productivity, quality, and worker satisfaction. Lately the idea has been introduced successfully into American industry and a number of health care settings.

A quality circle is a group of approximately 8 to 12 employees (workers) and supervisors who volunteer to meet regularly to discuss work and quality problems. They try to identify the causes and develop practical solutions, the supervisor acting as the leader of the circle. The underlying thought is that the employees doing the job often know best why productivity is low and quality poor, and often they have excellent ideas and answers. These circle solutions are then presented to management. The quality circle idea fits into the existing organizational structures, following the existing channels of communications and command. Since quality circles is an application of participative management, the concept can be introduced with success into any organization where administration's philosophy has been democratic, open, and participative. It is unlikely that they would produce results in an environment that practices autocratic and highly centralized management.

General Supervision

This democratic participative approach to directing subordinates leads to what we have already referred to as general, or loose, supervision when it comes to *routine assignments* and carrying out the daily chores involved in each employee's job. General supervision, as we know, means to let the subordinate work out the details of the job, to let the employee make decisions of how best to do it. Through this process, workers will gain great satisfaction from being on their own and from having a chance to express themselves and make decisions. Instead of having a specific detailed list of orders to comply with, the supervisor will just generally indicate what needs to be done and might make a few suggestions as to how to go about it. In so doing, the supervisor assumes that given the proper opportunity, the average employee wants to do a good job. The supervisor is primarily interested in the results. Once the subordinate is told what is to be accomplished and goals are established and limits defined, the employee is left on his or her own. Obviously, this kind of thinking and supervision can only lead to higher motivation and morale and ultimately better job performance. It gives employees the opportunity to satisfy their needs for self-expression and being their own boss.

Explaining Directives. The supervisor who practices general supervision creates an atmosphere of understanding and mutual confidence in which the employee will always feel free to call on the boss whenever the need arises without fear that this would indicate incompetence. By the same token, the supervisor takes great pains to explain to the workers the reasons for general directives and why certain things have to be done. By explaining the purpose behind the directives, the employee will be able to understand the environment of the activities. This will make the employee better informed; the better informed the subordinate is, the better he or she will be able to perform the job.

Indeed, it is a common complaint in many enterprises that subordinates are kept in the dark most of the time and that supervisors hoard knowledge and information that they ought to pass on. In most instances, it is exceedingly difficult to issue directives so completely as to cover all particulars. If the person who receives the directive knows the purpose behind it, however, he or she is in a better position to carry it out than one who does not know. This will enable the worker to put the environment in total perspective and to make sense out of it, so that he or she can take firm and secure action. Without such knowledge, the employee might find himself or herself in an anxiety-producing situation. Also, subordinates may run into unforeseen circumstances, and, if they know why the directive was given, they will probably be able to use their own good judgment and carry it out in a manner that will bring about proper results. They could not possibly do this if they were not well informed.

There is an often-told story illustrating the importance of explaining directives. A foreman had a crew of workers dig holes at random in the factory yard. Each time two men had dug a hole four feet deep, the foreman was called over to inspect the hole, after which he ordered the men to fill it up again. After the lunch break, the work crew refused to do the job because they thought it completely useless. At that point, the foreman explained the purpose, telling them that the blueprints for an old water main line had been lost and that they were searching for the water main. With this explanation the workers were happy to return to their job. It is obvious that the supervisor could have saved himself some trouble had he explained the reason for the job in the beginning. As each hole was dug, the workers could have searched for the water main themselves and the supervisor could have avoided the inspection.

This story should not blind us to the fact that sometimes a supervisor can overdo a good thing and, instead of clarifying the situation, provides so much information that ultimately the subordinate is utterly confused. Explanations should include only enough information to get the job done. If the directive involves a very minor activity and not much time is available, the explanation will probably be very brief. Supervisors, of course, must use their own judgment in deciding how far they will go in explaining their directives. They will take into consideration such factors as the capacity of the subordinates to understand, the training they have had, the content of the directive, the underlying managerial attitude, and the time available. After evaluating these factors, the supervisor will be in a better position to decide what constitutes an adequate explanation.

General Supervision Compared With "No Supervision." It should be recalled that general supervision is not the same as no supervision at all. General supervision requires that the employee be given a definite assignment. But this assignment is definite only to the extent that the employee understands the results expected. It is not definite regarding the specific instructions that state precisely how the results are to be achieved. General supervision does not mean that subordinates can set their own standards. Rather, the supervisor will set the standards, but will make them realistic, high enough to be a challenge, yet not higher than possibly can be achieved. Although general supervision excludes direct pressure, employees know that their efforts are being measured against these standards, and this knowledge alone should lead them to work harder. By setting the standards reasonably high, the supervisor does apply a degree of pressure, but the pressure is quite different from that exerted by "breathing down someone's neck."

General supervision requires a continuous effort on the supervisor's part to develop the potential of the employees. Everyone knows that active learning is more effective than passive learning. Employees learn more easily when they work out a solution for themselves than if they are given the solution. It is a known fact that employees learn best from their own mistakes. In general supervision, the supervisor spends considerable time teaching employees how to solve problems and make decisions as problems arise in the work situation. Continuous training of employees is an absolute necessity in general supervision. The better trained the employees become in basic problem-solving methods, the less need there will be for supervision. In fact, one way to judge the effectiveness of a supervisor is to see how the employees in the department function when the boss is away from the job.

General supervision, however, is a way of life that must be practiced over a period of time, and the supervisor cannot expect instantaneous results if general supervision is introduced into a situation where the employees have been accustomed to close supervision. It will take time before the results can be seen. The general supervisor is just as much interested in results as any other kind of supervisor, but he or she is also interested in the individual development of the employees, which differentiates him or her from the autocratic supervisor.

Although the supervisor may be a firm believer in general supervision and will practice it whenever possible, under certain conditions firmness, fortitude, and decisiveness must be shown. There may be occasions and certain employees who just do not seem to thrive under loose supervision. This, however, is the exception and not the rule. Although general supervision is not a cure-all for every problem, all research studies seem to indicate that it is more effective than close supervision in terms of productivity, morale, and achievements. General supervision permits the employee to acquire pride in the work and in the results achieved. It helps develop the employee's talent and capabilities. It permits the supervisor to spend less time with the employees and more time on overall management of the department. General supervision provides the motivation for the employees to work on their jobs with enthusiasm and energy, thus deriving full satisfaction from their work.

Influencing and Managing Change

The supervisors' influencing function is extremely important whenever they are faced with the introduction of a change. Since every enterprise operates in a larger context and the environment is dynamic, change is inevitable and is a part of everyday life. In fact, the growth of most undertakings depends largely on the concept of change.

Although all organized activities are subject to some change, the degree and complexity of change vary considerably from one activity to another. This is particularly so in the field of health care, in which the speed and complexity of changes have continuously increased in the last few decades and will continue to do so in the future. There is little doubt that most of these changes have been beneficial. Hospital floors are filled with patients benefiting from one new breakthrough or another. Indeed, the health care center as a social system produces an ever-shifting equilibrium of forces because of the amazing advances in medical sciences and technologies. The supervisor's own department is a small social subsystem, interdependent with the larger system of the health care center. Any change imposed from without is likely to shift the equilibrium of forces within each individual department, as well as within the organization as a whole.

Moreover, it is the departmental supervisor who is in the forefront of change, since he or she is the one who in the daily working situation has to make it a reality. The supervisor must "sell" the idea of change to the subordinates. Most of the time the supervisor has had little to do with the decision to make the change or with its timing. It originated higher up in the administration or somewhere else. Hopefully, however, the supervisor understands and accepts the change because it is now his or her role and duty to introduce it, explain it to the subordinates, and feed back their reactions to the superiors. Of course, the supervisor will encounter reactions from the employees that range from ready acceptance to outright rejection and hostility, with varying degrees of everything in between.

Most people pride themselves on being modern and up to date, and most gladly accept and welcome changes in material things. But when it comes to changes in jobs and interpersonal relations, there is a tendency to resist them. This is unfortunate because if an enterprise is to survive, it must be able to react to the prevailing conditions by changing itself and by issuing directives that will incorporate and realize the necessary changes. Since resistance to change is a common phenomenon, it is essential for the supervisor to learn about the causes for this resistance and what can be done to help the employees accept necessary changes.

Reasons for Resistance to Change

There are many reasons for internal inflexibilities and resistance to change. One of the important internal inflexibilities is psychological. Supervisors and employees may develop patterns of thought and behavior that are resistant to change. Supervisors are often frustrated in instituting a change by the unwillingness or inability of people to accept change. To overcome these inflexibilities the supervisor must realize that it requires patient selling of the idea, careful dissemination of information, good leadership, and development of a tradition of change among the members of the department. The supervisor must not fail to realize that even a trifling change may cause deep reactions within some of the employees of the department.

This difficulty is further complicated because of *distorted perceptions.* For example, employees may believe that a new organizational arrangement will result in loss of control or influence. This belief will cause resistance to change. The fact that the new structure will in no way reduce their influence does not diminish their resistance as long as they perceive a threat and feel threatened or attacked.

To a large degree these sources of resistance to change center around a few major considerations, such as uncertainty about the effects of change and unwillingness to give up existing benefits because the costs of change will not be made up by the rewards. It is also possible that the change may be fraught with weaknesses that have been overlooked or brushed aside.

One reason for resisting change is that it disturbs the equilibrium of the current state of affairs. The assumption is that before the change the employee exists within an environment in which his or her *need satisfaction* has reached a high degree of stability, and the change may prevent or decrease the satisfaction of these needs. Therefore, it is natural for the employee to do whatever possible to thwart the introduction of the change.

A second reason for resisting change is that any change is seen as a potential threat to the employee's *security*. The subordinate must give up the known familiar routine for something new and unpredictable. For example, new apparatus in the laboratory could make some of the technologists' previous skills superfluous. This could undermine their sense of occupational identity. The change may require the technologists to upgrade their skills, and they are not sure that they can master the new responsibilities. At the outset, any new ideas and methods almost always represent a threat to the security of the individuals involved in the change. Usually people fear change because they cannot assess or predict what it will bring in terms of their own position, activity, and future. It makes no difference whether the change is actually threatening or not. What matters is that the subordinate believes or assumes this.

A third reason for resistance to change is that the change may threaten the employee's *status* within the organization. The employee may fear that his or her status will be lowered and someone else's raised. Such fears have, for example, caused many new computer installations to be used less effectively than anticipated or to be slowed down in their effects on the overall organization. This was because employees in the controller's office where the computer is housed, started to gain a different status in the organization once the computer became their domain. Its introduction caused what appeared to be threatening changes in the reporting relationships and status of numerous employees.

Often threats of an *economic* nature provide an additional reason for resistance to change. The subordinate may fear that the change will affect his or her job economically. Hundreds of years ago, hand weavers in the Low Countries of Europe tried to destroy mechanic looms by throwing their wooden clogs (sabots) into the machinery (sabotage) because they feared that the machines would destroy their jobs and income. The same fears still prevail today when it comes to the size of the paycheck.

In general, we may say that the changes affect different people in different ways. A change that causes great disturbance to one person may create little disequilibrium for another. The type and severity of the reaction that occurs in a particular situation will depend on the nature of the change and the person concerned.

The important thing for the supervisor to recognize is that changes do disturb the equilibrium of the employee and that when individuals become threatened they develop behaviors which serve as barriers to the threat. Therefore, it is the supervisor's duty to facilitate the inevitable process of adjustment when changes are necessary. Let us see how this can be done.

Facilitating Change

A model for facilitating change that is frequently cited was developed by Kurt Lewin.* This model is concerned with changing the attitudes, skills, and knowledge of individuals and suggests three elements: a period of *unfreezing* old attitudes; *changing*, moving to a new attitude; and *refreezing*.

The supervisor should always remember that employees seldom resist change just to be stubborn. From the foregoing discussion, we learned that there are valid reasons for resistance. Subordinates resist because the change affects their equilibrium socially, psychologically, and possibly economically. With the proper attitude and the right techniques, however, the supervisor can facilitate the introduction of change to a great extent. Involving subordinates in change discussions and decisions will help to overcome the various types of resistance.

One of the factors that is particularly important in gaining acceptance of change is the relationship which exists between the supervisor who is trying to introduce the change and the employee who is subject to the change. If a relationship of mutual confidence and trust exists between the two, the employee is much more likely to go along with the change than otherwise.

The supervisor should assume that a considerable amount of time is necessary to implement a change; a rigid timetable for change is unrealistic. The change must be planned far in advance, and its impact on each position and job should be anticipated. Even if the change is well thought out and carefully planned, some ramifications will probably be overlooked. The supervisor must leave room to discuss and accommodate them.

Explanation

Of course, the most important aspect in facilitating the introduction of change is the supervisor's duty to *explain* the change to the employees in advance. This should begin long before the change is to be initiated. There should be ample time before the changeover to familiarize the employees with the idea, allow them to think through the implications and ramifications, and ask questions for more clarification. In other words, there must be sufficient time for feedback and additional communication.

---

*Kurt Lewin, "Frontiers in Group Dynamics: Concept, Method, and Reality in Social Science; Social Equilibria and Social Change," *Human Relations*, Vol. 1, No. 1 (June, 1947): 5-42; also see Edgar H. Schein, "Management Development as a Process of Influence," *Industrial Management Review*, Vol. 2, No. 2 (May, 1961): 59-77.

In explaining the change, the supervisor should put himself or herself into the subordinates' position and discuss its pros and cons from their point of view. This discussion should explain what will happen and why. It should clarify the way in which the change will affect the employee and what it means to that person. It should show that the change will leave the employee no worse off or even improve the present situation. All of this information should be communicated to the entire department, those employees who are directly involved, as well as those who are indirectly involved. Overstatements are ill-advised, however, and it is essential to be absolutely truthful. The supervisor cannot afford a credibility gap.

The supervisor must also try to communicate, explaining to the employees what they consciously and subconsciously want and need to know in order to resolve prevailing fears. Only then can employees assess and understand what the change proposal would mean in terms of their positions and activities. The supervisor must help the subordinate understand the need for the change. This will be easier if the supervisor has always been concerned with setting the proper stage and giving the proper background information for all of the directives. In such a case, the employee is thoroughly acquainted with the underlying factors and is more likely to view the change as a necessary adjustment in a dynamic environment. The subordinate might ask a few additional questions about it, but then can quickly adapt to it and resume his or her previous behavior. The subordinate who has been informed of the reasons for change knows what to expect and why. Instead of blind resistance, there will be intelligent adaptation to the instructions, and instead of insecurity, there will be a feeling of security. In the final analysis, it is not the change itself that leads to so much misunderstanding, it is more the manner in which the supervisor introduces the change. In other words, resistance to change that comes from fear of the unknown can be minimized by supplying appropriate information.

Participation

Another effective way of reducing the resistance to change is to permit participation in planning the change. No doubt those who are affected by the change may have something to contribute, since they are close to the situation and can see some weaknesses in the change proposal that management might have overlooked. Furthermore, playing a part in planning the change will remove most of the fears and threats that normally would be the causes for resistance.

This participation may be in the form of consultation whereby criticism and suggestions are sincerely solicited from the employees in connection with the contemplated change. In face-to-face conversations, the supervisor discusses problems, asks questions, and tries to get the employees' ideas and reactions. Hopefully, management will then incorporate as much of this into the change as possible, and the employees will consider themselves a partner in the change. A change imposed from above without participation is likely to generate resentment.

A more advanced stage of participation occurs when the supervisor lets the employees make the decision themselves. The supervisor defines the problem and sets the limits, but lets the subordinates develop the alternatives and choose between them. If several employees are involved, this group decision making is an effective means for overcoming resistance to change. Such an approach recognizes that if the employees who are threatened by a change have the opportunity to work through the new ideas and methods from the beginning and can be assured that their needs will be satisfied in the future, they will accept the new ideas and methods as something of their own making and will give them their support. Group decision making also makes it easier for each member to carry out the decision once it is agreed on, and the group will put strong pressure on those who have reservations or who do not want to go along.

Both kinds of participation should be encouraged because they help to facilitate the introduction of change. Of course, in trying to implement change in the department, the supervisor will make use of all means available—persuasion, discussion, participation, and group decision making. Participation is not always possible; in extreme situations, it may be necessary to make unpleasant changes unilaterally, impose them, and then help the subordinates understand and accept them.

Summary

The influencing function of the manager forms the connecting link between planning, organizing, and staffing on one side and controlling on the other. Issuing directives is perhaps the most important part of the influencing function because without them nothing or at best very little would be achieved. Certain prerequisites ensure that a directive will be properly carried out. A good directive must encompass the formula of who, what, where, when, how, and why. The directive should be accomplishable, intelligible, properly phrased, and compatible with the objectives of the enterprise. In addition, a reasonable amount of time should be permitted for its completion.

In issuing directives, the supervisor may employ two major techniques: the autocratic technique, which brings about close supervision; or the consultative technique, characterized by general supervision. There are certain occasions, employees, and conditions under which the autocratic technique is probably the more effective one; but for most situations it is far better for a supervisor to apply consultative techniques to produce the highest motivation and morale among employees. This means that in the case of new assignments the supervisor will consult with the employees as to how the job should best be done. Their contributions to the decision are elicited. In those directives which are primarily concerned with routine assignments and the daily performance of the job, the supervisor will employ a form of general supervision instead of close supervision. In so doing, the supervisor gives the employees the freedom to make their own decisions on how the job is to be done, after the goals and standards to be achieved have been set. This also gives employees the freedom to use their own ingenuity and judgment, and experiences of this type offer continuous ground for further training and improvement. In addition, it motivates employees to the extent that they find satisfaction in their jobs. All indications are that general supervision produces better results than close supervision.

Since the health care field is dynamic, necessitating continuous and often substantial changes, the supervisor is confronted with the problem of how to introduce change. To successfully cope with the average employees' normal resistance to change, the supervisor must realize that there are social, psychological, and possibly economic reasons for this resistance. By involving employees in change discussions and decisions the various types of resistance can be overcome. In the final analysis, the supervisor is in the front line, and it is his or her responsibility to accommodate change and make it become reality.

20

Motivation

Clearly, influencing is a crucial function, the one that deals most intimately with the human being. Thus, to understand this function we must understand something about what makes the human being tick, what motivates a person, and more basically what underlies a person's motivations. Motivation is the force that arouses, moves, energizes, directs, and sustains human behavior. It is important for contemporary managers to understand the basic motivational processes. This knowledge will enable them to deal better with their employees and environment. Understanding motivation will facilitate the achievements of high levels of job satisfaction and job performance.

Theories of Motivation

Motivation has been a major concern for managers and psychologists, and many theories* have been developed explaining how people are motivated. There are a number of different ways to interpret the concept of motivation; two of the major categories of contemporary motivation theories are the content theory and the process theory.

Content theory centralizes on the question of what it is that moves, energizes, and starts behavior of an individual. This theory discusses the concept of needs or motives that drive people and the incentives that cause people to behave in a particular manner. Three of the most publicized content theories of motivation are Maslow's hierarchy of needs; McClelland's achievement, affiliation, and power needs; and Herzberg's two-factors approach of satisfiers and dissatisfiers. Each of these three content theories tries to explain individual behavior from a slightly different perspective.

Process theories try to provide a theory of why people choose a particular behavior to accomplish a goal. Equity and expectancy are the two

---

*For more details see Richard M. Steers, *Introduction to Organizational Behavior* (Santa Monica, Calif.: Goodyear Publishing Co., Inc., 1981), 51-77, 149-177; Kae H. Chung, *Motivational Theories and Practices* (Columbus, Ohio: Grid, Inc., 1977); Terence R. Mitchell, *People in Organizations*, 2nd ed. (New York: McGraw-Hill Book Co., 1982); Keith Davis, *Human Behavior at Work: Organizational Behavior*, 6th ed. (New York: McGraw-Hill Book Co., 1981).

major process theories. The first approach stresses the equity of effort in relation to the results, and the other theory emphasizes the importance of the likelihood of success of the expected results.

Model of Motivational Processes

A generalized and oversimplified model of basic motivational processes is presented in Figure 20-1. This model shows four basic parts of the process: (1) needs, (2) desires, expectations, perception, values, attitudes; (3) behavior; (4) goals; and (5) feedback. At any point in time individuals are likely to have a mixture of needs, desires, and expectations. For instance, one subordinate may have a strong need for achievement and a desire to earn more money; this person expects that doing the job well will lead to the desired rewards. This expectation is likely to cause behavior that is directed toward specific goals. Achieving the goals serves as feedback on the impact of this behavior and reassures this individual that the behavior is correct; it satisfies the needs and expectations. Or it may tell the person that the present course of action is incorrect and should be altered. This model of motivation obviously is oversimplified because it does not take into account all influences on motivation; however, it shows the basic cyclical nature of the process. People are forever restlessly striving to satisfy a variety of needs and expectations, and the success of one effort triggers the pursuit of another need and desire. Once one need has been met, another need or desire emerges and stimulates further action.

Figure 20-1. Model of the motivational process.

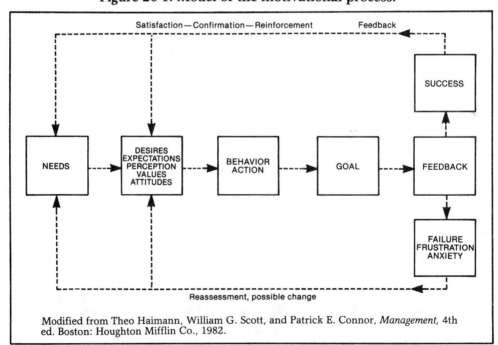

Modified from Theo Haimann, William G. Scott, and Patrick E. Connor, *Management*, 4th ed. Boston: Houghton Mifflin Co., 1982.

Maslow's Hierarchy of Human Needs

One of the approaches to employee motivation is based on individual human needs. Every action is motivated by unsatisfied needs. These unsatisfied needs cause humans to behave in a certain manner and to try to achieve certain goals in hopes of reducing the tensions that arise from unmet needs. A person eats because hunger creates the need for food. Someone else has a strong need for achievement and strives for advancement within his or her field of work. In other words, there is a reason for everything that people do. People are always striving to attain something that has meaning to them in terms of their own particular needs. It is often observed that humans never seem satisfied. They are continuously fulfilling needs. After the successful fulfillment of one need, they will start on another round of pursuits. Indeed, we can say that life is a process in which needs constantly arise and demand satisfaction.

Probably the most widely known and accepted theory of needs and motivations is the model designed by Abraham H. Maslow.* He developed a model consisting of *deficiency needs* and *growth needs*. Deficiency needs are those needs which must be satisfied if the individual is to be healthy and secure. These are the physiological needs for food, water, clothing, shelter, etc.; needs for safety; and the feeling of belonging, love, and respect from others. Growth needs refer to development and achievement of one's potential. We should not think that all needs are of the same order of importance, however. There are many different kinds of needs, and some produce stronger motivation or demand more immediate satisfaction than others. Maslow suggests that these needs are arranged in a hierarchy. (See Figure 20-2.)

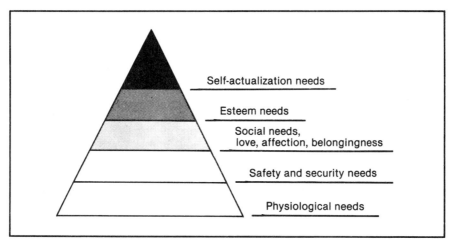

Figure 20-2. Hierarchy of needs.

*Abraham H. Maslow, "Theory of Human Motivation," *Psychological Review* 50 (1943): 370-396; Abraham H. Maslow, *Toward a Psychology of Being,* 2nd ed. (New York: Van Nostrand, 1968); Abraham H. Maslow, *Motivation and Personality,* 2nd ed. (New York: Harper & Row, Publishers, Inc., 1970), Chapter 4.

Maslow's model contains five levels of needs that can be visualized as forming a pyramid. The most basic needs are *physiological needs.* These are the biological needs that everyone has for food, shelter, rest, recreation, and so on. Normally, wages and salary enable an individual to obtain the necessities and comforts of life that are vital to fulfilling these physiological needs.

When the physiological needs are reasonably satisfied, needs at the next higher level begin to dominate. These are usually called *safety needs.* The second level stresses the needs for a safe physical and emotional environment. They are the needs we have for protection against danger and threat. Such needs are natural reactions to insecurity. We all desire more control over and protection from the uncertainties of life. In a work environment, these uncertainties would produce safety needs caused by fear of arbitrary management action, loss of job, favoritism, discrimination, unpredictable administration of policy, and so on. Most enterprises today offer various programs that are designed to satisfy and fulfill these safety or security needs. For example, most enterprises have medical and other insurance plans, provisions for retirement benefits, provisions for unemployment compensation, seniority, etc.

Once the physiological and safety needs are satisfied, *social and belongingness needs* become important motivators. Social needs consist of belonging, association, acceptance by one's peers, and giving and receiving friendship and love. These needs are often identical with the needs people have for a feeling of group identity, being part of a group, and being accepted and respected by their peers. A supervisor must be aware of the existence of these needs, which can be fulfilled by the organization's informal groups. As we know, tightly knit, cohesive work groups will generally enable employees to gain greater on-the-job satisfaction and produce a better climate for motivation. This is why the supervisor should look at the positive aspects and strengths of informal groups. Often supervisors incorrectly go to great trouble to control and interfere with the natural "grouping" tendency of human beings. This is ill advised. When a person's social needs are thwarted and frustrated, this individual will behave in ways that are likely to hurt organizational objectives. The manager should always realize that social needs are fulfilled to a large extent by informal groups and informal organization, as discussed in Chapter 15.

Once the first three needs, also known as *deficiency needs,* have been satisfied, people will generally attempt to satisfy *growth needs.* These are the needs for esteem and self-actualization.

Esteem needs focus on one's desire to have a worthy self-image and receive recognition from others. The needs for *esteem* are both self-esteem and esteem from others. Self-esteem includes the need for self-confidence, independence, achievement, competence, and knowledge. These needs are often fulfilled by mastery over part of the environment, for instance, by knowing that you can accomplish a certain task. But a person also needs the esteem and recognition of others for his or her accomplishments. These needs relate to reputation, need for status, recognition, appreciation, and the deserved respect of colleagues. Many jobs in industrial settings offer little opportunity for satisfaction of such needs. Most positions in the health care field are much more conducive to the achievement of these needs. Of course, it is desirable that both aspects of the need for esteem are fulfilled. Frequently, however, the esteem of self comes before esteem from others.

The highest level of needs is the need for *self-actualization, self-fulfillment,* or *self-realization.* These are the needs for realizing one's own potentials, continued self-development, being creative in the broadest sense of the term. It has often been said that this is the need "to become what one is capable of becoming." Unlike the other four needs, which probably will be satisfied, self-actualization is only seldom fully achieved. It is a process of becoming, and as one gradually approaches self-fulfillment this process is intensified and sustained. Conditions of modern life give many people little opportunity to fulfill this need. Most employees are continuously struggling to satisfy the lower needs; they must divert most of their energy to satisfy them. Therefore, the need for self-fulfillment frequently remains dormant and unfulfilled.

It is interesting that there seems to be a relationship between the hierarchy of needs and age. Physiological and safety needs are paramount in the life of an infant. As a child grows up, love needs become more important. When the adolescent reaches young adulthood, needs for esteem seem to dominate the field. If the person is successful in life, then the move to self-actualization later in life is likely. Such a step does not necessarily follow because pressing circumstances may arrest the route of progress at the esteem level or at lower levels. And, as we shall see later, this situation is often the basis of conflict between organizational and individual goals.

Maslow's hierarchy of needs has been and still is popular among and appealing to managers. Since it is the supervisor's job to create a climate in which employees can satisfy the multitude of needs, this theory makes clear recommendations to management. Some of the specific dynamics of Maslow's theory may still be in question; nevertheless, Maslow's hierarchy was the first clear statement urging managers to recognize the importance of higher order needs. It caused a shift from the traditional lower order motivators to higher motivators. It is likely that most healthy and normal employees have satisfied the lower order deficiency needs (they are not hungry, feel reasonably secure, and have sufficient social relationships); therefore, supervisors should emphasize a working climate conducive to satisfying the higher order growth needs. That means supervisors should stress some variety of duties, delegation of authority, autonomy, and responsibility so that employees can more fully realize their potential, their growth needs.

McClelland's Needs

David McClelland's research* in organizational behavior led to what he has termed and is now commonly known as *need for achievement (n Ach),*

*D. C. McClelland, J. W. Atkinson, R. A. Clark, and E. L. Lowell, *The Achievement Motive* (New York: Appleton-Century-Crofts, 1953); D. C. McClelland, *The Achieving Society* (Princeton, N.J.: Van Nostrand, 1961); D. C. McClelland, "Toward a Theory of Motive Acquisition," *American Psychologist* 20 (1965): 321-325; D. C. McClelland, *Power: The Inner Experience* (New York: Irvington Publishers, Inc., 1979); D. C. McClelland, "Power Is the Great Motivation," *Harvard Business Review,* Vol. 54, No. 2 (1976): 100-110.

need for affiliation (n Aff), and the *need for power (n Pow).* The n Ach is a need for personal challenge and accomplishment. It involves the desire to assume personal responsibility and pursue reasonably difficult goals, a preoccupation with the task, and feedback as to accomplishment. This n Ach can be learned from early childhood on and can be taught to adults. McClelland defines it as "behavior toward competition with a standard of excellence." The need for affiliation is the need for human companionship, support, and reassurance. People with a strong n Aff look for approval and reassurance from others, are willing to conform to the norms and wishes of others, and are sincerely interested in the feelings of others. The third need is the need for power, or need for dominance. It is a need to influence others and to lead and control them.

Levels of Aspiration

A person's level of aspiration is closely related to the hierarchy of needs. An individual's level of aspiration causes his goals to shift as various needs are satisfied. That is, once the needs on one level are satisfied, there is a tendency for the individual to aspire to higher levels. Suppose an individual is highly motivated by the need for achievement, and attitudes and personality cause this person to look for satisfaction of the need by working as a nurse in a health care center. Such a person will not be satisfied for any length of time by a low-level supervisory position. Once the position has been attained, this individual is likely to strive for the next higher position, for instance, assistant director of nursing service. After achieving the top position within the service, the objectives may shift to higher positions within the overall administration of the hospital; for instance, this person may seek to become an associate administrator or even the chief administrator. Or the objectives may shift to something outside the hospital, such as governmental activities that present possibilities for the satisfaction of the achievement needs. This endless search for alternatives to satisfy increasing aspirations is an important aspect of human motivation. If an organization can provide an individual with a wider range of need satisfactions, this person's commitment to the organization will be greater.

Herzberg's Two-Factor Motivation-Hygiene Theory

Another approach to motivation seen as a need classification system was developed by Frederick Herzberg.* Herzberg, a psychologist, has done a great deal of research on job satisfaction and developed a number of conditions on which satisfaction is based. He distinguishes between those factors in the work situation which are unlikely to motivate employees (hygiene factors) and those which tend to motivate employees (motivators). In essence he states that the hygiene rewards or outcome satisfy what is commonly known as

---

*Frederick Herzberg, "New Approaches in Management Organization and Job Design" in *Industrial Medicine and Surgery* 31, No. 11 (November, 1962): 477-481.

lower order needs, whereas the motivators satisfy higher order needs. Herzberg identified the following as hygiene factors and another group as motivators:

Hygiene Factors	*Motivators*
The organization's policy and administration	Achievement
Technical supervision	Recognition
Salary	Work itself
Interpersonal supervision	Responsibility
Working conditions	Advancement

He measures satisfiers and dissatisfiers in terms of the frequency with which they appear and the duration of the period during which they produce either a significant improvement or reduction in job satisfaction. (See Figure 20-3.) The five hygiene factors are environmental. When they are at an unacceptable level, dissatisfaction will occur. When they are at an acceptable level, satisfaction results. The factors most frequently involved in events causing job dissatisfaction (dissatisfiers) are company policy and administration, supervision, salary, interpersonal relations, and working conditions. When these factors are negative or lacking, they are considered to be dissatisfiers. Even when they are positive and appropriate, these factors do not tend to motivate people; it is almost as if they are expected. When positive, they are *satisfiers*. This, however, does not mean that these factors are unimportant. They are essential because their fulfillment or absence is either satisfying or dissatisfying.

If managers really want motivated employees, they should use *motivators*. Herzberg's study indicates that the most frequently mentioned factors in improved job satisfaction are achievement, recognition, work itself, responsibility, and advancement. These are the factors which, if present, truly motivate people. It is the opportunity for advancement, greater responsibility, the possibility of promotion, growth, achievement, and interesting work that make a job challenging, meaningful, and really motivating to subordinates. Such factors are obviously associated with the higher order needs of people.

Herzberg's findings have important implications for the supervisor. Although management strives for good organizational "hygiene" through sound wage administration, enlightened supervision, pleasant working conditions, appropriate fringe benefits, and so forth, these factors alone normally do not produce a motivational climate. If properly fulfilled, we merely minimize dissatisfaction; but they are not motivators. What is actually required, therefore, is a two-way effort that is directed first at the hygiene factors and then at the development of motivation. In addition to the need to avoid unpleasantness that comes from largely dissatisfying conditions, the supervisor must produce positive motivation through a more sophisticated set of factors, which is closely related to the concept of self-actualization. Although it is difficult to apply these motivators in many jobs, most positions in the health care setting provide ample opportunity to stress them.

Figure 20-3. Factors affecting job satisfaction.

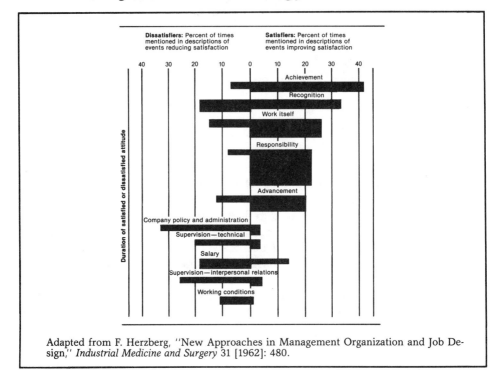

Adapted from F. Herzberg, "New Approaches in Management Organization and Job Design," *Industrial Medicine and Surgery* 31 [1962]: 480.

Perceptions, Values, and Attitudes

As we have said, all human behavior is motivated by unsatisfied needs. These needs spring from causes that are deep within the person and, together with other motives, attitudes, and behaviors, form the configuration usually called the *personality*. From this point of view, motivations that contribute to personality can be defined as a potential to act in order to satisfy those needs which are not met. The term *potential to act* implies that some motives are stronger than others and hence more likely to produce action. The strength of motivation is determined by the strength of a particular need, the probability that the act required to satisfy that need will be successful and the rewards forthcoming. Obviously, an individual is more likely to act if the motive is stronger and if the probability for success is high and the reward is significant.

But other factors are also involved in producing human behavior or action. Motives do not stand alone. Closely related to them and significantly affecting their strength are *perceptions, values,* and *attitudes*.

We are constantly subjected to a large number of stimuli from our environment; all of them compete for our attention. In our daily working environment there are noises, sights, sounds, smells, supervisors' instructions, physicians' directives, co-workers' remarks, paging over the loudspeaker, people walking by, phones ringing, posted signs, and so on. All of these and many more vie for our attention. The individual therefore has the problem of how to make sense out of all of them, how to organize and interpret the more important ones, and how to respond to them.* *Perception* is the process by which this is done; it is the process by which the individual screens, selects, organizes, and interprets them so that an appropriate response can be made. This does not necessarily lead to an accurate portrayal of the environment, but to a unique picture, influenced by the perceiver's needs, desires, values, disposition, and frame of reference. It is a personal construction for which the individual has selected certain objects for a major role perceived in an individual manner.

Through the process of *perceptual selectivity* certain of these stimuli catch our attention and are selected, whereas others are screened out. Once a particular object has been noticed by individuals, then they attempt to make sense out of it by organizing it according to their frame of reference and needs. This is known as the process of *perceptual organization.* Once meaning has been attached to a certain stimulus, the individual can reach an appropriate response. A number of *barriers* to accurate perception of others, however, can enter into these perceptual processes. Examples of barriers are the frame of reference, stereotyping, the halo effect, biases, perceptual defense, etc. (See Chapters 5 and 17.) All of the perceptual processes affect our attitudes and behavior at work.

Attitudes and values also play a role in all behavior. Attitudes are different from values. *Values* are broader, general, more encompassing concepts than attitudes; for example, most of us value freedom and equality. Our values of equality can be translated into our attitude toward minority groups. "Besides being broader, values carry with them an 'oughtness' component. They are frequently defined as ideas about how everyone *should* feel or behave."†

Attitude can be seen as "*a predisposition to respond in a favorable or unfavorable way* to objects, persons, concepts, or whatever."* It is the way an individual tends to interpret, understand, or define a situation or relationship with others. Attitudes constitute one's feelings about something, an individual's likes and dislikes directed toward persons, things, situations, or a combination of all three. Attitudes are more than casual opinions, since they are heavily charged with emotional overtones. Attitudes may include feelings, as well as intellectual elements. They also include evaluations and value judgments. Attitudes differ in kind, strength, and the extent to which they are open or hidden. Basically, they are revealed in two ways: either by the individual's expressed statements or behavior. An individual may express dislike for the hospital he or she works for or may merely demonstrate this attitude by being absent excessively. Although we cannot see perceptions, values, and attitudes, their consequences can be observed in the behavior.

---

*Much of this is based on Richard M. Steers, *Introduction to Organizational Behavior* (Santa Monica, Calif.: Goodyear Publishing Co., Inc., 1981), 97-124.

†Terence R. Mitchell, *People in Organizations*, 2nd ed. (New York: McGraw-Hill Book Co., 1982), pp. 127-128.

Factors Determining Attitudes

There are an infinite number of factors that determine and influence an individual's attitudes. A major influence is a person's *biological,* or *physiological, makeup.* Such factors as sex, age, height, race, weight, and physique are important in determining the attitudes that contribute to overall personality structure. In addition, many psychologists believe that the very early years of life are crucial to attitudinal development. Freudian psychologists, in particular, believe that early childhood is the most critical period of all in what a person actually becomes. This theory is often referred to as *childhood determinism;* it maintains that such factors as feeding patterns, training patterns, and home conditions in early childhood are the primary determinants of personality structure.

Another area that influences a person's attitudes and personality is his immediate *environment.* Factors such as education, employment, income, and many other experiences which confront an individual as he or she goes through life will influence what this person is and eventually becomes. Furthermore, one should never forget that the *broader culture* of our society also influences a person's attitudes. In this country, we believe in competition, reward for accomplishment, equal opportunities, and other values that are part of our democratic capitalistic society. Individuals learn from their early years to strive for achievement, think for themselves, and work hard and that these are roads for success. All such cultural influences affect a person's attitudes and thus behavior. Of course, an infinite number of other factors also influence attitudes and personality. We have only touched on the more obvious ones.

Attitudes and Behavior

No matter what factors have caused their development, however, attitudes become deep-seated attributes of the individual's makeup. They are learned and acquired through all life's experiences. As stated above, they do not have to be rational or logical. Attitudes tend to last for a long time. We hold firmly to our attitudes and resist forces that attempt to interfere with them. Attitudes can change, but they change very slowly. Attitudes do not exist only within individuals, but are also generated within groups. In the discussion of informal organizations, it was stated that often individuals gladly accept as their own the attitudes of the group to which they belong.

Needs and motives do not stand alone as determinants of behavior. They are also influenced by the underlying attitudes and values of a person. This is shown in Figure 20-1. Indeed, we can say that *values and attitudes will determine the route a person takes for the satisfaction of his or her needs.* Although basically the same needs appear in every person, an individual's attitudes will vary greatly and will affect his or her unique responses to his or her needs. In other words, attitudes help determine what motivates a person to take a certain action in order to fulfill a certain need. For example, many people may have a strong need for achievement. But differing attitudes and values will motivate one individual to seek fulfillment of need by working in a hospital, another by working in a government agency, another by working in industry, and a fourth person may seek fulfillment by teaching in a university or going into politics.

Motivation vs. Frustration

If the individual's chosen route results in goal accomplishment, the need will be satisfied and the attitudes reinforced. In other words, accomplishment of the goal works as "feedback" to let the individual know that the needs are satisfied and the attitudes are reinforced. What happens, however, if the chosen course of action does not result in goal accomplishment? What happens when we wish to pursue a certain course of action but are prevented from doing so? This obstruction may be caused externally or internally.

Generally, actions that do not succeed in obtaining goals result in blocked satisfactions, frustration, and anxiety. As shown in Figure 20-1, feedback notifies the individual that his or her needs are not being fulfilled. In other words, there is stress: frustration and anxiety instead of need satisfaction. Basically, there are five ways in which people commonly resolve the problems of conflict and frustration. The best way is problem-solving behavior, but there are also other methods, such as resignation, detour behavior, retreat, or aggression.

Problem-solving behavior is usually the most desirable way of meeting frustration. It is advantageous if a person can look at personal problems objectively and base his or her decisions on reasoned analysis of the situation. Unfortunately, many people are not capable of doing this and it is the supervisor's duty to help the employees learn problem-solving behavior. Suppose, for instance, that an LPN is eager to advance to a better position, but all better positions demand the RN degree as a prerequisite. Of course, the LPN is frustrated because she is beating her head against a wall. In this instance, reasoned analysis of the situation and a thorough discussion with her supervisor could encourage the LPN to go to school and obtain the RN degree, which will enable her to move up within the hierarchy of nursing services. Such a route would constitute intelligent problem-solving behavior.

Another way to solve a conflict situation is by *resignation*. Suppose the same LPN were to say to herself, "What else can I do? I have to stick it out." She seems resigned to her lot. She will keep on working for the hospital but may no longer consider herself a part of it. Once an employee has given up in the face of obstacles, it is difficult to build up morale to the point where hospital and departmental goals are really important. Some employees simply stay on the job listlessly until they are able to retire. Such employees who have resigned themselves to their lot are usually passive and resistant to change. They are difficult for the supervisor to deal with because new ideas do not excite or stimulate them. Hopefully, the supervisor can help such subordinates use problem-solving methods of reasoned analysis and objective evaluation. If, however, the supervisor does not succeed in this respect, the boss may try to restimulate the employee to strive either for old goals or toward some new and desirable goals. The supervisor knows that the result of resignation is usually inferior performance on the job, lowering of morale, and a climate that is not conducive to the best performance of the department.

A third way to solve a frustrating situation is to resort to *detour behavior.* Since the direct way of reaching the goal is barred, the employee will try to find another way to get there. Such detours, however, are often obscure and sometimes devious. For example, one kind of detour behavior is self-induced illness. Children learn early in life that being sick gives them an acceptable excuse for getting out of doing an unpleasant task. Similarly, employees will often have painful and real physical disorders to evade a conflict situation. Of course, some people can stand conflict and frustration better than others. But sooner or later the strain begins to tell, and some sort of conflict resolution is necessary.

Leaving the field (retreat) is a fourth way to meet the problems of conflict and frustration. Most people at one time or another have looked at their jobs and have wished that they could quit right there and then. They may believe that they are not getting the satisfaction they thought the position would bring, that no one realizes the difficulties involved in the job, that their supervisor does not appreciate all the things they are doing, and so on. Certainly, in most people's lives there are occasions when feelings of this sort prevail. And in many instances, an employee does quit the job and take another position, possibly even in another town. Whether this reaction to frustration is good or bad, however, will depend on the major source of the conflict and frustration. If the major source is in the employee's personality and the conflict does not stem from the working situation, then, of course, leaving the field would not be the right answer. In other words, if the frustration is due to the person's own peculiar psychological makeup, such a change probably will not bring about the desired result. If, however, the conflict is because of an unfavorable work situation, then leaving the field, quitting, or even leaving the city may represent a real solution to the problem. Often it is difficult for the individual to determine whether or not this is the case. Of course, it is not always necessary to quit the job or move to another city in order to "leave the field." Leaving the field may show itself simply by "daydreaming," spending a lot of time in the washroom, a high rate of absenteeism, alcoholism and drug abuse, or some other form of symbolic escape. Obviously, all of these forms of leaving the field will cause the supervisor additional problems.

Aggression is the fifth way in which people may meet the problem of severe frustration. Sabotage, for example, is one common form of aggressive behavior. By aggression we mean not only hostile behavior aimed at harming other people or inanimate objects, but also merely the tendency to commit acts of aggression. This tendency may manifest itself in thoughts or words or even in feelings that have not as yet been put into words. The supervisor should always remember that frustration and aggression are closely tied together and that all aggressions stem from some kind of frustration. Of course, as we have said, some individuals can stand more frustration than others and are not as easily moved into aggressive behavior. Moreover, many minor frustrations that could lead to aggressive behavior do not because we hold back and inhibit them. Obviously, the job of the supervisor is to see that frustration is minimized. The supervisor should try to anticipate the sources of frustration and attempt to eliminate them. If this cannot be done, however, then the best the supervisor can do is see that the causes of frustration are not aggravated. Often patient listening will help to ease employee tensions, and it may enable the subordinate to seek the real source of the frustration. Or a good counseling interview may also alleviate a frustrating situation.

Conflicts Between Individual and Organizational Goals

Although there are many causes of frustration, a major cause arises when individual needs and goals conflict rather than coincide with those of the organization or, to be more specific, with those of the department. Much has been written about the conflict between the individual who seeks activity and independence and the climate in a bureaucratic formalized organization that stifles a person's natural desire for freedom and self-determination. The consequences of such a climate manifest themselves in high turnover, waste, lower productivity, slowdown, lack of innovative and creative behavior, non-acceptance of leadership, and so on. The most serious consequence of a bureaucratic organization, however, is that it blocks the individual from attaining satisfaction of his or her needs. In this day and age, administrators are becoming more aware of these consequences and of the necessity for an organization to provide a climate that will enable those who work within it to find personal satisfaction. In fact, the need for an appropriate organizational climate is increasing because of the rising expectations of employees. This is especially true in the health care field where we are confronted with an ever-advancing and more sophisticated area of activity. The highly skilled and educated employees are to a large degree professionals, who expect to fulfill a multitude of their needs right on the job. Since such employees tend to take high wages and appropriate fringe benefits for granted, it should be apparent that the key to long-term motivation for them rests in the satisfaction of the higher level needs, that is, their esteem and self-fulfillment needs. It is management's duty to develop an organizational climate that will produce effective motivation and satisfaction of these needs, thereby helping to resolve the conflict between individual and organizational goals. Therefore, the supervisor's knowledge of the basic motivational processes is necessary because it will facilitate high levels of job satisfaction and minimize conflicts.

Summary

Influencing is the managerial function in which the supervisor creates a climate that enables subordinates to find as much satisfaction as possible while getting the jobs done. Influencing is that function which is particularly concerned with behavioral responses and interpersonal relations. Only by appropriately influencing will the supervisor instill in the department's employees the motivation to go about their jobs with enthusiasm and also to find personal fulfillment of their needs. Therefore, it is necessary for supervisors to understand basic motivational processes.

This chapter deals with the concept of motivation, which is the force that arouses, energizes, directs, and sustains human behavior. Various approaches and developments in the study of motivation by psychologists were presented.

All human behavior is caused by unsatisfied needs. These needs eventually stimulate the formation of goals that motivate people to take certain actions. Motivation, however, is caused not only by unmet needs, but it is also largely influenced by an individual's perceptions, values, attitudes, and entire personality.

An individual's attitudes are formed beginning in early childhood. They affect and are affected by an infinite number of factors in the person's life. Attitudes will determine the individual route a person takes for the satisfaction of those needs. Although they vary in strength, most needs are basically the same in all people. Thus, Maslow speaks of a hierarchy of needs; in ascending order they are physiological, safety, social, esteem, and self-fulfillment. A person's level of aspiration is closely related to this hierarchy of needs.

Maslow's individual needs are arranged in a hierarchy and people generally move from one level to the next. McClelland focuses on describing various other human needs: achievement, affiliation, and power. Herzberg, in his two-factors approach, stresses the importance of motivators vs. hygiene factors; he shows that the more important forces of employee motivation lie in job-related factors and not hygiene factors.

A person who is able to understand his or her needs and attitudes fairly well will be able to choose courses of action that result in achievement of goals. Goal accomplishment serves as a feedback to the individual; the need is satisfied and the underlying attitudes are confirmed. If a goal is not attained, however, conflict often sets in. This is because action that does not succeed results in blocked satisfaction and frustration and anxiety. By and large, most people react to conflict and frustration in one of the five following ways: problem-solving behavior, resignation, detour behavior, retreat, or aggression.

It is the supervisor's duty to minimize frustrating situations, especially if these result from a conflict between individual and organizational goals. One way to minimize such conflict situations is to realize that in the work environment a number of factors influence the realization of an employee's expectations. Some of these factors are merely satisfiers and dissatisfiers (Herzberg's hygiene factors), whereas others are motivators and are able to fulfill the higher level needs and goals of people. These motivators include opportunity for advancement, greater responsibility, chance for promotion, growth and achievement, and an interesting and challenging job. Supervisors, in their desire to create a good organizational climate, must see to it that in addition to satisfying hygiene factors, as many of these motivators as possible are at work.

21

Leadership

Leadership is a most popular and important topic in organizational behavior. It is a key process in any organization, and an organization's success or failure is largely attributed to it. It is an essential component of the organizational climate; we have mentioned the term leadership on numerous occasions throughout this text, but merely in passing. Ultimately, management leadership is responsible for establishing the kind of climate that facilitates motivation and the successful performance of the influencing function.

The concept of leadership is controversial and not well understood; it is still being widely researched and investigated. It is of utmost importance because every organization is concerned with attracting and developing people who will be effective leaders. Leadership plays an important role in organizational life. It fills in many areas not covered by organizational design or manuals. It facilitates coordination and brings about organizational effectiveness.

We can define leadership as a process by which people are imaginatively directed, guided, and influenced in choosing and attaining goals. It is helpful to look at leadership in an organizational setting as something "one person does to influence others."* Leadership can also be defined as "the influential increment over and above mechanical compliance with the routine directives of the organization."† It is the process in which one person influences others to do something of their own free will, rather than of fear of the consequences if they do not do it or because they are forced to do it. This aspect is different from other processes, such as influence by authority or power. In any organized activity, a leader mediates between organizational and individual goals so that the degree of satisfaction to both is maximized. A manager, of course, also plays this mediating role but not necessarily in the same manner that a leader does. Although the terms manager and leader are often used interchangeably, leadership is not synonymous with managerial ability. A manager can do a reasonably good job of managing without being a

---

*Richard M. Steers, *Introduction to Organizational Behavior* (Santa Monica, Calif.: Goodyear Publishing Co., Inc., 1981), 253.

†D. Katz, and R. L. Kahn, *The Social Psychology of Organizations*, 2nd ed. (New York: John Wiley & Sons, Inc., 1978), 528.

leader. Since the manager's job is getting things done through people, it is obvious that a person who is also the leader of the employees will be a much more effective manager. But what enables a person to be a leader? What qualities are present in a leader, as well as a manager, and what other prerequisites must prevail?

Leadership Theories

Much has been written and said about leadership ever since the days of antiquity when emphasis was focused on the person as a leader to the exclusion of everything else. Many theories have been formulated as to what constitutes a good leader and what enables some people to be a leader and not others. We shall look at a few of these theories briefly.

The Early Genetic Theory

For hundreds of years observers recognized leadership as the ability to influence people in such a manner that they willingly strove toward an objective. It was believed that this ability was something apart from official position. It was held that certain people were born to be leaders, having inherited a set of unique traits or characteristics which could not be acquired in any other way. This view, also known as the "great man" theory of leadership, concluded that leadership was inherited simply because it emerged frequently within the same prominent families. In reality, however, strong class barriers made it impossible for anyone outside these families to acquire the skills and knowledge required to become a leader. This is when the approach in inherited leadership characteristics lost ground, although the significance of certain leadership traits remained in the picture.

The Trait Theory

As social and economic class barriers were broken down and leaders began to emerge from the so-called lower classes of society, the early genetic theory was modified. This modification was largely because beginning in the middle 1930s behavioral scientists began to contribute to the literature on leadership. The first contribution was made by writers who, rather than considering leadership only a function of inherited characteristics, held that it could also be acquired through experience, education, and training. Efforts were made to identify the traits great leaders throughout the ages had in common. These writers tried to focus on all the traits, whether inherited or acquired, that were found in individuals regarded as leaders. Lists of qualities that recognized leaders had in common were compiled. These traits frequently included physical and nervous energy, a sense of purpose and direction, willingness to accept the consequences, enthusiasm, friendliness and affection, integrity, technical mastery, decisiveness, assertiveness, initiative, intelligence, teaching skill, and faith.

The inadequacy of this approach soon became obvious, however. Seldom, if ever, did any two lists agree on the essential leadership characteristics. Furthermore, the lists were confusing because they used different terminology and had different numbers of characteristics. Nevertheless, the trait approach was widely accepted for a long time. It was extremely plausible because studies of various successful leaders almost always indicated many similar personality and character traits; however, the intensity and degree of the traits varied. Moreover, no satisfactory answer could be reached about which traits were most essential for leadership, or whether a person could be a leader if certain traits were lacking. Nor was there any suggestion of how to isolate and identify all the specific traits common to leaders. A further weakness of the trait approach was that it did not distinguish between those characteristics which were needed for acquiring leadership and those which were necessary for maintaining it.

Although the trait approach is partially discredited today, a considerable body of research shows that leaders *do* have in common certain general characteristics. Some of these are intelligence, communication ability, sensitivity to group needs, and those mentioned above. Such traits are interwoven in the personality of the leader, but they should always be considered relative to the situation and followers and members of the group. For example, the most intelligent person in the group will not necessarily emerge as the leader. Instead, the leader is more likely to be the person with the optimal combination of these traits for the particular situation of the group. Although the trait approach helped to a large measure in understanding leadership, one has to look farther than just personality traits.

The Situational Approach

Another major shortcoming of the trait approach is that it does not pay enough attention to the influence of situational factors and the nature of the followers. In their search for the "universal traits" of leaders, behavioral scientists discovered the importance of situational factors that make it easier for certain persons to acquire positions of leadership.* This approach, also known as the contingency model of leadership effectiveness, points out the interdependence between leadership style and the demands of the situation.

The proponents of the situational approach do not deny that the characteristics of individuals play an important part in leadership, but they point out that leadership is also the product of situations in particular groups. Leadership in one group will differ from leadership in another group; in one situation a certain person might evolve as the leader, whereas in a different situation someone else would emerge as the leader. For example, on a sinking boat a person with strong swimming ability may emerge as the leader, but in a

---

*Fred Edward Fiedler, *A Theory of Leadership Effectiveness* (New York: McGraw-Hill Book Co., 1967).

political meeting someone with good speaking ability may rise to the top. In other words, the leadership characteristics needed are a function of the specific situation in which the group finds itself.

In their desire to deemphasize the traits approach, however, some behavioral scientists may have gone overboard in emphasizing the situation. In so doing, they may have ruled out the possibility that at least some characteristics *predispose* people to attain leadership positions or at least increase their chances of becoming leaders; *both* characteristics and the situation are involved in the concept of leadership.

The Follower Approach

A still better understanding of leadership incorporates the function that groups and followers have to fulfill. This approach maintains that the followers must also be studied because essentially it is the follower who perceives the leader and the situation and accepts or rejects leadership. Proponents of this approach further maintain that it is the followers' persistent motives, point of view, and frame of reference that will determine what they perceive and how they react to it. The follower approach emphasizes the importance of the group situation at a particular point in time, but does not fail to take into consideration the fact that certain characteristics will help one person emerge as the leader rather than another person. The satisfaction of the followers' needs is an important aspect, however.

More specifically, the group and follower approach stresses the idea that the leadership function must be analyzed and understood in terms of a dynamic relationship, a social exchange process between the leader and the followers. They bring to the situation their personalities, needs, motivations, and expectations. The leader appears to the followers as the best means available for the satisfaction of their needs, whether those needs are emotive or task oriented. The group members will follow the leader because they see in that person the means for personal fulfillment. A leader is essential for influencing a group to act as a unit to move toward task accomplishment. The members look at this individual as their leader not only because he or she possesses certain characteristics, such as intelligence, skill, drive, and ambition, but also because of his or her functional relationship to the members of the group.

Of course, a leader may also arise in the reverse fashion. Instead of answering groups needs, the leader's own personal need satisfaction may cause him or her to seek out leadership of the group. That is, the leader may want to accomplish an objective which can only be attained if he or she can direct the activities of other people. This situation is more typical of a manager formally appointed to a managerial position within an organization.

Conclusions

All three variables play a role in the leadership process: personal characteristics, the situation, and the followers. The leader is an individual perceived in harmony with the needs of the group and responsive to the group situation. But because leaders must always be recognized as such by group consensus and because managers who are appointed do not necessarily reflect subordinate group choice, they are not generally regarded as leaders at the outset. They may become true leaders of the group but they do not start out as such. Obviously, it is desirable from an influencing standpoint that subordinates quickly accept the manager as a leader and not merely as the head of their department.

Leadership Style

Leadership style is of utmost importance because it influences acceptance of managers by subordinates. Generally, leadership styles can be classified into three broad categories: autocratic, democratic, and free rein.

Autocratic Leadership (Theory X)

Autocratic leadership usually reflects tight supervision, a high degree of centralization, and a narrow span of supervision. The autocratic style is repressive and normally withholds communication other than that which is absolutely necessary for doing the job. Autocratic management makes decisions unilaterally and does not consult with the members of the department. Therefore, the autocratic style of leadership minimizes the degree of involvement by subordinates.

In more specific terms, autocratic leadership is described by Douglas McGregor as Theory X.* According to McGregor, a manager who fits into Theory X leans toward an organizational climate of close control, centralized authority, authoritarian practices, and minimal participation of the subordinates in the decision-making process. As we already know, the reason why a Theory X manager accepts this combination is that he or she makes certain assumptions about human behavior. Theory X assumptions, according to McGregor, are as follows:

(1) The average person dislikes work and will avoid it to the extent he or she can.
(2) Most people have to be forced or threatened by punishment to make the effort necessary to accomplish organizational goals.
(3) The average individual is basically passive and therefore prefers to be directed, rather than take any risk or responsibility. Above all else he or she prefers security.

---

*Douglas McGregor, *The Human Side of Enterprise* (New York: McGraw-Hill Book Co., 1960), Chapters 3 and 4.

Democratic Leadership (Theory Y)

The democratic style emphasizes a looser kind of supervision and greater individual participation in the decision-making process. Authority is delegated as far down as possible, and a wide span of management is advocated. A free flow of communication is encouraged among all members of the department so that a climate of trust and confidence can be established.

In McGregor's terms, the democratic style is represented by Theory Y. The Theory Y manager operates with a completely different set of assumptions regarding human motivation. He maintains that an effective organizational climate utilizes more general supervision, greater decentralization of authority, little reliance on coercion and control, democratic techniques, and consultation with subordinates on departmental decisions. The assumptions on which this type of organizational climate is based include the following:

(1) Work is as natural to humans as play or rest and, therefore, it is not avoided.

(2) Self-motivation and inherent satisfaction in work will be forthcoming when the individual is committed to organizational goals; therefore, coercion is not the only form of influence that can be used to motivate.

(3) Commitment is a crucial factor in motivation, and it is a function of the rewards coming from it.

(4) The average individual learns to accept and even seek responsibility given the proper environment.

(5) The ability to be creative and innovative in the solution of organizational problems is widely, not narrowly, distributed in the population.

(6) In modern businesses and organizations the intellectual potentials of employees are only partially utilized.

McGregor underscores the notion that Theories X and Y are beliefs held by management about the nature of humans. As such, they constitute the foundation on which the organizational climate is built. The supervisor who follows Theory X has a basically limited view of people and their capabilities. He or she believes that individuals must be controlled, closely supervised, and motivated on the bases of money, discipline, and authority. Thus, the autocratic manager believes that the key to motivation is in the proper implementation of approaches designed to satisfy the lower level needs of people.

The Theory Y supervisor, however, has a much different opinion of the capabilities and possibilities of people. He or she believes that if the proper approach and conditions can be presented, people will exercise self-direction and self-control toward the accomplishment of objectives. The Theory Y manager recognizes that the supervisor's activities must fit into the scheme of each employee's own set of needs. He or she also believes that the higher level needs of people are more important in terms of personality and self-development.* Thus, the supervisory skills are used to try to enable employees to achieve on the job at least partial satisfaction of their needs for esteem and self-actualization.

Of course, this confronts the supervisor with the question as to which management philosophy and organizational climate will produce the best results. On the surface one is inclined to say that Theory Y would be more desirable than Theory X because it appears humanistic and less harsh. Also it is more optimistic about human motives at work.

Theory Z Approach

A different managerial approach that has been widely discussed lately is the Theory Z approach, influenced by practices in the Japanese industry. The success of the Japanese industry in respect to productivity and quality has been attributed to a managerial philosophy about people and organizations that is different from ours.† The Japanese organizational climate is based on lifetime employment, slow evaluation and promotion paths, nonspecialized careers, consensual decision making, collective responsibility, informal controls, and a holistic concern toward the firm. This is contrary to many current practices in the United States, such as short-run employment expectations, rapid evaluation and promotions, specialized careers, individual decision making and responsibility, and explicit controls. Theory Z is an approach that would incorporate some of the Japanese ideas into our present system as a possibility for increasing productivity and job satisfaction. Quality Circles discussed in Chapter 19 are an outgrowth of the Japanese approach to management.

Free-Rein Leadership

The free-rein style goes beyond democratic leadership and Theory Y. It is often called *laissez-faire leadership* because the climate of the organization is such that people are left almost entirely alone to do their jobs. On the assumption that individuals are self-motivated, a minimal amount of supervision is imposed. Although the manager is available as a consultant to help out if need be, the individuals have enough authority to provide their own solutions.

---

*For those who would like to read more about theories of changing organizational climates: Rensis Likert, *The Human Organization* (New York: McGraw-Hill Book Co., 1967), 14-24 and 120-121; also see Robert R. Blake and Jane Srygley Mouton, *The New Managerial Grid* (Houston: Gulf Publishing Co., 1978.)

†William G. Ouchi and Alfred M. Jaeger, "Type Z Organization: Stability in the Midst of Mobility," *Academy of Management Review* 3 (April 1978): 305-314; William G. Ouchi, *Theory Z: How American Business Can Meet the Japanese Challenge* (Reading, MA: Addison-Wesley Publishing Co., 1981).

Making a Choice

Obviously, no single leadership style is appropriate for all situations. A leader must be able to call on a whole range of responses. A good manager knows when to use one or another style of leadership. Obviously, each of these three styles has a place in the practice of management. Free-rein is probably the most useful in an organization of professional people who desire and have shown the capacity for independent work. This would apply, for instance, to research scientists, professors, and so on. The democratic style seems to be appropriate when a relatively unfettered environment is necessary under which skilled and educated people seem to thrive. This would probably include most activities performed in any health care center. It would be wrong to state, however, that a democratic leadership style is beneficial for all organizations, regardless of the nature of their activities and skill levels of their employees. In some situations, even the autocratic leadership style will produce good results, especially among unskilled subordinates who are poorly prepared to participate in decision making and who might be uncomfortable if urged to do so.

In conclusion, it is proper to state that leadership style must be adapted to each specific situation. It seems that in general a more democratic open style achieves greater leader acceptance than an autocratic one. Such a style is more humanistic and more optimistic, which also makes it more acceptable to most employees. In addition, much of the research evidence indicates that the Theory Y democratic leadership approach is more likely to achieve better results. Nevertheless, it is a sign of a good manager and a good leader to be able to utilize any one of these three techniques whenever the need or occasion arises. Employing the appropriate style will largely determine the degree to which the leader can influence others in the performance of a common task, and this is what leading is all about.

Leadership Roles

No matter which leadership style is chosen, it will require the manager to assume definite leadership roles. Most of us have had the occasion to observe individuals and the different roles they play in groups. One person may organize the group to achieve goals, whereas another plays the "devil's advocate," raising a stream of objections, and yet someone else is a "synthesizer" who puts together the ideas of all group members. These roles and many others are essential for group life. They fulfill the needs of the individual members of the group and are vital to the group's accomplishment. Of course, the group's leader is not expected to assume all of these roles, but he or she is expected to fulfill some of them. Generally, leadership roles fall into two broad classifications: task-oriented roles and emotive leadership roles.

Task-oriented roles are those used by the leader to organize and influence the group to achieve specified objectives. Usually in an organized activity these objectives are imposed on the group from above. In groups that arise spontaneously, however, tasks and objectives are generated from within the group itself. In both instances, the leader must facilitate the accomplishment of the group's goals. That is, the leader plays the role of getting the group to fulfill its tasks.

Emotive leadership roles are just as important as task roles. They are employee centered and provide satisfaction for the individual needs of the group's members. The emotional needs of people are of a social and psychological nature. A leader in the emotive role helps members of the group to gain satisfaction of these needs and at the same time prepares the way for task performance.

Frequently, the ideal leader is one who plays both roles effectively. But leadership of a group can be shared without diminishing the group's performance or morale. In such a case, one person plays the task role and another takes the emotive role. This would not be an unusual situation in a large institution. The formal organization of such an institution often forces a supervisor to be primarily concerned with getting the job done. He or she must concentrate largely on task leadership. Under these conditions, however, the groups will probably select another individual, the informal leader, who will function in the emotive role. The supervisor, of course, should not object to the informal leader's role. Rather, the supervisor should realize that it is a necessary part of the leadership process, one that fulfills important human needs and is an essential component of high employee morale. (See Chapter 22.)

Summary

Obviously leadership is a most important topic in organizational behavior. Leadership is a process by which one person tries to influence others in the performance of a common task; it is a process by which subordinates are imaginatively directed, guided, and influenced in choosing and attaining goals. One cannot equate the term leadership with that of management; a person does not have to be a leader to be an adequate manager, but it would be far more desirable if the supervisor of the department were also the leader.

Much research has been directed to the leadership phenomenon. The earlier genetic theory maintained that leadership was a function of specific characteristics with which a leader was born. Later the genetic approach was altered to state that leadership was a function of numerous personal traits which could be acquired, as well as inherited. More recent studies point out that the situation has a significant bearing on who emerges as a leader. Furthermore, the follower approach adds to the concept of leadership the importance of the perception of the followers and the group that they constitute. By and large, a person must be accepted by his group as a leader before he or she can actually function as one. Thus, it is important for each manager to adopt a leadership style that facilitates such acceptance.

There exist three broad categories of leadership style: autocratic (Theory X), democratic (Theory Y), and free-rein styles. Managers will use these styles in their efforts to emerge as a leader. A manager who is appointed to a position of organizational authority is not generally perceived as a leader at the outset. Hopefully, however, this person will emerge as a leader of the subordinates, thus becoming a much more effective manager as well.

In the leadership process it is necessary to fulfill both the task role, that is, influencing the group to achieve its goals, and the emotive role of satisfying the emotional needs of group members. If it is impossible for the leader to fulfill the emotive role, however, one should not object if an informal leader is chosen by the group to substitute for him or her in this role.

Although much about leadership remains to be studied, the research into this concept has given us a better understanding of the types of behavior needed in different settings and the importance of leadership for organizational effectiveness.

22

Morale

The supervisor's skill and understanding of motivation and leadership have a great bearing on the morale of the subordinates. Writers sometimes distinguish between morale and satisfaction; they connect satisfaction with an *individual's* needs and attitudes, whereas morale pertains to the spirit of a *group.* Although this distinction is precise, it is largely academic, since the factors and methods used in measuring group morale are usually the same as those used in measuring an individual's satisfaction.

The Meaning of Morale

Although there are many definitions for morale, a particularly useful one is to describe it as a state of mind and emotion affecting the attitudes, feelings, and sentiments of individuals and groups toward their work, environment, administration, and colleagues. Some writers do not speak of morale of the individual, but refer to job satisfaction, emphasizing the satisfaction of needs. Others stress the social aspects of groups and friendships, and some are particularly concerned with attitudes toward co-workers, the organization, and supervision. Morale is not a single feeling. It is a composite of feelings, satisfaction, sentiments, and attitudes. When morale is high, the employees are likely to strive hard to accomplish the objectives of the enterprise; conversely, low morale prevents or deters them from doing this.

The Nature of Morale

Supervisors often make the mistake of speaking of morale as something that is either present or absent among their employees. But morale is always present and by itself has neither favorable nor unfavorable meaning. Morale can range from excellent and positive through a large number of intermediate degrees to poor and completely negative. If the attitude of the subordinates is poor, then the morale is also poor; but if the subordinates' state of mind and emotion affecting their willingness and dedication to strive hard for the best possible patient care is high, then we speak of high morale. Employees with high morale find satisfaction in their position in the enterprise, have confidence in their own and associates' ability, and show enthusiasm and a strong desire for voluntary cooperation in achieving the hospital's objectives to the fullest extent of their ability.

But high morale of this type cannot be ordered. It can only be created by introducing certain conditions into the work situation that are favorable to its development. High morale is not the cause of good supervision and human relations; rather, it is the result of good motivation, respect and dignity of the individual, realization of individual differences, good leadership, effective communication, participation, counseling, and many other human relations practices. In other words, the state of morale will reflect how appropriately and effectively the administration practices good human relations and good supervision.

The Range of Morale

Every manager, from the top administrator down to the supervisor, should be concerned with the level of morale in the organization. A good supervisor is aware that it is a supervisory function to elicit and maintain the morale of the subordinates at as high a level as possible. It is the immediate supervisor who, in the day-to-day contact with the employees, influences and determines the level of morale more than anyone else. Raising morale to a high level and maintaining it there is a long-run project and cannot be achieved solely on the basis of short-run devices such as pep talks or contests. The supervisor will also find that although good morale is slow to develop and difficult to maintain, it can change quickly from good to bad with many shadings in between. Indeed, the level of morale varies considerably from day to day and is far more changeable than the weather. Morale, moreover, is contagious. The higher the degree of individual satisfaction of group members, the higher the morale of the entire group. This in turn tends to raise the overall level of morale even higher, since individuals get personal satisfaction from being in a high-morale group. Although favorable attitudes spread, unfavorable attitudes among employees spread even more quickly. It seems to be human nature to quickly forget the good and remember the bad.

Of course, management is not alone in their desire for a satisfactory level of morale. Each employee of the institution is likewise concerned because bad morale is simply not as satisfying as good morale. A state of bad morale creates an unpleasant environment for the employees of the hospital, and they have as much at stake as the administration. Good morale, on the other hand, will make the employee's day at work a pleasurable and satisfying experience and not a misery. The employee will find satisfaction in working with the supervisors and associates. High morale is also important to the hospital patient and the patient's family. They will quickly sense whether the employees of the institution are operating on a high or low level of morale, and they will respond accordingly. But what, we may ask, determines the level of morale?

Factors Influencing Morale

Since morale is a composite of feelings, sentiments, attitudes, satisfaction, well-being, and happiness, almost anything can influence the morale of the employees. Some of these factors are within the control of the supervisor, whereas others are not. Although there are an infinite number of morale determinants, they can generally be classified into two broad groups: those factors which have their primary source in situations that are external to the institution, and those factors whose source lies mostly within the daily supervisory practices and environment of the job.

External Factors

External factors affecting morale, those which are connected with events and influences outside the work environment and institution, are generally beyond the scope of the supervisor's control. Although they are external in origin, these factors nevertheless concern the supervisor, since everyone takes his or her problems to work and does not leave them in the car or on the parking lot. Examples of external factors are family problems, financial worries, associations with friends, a breakdown of the car, sickness in the family, and so forth. Obviously, what happens away from the job may change the employee's feelings quickly; an argument before leaving home may set the emotional tone for the rest of the day. The headlines in the morning paper may be depressing, or they may be conducive to high morale.

These external factors can generally be dealt with only indirectly, primarily in the form of a nondirective counseling interview as discussed in Chapter 17. The supervisor should try to sense such factors because they are reflected in the work attitudes of the subordinates. If something has happened to lower an employee's morale and if the supervisor is familiar with the cause, he or she should try to get the employee to forget the incident as quickly as possible by supplying an antidote. One of the best ways to erase the effects of an occurrence that depresses morale is to encourage the employee to talk about it freely. In so doing, the supervisor will find out what is happening and why and may be able to devise effective means of action to raise the morale. But aside from a nondirective counseling interview, for which the supervisor may not have time or in which the employee may not wish to participate, there is little a supervisor can do to cope with outside factors affecting morale. The supervisor must remember that he or she or the institution is not always the cause of shifts in the level of morale.

Internal Factors

A large number of important factors that affect the morale of employees are within the realm of the supervisor's activities. These include incentives, working conditions, and, above all, the quality of supervision. When considering incentives, the first thing that comes to mind is pay. Of course, wages are exceedingly important, but aside from wages and fringe benefits, many other things are essential to the employee. Considerations such as job security, interesting work, good working conditions, appreciation of a job well done, chance for advancement, recognition, prompt and fair treatment of grievances, etc., are all necessary components of a high-morale environment.

(See Chapter 20.) None of these will take the place of appropriate compensation in dollars and cents. But assuming that the pay reflects the going rate, the additional factors mentioned above play a significant role. For example, although reasonable monetary incentives may be provided and the quality of supervision is high, morale can still sink quickly if, for example, working conditions are neglected. The important factor is that an honest attempt is made to improve working conditions whenever possible. In many cases employees work under undesirable conditions and still maintain high morale, as long as the supervisor has made a serious effort to correct the conditions.

The Supervisor's Attitude

Aside from these on-the-job factors influencing morale, the most significant influence is exercised by supervisors in their immediate, day-to-day relationship with employees. The boss's overall manner of supervision, directing, leadership, interpersonal skills, and general attitude will, more than anything else, make for good or bad morale. Employees will put forth their best efforts when given an opportunity to obtain their need satisfactions through work they enjoy and that at the same time achieves the department's objectives. Such job satisfaction will raise and keep morale at a high level. It can only be maintained if the supervisor lets the employees know how significantly they contribute to the overall goals of the hospital and how their work fits into the overall effort. Morale can also be maintained if the boss gives them a feeling of accomplishment in their work and allows them to be on their own as much as possible. The supervisor who practices democratic supervision, as discussed in previous chapters, is likely to reduce the undesirable features of a job and create an environment in which the employees derive genuine satisfaction from the work they do every day. In addition, the supervisor should not forget the importance of social satisfactions on the job. The employees should have an opportunity to develop friendships and work as a team. In other words, one must not forget the positive contributions that informal groups and informal organization make.

The supervisor should bear in mind that the employees' morale is affected not only by what the supervisor does, but also by how it is done. There is little doubt that if the supervisor's behavior indicates a feeling of superiority to the employees or they are suspicious of the employees' motives and actions, only a low level of morale can result. The supervisor should not forget how little it takes to make one's own spirits rise or fall. A word of appreciation from the boss or even from the hospital administrator can change the supervisor's outlook toward the whole work situation. He or she will become more cheerful and in all likelihood so will the employees.

The supervisor also knows that a frown or quizzical expression on the boss's face can have the opposite effect. The supervisor will begin to wonder what he or she did wrong, and morale will sink. Supervisors should remember that employees react the same way to them as they do to their bosses. Attitudes beget like attitudes. If the supervisor shows worry, the employees tend to follow suit. If he or she becomes angry, others become angry. When the supervisor appears confident in the operation of the department, employees will react accordingly and believe that things are going well. This does not mean that the supervisor should only see the good side of departmental operations and refuse to acknowledge difficulties and troubles. The supervisor should show the employees that as a leader he or she has the situation well in hand and that if anything goes wrong, he or she will give them an opportunity to correct the situation and prevent it from happening again.

Obviously, the supervisor can never relax his or her efforts to build and maintain a high degree of morale among the employees. Nor should the supervisor be discouraged if from time to time the morale drops. So many factors can cause such a change, some of which are beyond the supervisor's control. The supervisor can be reasonably satisfied when the employees' morale is high most of the time.

The Effects of Morale

The question arises as to how good or poor morale affects other variables, such as turnover, absenteeism, the rate of accidents, teamwork, and productivity. Much research has been done in this area, and some general conclusions can be drawn. Normally, higher morale reduces the rate of turnover and results in lower absenteeism. Probably the same holds true for a lowered rate of accidents, although some of them have no relation whatsoever to high or low morale. Let us look at the evidence for these conclusions a bit more carefully.

Morale and Teamwork

The term *teamwork* is often associated with morale. The two do not mean the same thing, however. Morale applies to the *attitudes* of the employees in the department, whereas teamwork is the smoothly coordinated and synchronized *activity* achieved by a small, closely knit group of employees. Although good morale is usually helpful in achieving teamwork, it is possible for teamwork to be high, yet morale low. Such a situation could exist in times when jobs are scarce and when the employees will put up with close and tight supervision for fear of losing their jobs. It is also conceivable that teamwork may be absent even though morale is high; in such a case, the employee, a solo performer, probably prefers individual effort and finds satisfaction in his or her own job performance.

Morale and Productivity

It is generally assumed that high morale is automatically accompanied by high productivity. Supervisors believe that as long as the morale of employees is high, their output will be accordingly high. They are aware that the willing cooperation of employees is almost always necessary to get continuous superior performance. Moreover, there is substantial research evidence to back up the contention that there is a positive relationship between overall morale or job satisfaction and productivity. Every supervisor also knows from personal experience that a highly motivated, self-disciplined group of employees will consistently do a more satisfactory job than a group forced to perform at a certain rate. It is therefore obvious that supervisors will do everything possible to keep morale high so that the department's output remains high.

More recent studies show that this general statement does not hold true in all situations, however. There is proof that the morale-productivity relationships can appear in many forms, namely, low morale and high productivity, high morale and low productivity, as well as high morale and high productivity and low morale and low productivity. Much depends on other factors, for example, the economic situation, the job market, how highly machine paced the job is, and so on. Thus, a supervisor cannot automatically depend on the positive relationship between morale and productivity.

Surveys of Current Morale

It is important for management to be familiar with the extent of job satisfaction or dissatisfaction of the employees of the health care center. Much of the foregoing discussion has assumed that the level of morale can be measured, but it should be realized that morale cannot be measured directly. Nevertheless, there are suitable indirect ways and means of determining the prevailing level of morale and its trends. Although some supervisors pride themselves on their ability to intuitively detect low or high morale, the wise supervisor will do better to approach this problem more systematically in either of two ways. One approach is through observation of activities, events, trends, and changes; the other method is to use what is commonly referred to as attitude, opinion, or morale surveys.

Observation

Observation is a tool that involves watching people and their reactions. Although this tool is available to every supervisor, it is often not fully utilized. If the supervisor does consciously and systematically observe the employees, however, their level of morale and major changes in it can be appraised. The manager should watch the subordinates' behavior and listen to what they have to say; he or she should observe their actions and notice any changes in their willingness to cooperate. The supervisor will probably find it fairly easy to recognize by observation the extremes of high and low morale. Finer means of measurement, however, may be required to differentiate among the intermediate degrees. Of course, personal observation can be used for obvious manifestations of morale, such as a facial expression or a shrug of the shoulder, but often they are difficult to interpret. It is also difficult to determine how far from normal the behavior must be in order to indicate a shift in morale. Thus, it takes an extremely sensitive supervisor to correctly conclude from indicators of this sort that a change in morale has taken place or is taking place.

Moreover, the supervisor may not be able to make the detailed observations necessary for accurate morale appraisal. Although the closeness of the day-to-day working relationship usually offers much opportunity for supervisors to become aware of morale changes, they are often so burdened with work that they do not have time to look, or if they do look, they do not actually see. At times, they may even be afraid to look for fear of what they might find. Although some supervisors may realize that changes are taking place, they are frequently inclined to ignore them. Only later, after a change in the level of morale is openly manifested, will they recall the first indications and admit to noticing them, but not giving them much thought at the time.

To avoid such situations, the supervisor must take care not to brush any indicators conveniently aside. The most serious shortcoming of observation as a yardstick for measuring current morale is that when the activities and events causing an observable lowering of morale are recognized, the change has probably already occurred. The supervisor, therefore, should be extremely keen in his or her observation in order to do as much as possible to prevent such changes before they take place or to speedily counteract them if they have already begun. Naturally, the closer the supervisor's relations are with the employees, the more sensitive he or she will be to these changes and the shorter will be the reaction time.

Attitude Surveys

Management needs sound information to make good decisions. Therefore, many institutions use attitude surveys as a way of finding out how employees feel about their jobs, their supervisors, the hospital as a whole, specific policies, and so on. Such surveys, also called opinion or morale surveys, provide valuable upward communications because they allow employees to express their feelings about their jobs. As a result, administration will know what the general level of satisfaction in the hospital is and which specific areas cause dissatisfaction. It is a valuable diagnostic tool for management to assess employee problems. The attitude survey shows employees that management is truly concerned and, at the same time, gives the employees an opportunity to vent their dissatisfactions. This in itself will improve morale. For surveys to be meaningful, however, administration must be committed to this undertaking. The survey must be properly designed and administered. Also, administration must be willing to follow through with action and communications of results.

Expressions of the opinions of employees are requested in the form of answers to written questionnaires. The questionnaires are prepared with the aid of the personnel department and the data processing center or some outside consulting firm. They may be filled out on the job or at home. Although there are many advantages to filling out questionnaires at home, a high percentage of those questionnaires are never returned. It is better to have more meaningful answers, however, even if the number of replies is smaller. Regardless of whether they are filled out on the job or at home, care must be taken that the questionnaires remain unsigned and that the replies be kept secret.

In a health care center, attitude surveys can cover the entire field of operations. At times it is feasible to limit the inquiry to only one large department, e.g., the nursing services, which usually accounts for half of all the employees. This, however, must be cleared with top administration, since too many surveys at frequent intervals would not be advisable. Once a hospital-wide survey is decided on, the administrator and all other managers must be prepared to endure criticisms because many dissatisfactions will probably be expressed. But more important than this is the fact that management must be prepared and willing to act on the complaints once they are revealed. Until the survey is taken, management can always plead complete ignorance, but after a survey, everyone knows that the administration has heard about the problems causing dissatisfaction. Hopefully, some of the complaints can be adjusted; at least a serious and honest effort must now be made. If the administration is not prepared or willing to act, it is far better not to take surveys. Once management asks the employees for their input and ideas and fails to take action, the employees will avoid expressing themselves in the future.

Taking the Survey and Analyzing Its Results

Questionnaires submitted to employees come in a variety of types (Figures 22-1 and 22-2). Since the data processing department will eventually be involved in the tabulation and correlation of the results, it is advisable to consult with them when designing the format of the questionnaire. Two general types are used most of the time. According to the format of the question asked we distinguish between *objective* surveys and *descriptive* surveys. An objective questionnaire asks the question and offers a choice of answers; there can be "multiple choice" questions or "true and false" questions. In objective surveys the employees mark the one answer that comes closest to their feelings. In a descriptive survey the question is asked, but the employees answer freely in their own words and ways. Since many employees have difficulty stating their opinions in complete sentences or even completing a started sentence, the best results are usually obtained by a form that enables the employees to check the box which seems to provide the most appropriate answer for them.

Once the forms have been filled out, the results must be tabulated and analyzed. This is usually done by the personnel department together with the data processing center or by an outside consultant. The analysis must be thorough and instead of simple straight-run statistics, it should produce more meaningful interpretations. For instance, instead of simply stating that 65 percent of the subordinates have frequent communication with their boss and 35 percent do not or that 75 percent of the respondents like their jobs and 25 percent do not, it would be better to state that of the 75 percent who like their jobs, 85 percent have frequent contact with their boss and 15 percent do not. At the same time, we can learn that among the 25 percent who do not care for their jobs, 55 percent claim that they have infrequent communications with

Figure 22-1. Opinion survey.

St. X Y Z Health Center

Dept. _____
Unit _____

    Each question may be answered in several ways, any one of which will give us the information we need. Check only *one* answer that most closely expresses your true feelings. DO NOT sign the form. Seal your questionnaire in the accompanying envelope and drop it in a box in the Personnel Department tomorrow or any day on or before July 15.

1. How would you rate the hospital as a place to work?
☐ Poor ☐ Not so good ☐ Better than most ☐ Good
2. Are you kept informed on the policies of the hospital and changes in them?
☐ Never ☐ Sometimes ☐ Usually ☐ Always
3. Do you feel that the policies of the hospital are fair to you?
☐ Never ☐ Sometimes ☐ Usually ☐ Always
4. Are you kept informed about what is going on at the hospital?
☐ Never ☐ Sometimes ☐ Usually ☐ Always
5. Where do you get most of your information about what is going on?
☐ Grapevine ☐ Local newspapers ☐ Bulletin boards ☐ Supervisor
6. Were you given a satisfactory introduction to and explanation of your new job before you started to work?
☐ No explanation ☐ Very little ☐ Fair amount ☐ Sufficient
7. Were you made to feel at home and at ease by your supervisor and fellow workers?
☐ Never ☐ Sometimes ☐ Usually ☐ Always
8. Do you like your job?
☐ Not at all ☐ Neither like it or dislike it ☐ Fairly well ☐ Very much
9. How well do you feel your experience and abilities are used in your job?
☐ Poorly ☐ Not so well ☐ Fairly well ☐ Very well
10. What do you think of your department head and supervisor?
Department Head
☐ Poor ☐ Below average ☐ Above average ☐ Very good
Why?
Immediate Supervisor
☐ Poor ☐ Below average ☐ Above average ☐ Very good
Why?
11. Are your duties and responsibilities clear to you?
☐ Never ☐ Sometimes ☐ Usually ☐ Always
12. Can you depend on your department head's and supervisor's promises?
☐ Never ☐ Sometimes ☐ Usually ☐ Always
13. Do your supervisor and department head give you full credit for suggestions you make about your job or department?
☐ Does not ☐ Seldom does ☐ Almost always does ☐ Always does
14. Do you get conflicting orders because of too many "supervisors"?
☐ Never ☐ Sometimes ☐ Usually ☐ Always
15. When your department head and supervisor criticize you or your work, is it done in a friendly and helpful way?
Department Head
☐ Never ☐ Sometimes ☐ Usually ☐ Always
Supervisor
☐ Never ☐ Sometimes ☐ Usually ☐ Always
16. Do your department head and supervisor give clear, exact, and easily understood instructions about your work?
Department Head
☐ Never ☐ Sometimes ☐ Usually ☐ Always
Supervisor
☐ Never ☐ Sometimes ☐ Usually ☐ Always

17. Does your department head or supervisor have a tendency to show favoritism?
Department Head
□ Does   □ Usually does   □ Seldom does   □ Never does
Supervisor
□ Does   □ Usually does   □ Seldom does   □ Never does
18. When changes are made in your work, are you usually given a reason for them?
□ Never   □ Sometimes   □ Usually   □ Always
19. Does your department head or supervisor take an understanding attitude toward your difficulties?
Department Head
□ Never   □ Seldom does   □ Usually does   □ Does
Supervisor
□ Never   □ Seldom does   □ Usually does   □ Does
20. If you are in trouble whether it is your fault or not, what are your chances of a fair hearing and getting a "square deal"?
□ No chance   □ Very little chance   □ Fair chance   □ Good chance
Why?
21. Do you feel that you can appeal to a higher authority if your immediate supervisor decides a point against you?
□ I do not   □ Reasonably so   □ Almost always   □ Always can
If not, why?
22. Is your job and future secure if you do good work?
□ No   □ Fairly secure   □ To a large extent   □ Very secure
23. Are your associations with your fellow workers and superiors as pleasant as they should be?
□ Not pleasant   □ Fairly pleasant   □ Almost always pleasant
□ Most pleasant
If not, why?
24. Do you feel that your fellow workers in your department are doing their fair share of the work?
□ Very few   □ About half of them   □ Most of them   □ All or almost all
25. Please list by number (1-10) items in the order of importance to you.
□ Physical working conditions   □ Doing something worthwhile
□ Opportunity for advancement   □ Liking of job   □ Job security
□ Satisfactory relations with co-workers   □ Wages
□ Knowing what is going on   □ Fair supervision   □ Credit for work done
26. What do you like best about your job?
27. What do you like least about your job?
28. Length of service at St. X Y Z Health Center (check one)
□ One month or less   □ 1 - 3 months   □ 3 - 6 months   □ 6 - 12 months
□ 1 - 5 years   □ 5 - 10 years   □ 11 years or more
29. Age (check one)
□ 16 - 20 years   □ 21 - 25 years   □ 26 - 34 years   □ 35 - 45 years
□ 46 - 50 years   □ 51 - 70 years
30. Employed   □ Part-time   □ Full-time

Please add any additional information that you feel would make the hospital a better place in which to work.

Figure 22-2. Employee opinionnaire.

Importance of this item to me

Columns: Agree | Don't Know | Disagree | Very Important | Important | Not so Important

1. My relationship with my immediate supervisor is clearly spelled out.
2. The deductions from my paycheck are adequately explained.
3. I am in favor of a no smoking area in the cafeteria.
4. The employees' lockers are conveniently located and easy to use.
5. The staff physicians are pleasant to work with.
6. My supervisor knows whether or not I am doing a good job.
7. I would be willing to rotate shifts more often.
8. I will accept the first chance to leave my job.
9. The hallways and stairways are spacious and clean.
10. My co-workers are usually friendly and courteous to other employees.
11. Compared to other cafeterias SMHC's meal costs are reasonable.
12. As long as I do a good job I will have a job at SMHC.
13. Do you think the employee who "yells the loudest" gets the "better pay."
14. I find the in-service training and education sufficient.
15. My work area is too small.
16. The pay at SMHC is competitive with other places for which I could work.
17. I consider the fringe benefits at SMHC to be good.
18. Considering the job I do, my pay is good.
19. The personnel policies have been clearly explained to me.
20. I know what responsibility I have should there be a disaster or fire.
21. My supervisor could have been more helpful in orienting me to my job.
22. I get a salary increase only when my supervisor feels like it.
23. There are many employees who abuse the sick leave policy.
24. More often than not I am criticized for the job I do rather than given credit for a job well done.
25. My job orientation was adequate.
26. I feel that administration is concerned about me and my fellow employees.
27. I find it more convenient to go to the canteen or bring my lunch rather than go to the cafeteria.
28. My work area is the cleanest area in which I have ever worked.
29. Whenever a complaint is filed it takes too long to get it settled.
30. The patients at SMHC are getting the best care available.
31. My supervisor encourages and assists me in improving my skills so I may have the opportunity to advance.
32. Many of my co-workers love to gossip.
33. The people I work with help each other get the job done.
34. My job is a challenge.
35. The cafeteria has a wide selection of food from which to choose.
36. SMHC should provide a day care center where young children would be taken care of during the working hours of the parent.
37. My supervisor is vague on instructions given me.
38. I think the Personnel Department is doing a good job.

Modified from a form developed by Saint Mary's Health Center, St. Louis and printed with their permission.

Importance of
this item to me

	Agree	Don't Know	Disagree	Very Important	Important	Not so Important
39. My supervisor really tries to explain new policy changes or new ideas.	☐	☐	☐	☐	☐	☐
40. Visitors are treated courteously.	☐	☐	☐	☐	☐	☐
41. The parking lots are secure.	☐	☐	☐	☐	☐	☐
42. I find that the noise in my work area is distracting.	☐	☐	☐	☐	☐	☐
43. My supervisor is an asset to SMHC and knows his/her job well.	☐	☐	☐	☐	☐	☐
44. My work area is well lighted and ventilated.	☐	☐	☐	☐	☐	☐
45. I am interested in extracurricular activities such as team sports, social outings, baseball and football games, etc.	☐	☐	☐	☐	☐	☐
46. My job description clearly spells out the work I am doing.	☐	☐	☐	☐	☐	☐
47. I would recommend SMHC to my friends and relatives if hospitalization is needed.	☐	☐	☐	☐	☐	☐
48. There exists some jealousy between my co-workers.	☐	☐	☐	☐	☐	☐
49. My work is tiring—I am exhausted at the day's end.	☐	☐	☐	☐	☐	☐
50. If an employee is dismissed at SMHC there is always just cause.	☐	☐	☐	☐	☐	☐
51. My supervisor treats me with respect and listens to my suggestions.	☐	☐	☐	☐	☐	☐
52. I would rather "time in" and "time out" with a time clock than with a time sheet.	☐	☐	☐	☐	☐	☐
53. No one ever has a chance for promotion from within the ranks.	☐	☐	☐	☐	☐	☐
54. My supervisor doesn't have enough time to spend with me when I have a problem.	☐	☐	☐	☐	☐	☐
55. Safety is stressed in my work area.	☐	☐	☐	☐	☐	☐
56. My work group always has all the supplies it needs to get the job done.	☐	☐	☐	☐	☐	☐
57. Parking facilities at SMHC are adequate.	☐	☐	☐	☐	☐	☐
58. My supervisor is fair in any disciplinary action that is taken.	☐	☐	☐	☐	☐	☐
59. Most news reaches me through the grapevine and not through the regular channels.	☐	☐	☐	☐	☐	☐

60. *Do not sign* the opinionnaire. However, please check one of the following boxes so that the results of this opinion survey will be more meaningful.

I am a member of the:

Nursing Services   ☐

Professional Care Division
(Pharmacy, clinical labs, medical records, dietary, rehabilitation, therapy, radiology, nuclear medicine, social service, central supplies)   ☐

Administrative Services
(Executive offices, data processing, general clerical, admitting, public relations, purchasing, switchboard, volunteer services, accounting, personnel, etc.)   ☐

Plant Operation and Maintenance Services
(Engineering, maintenance, housekeeping, laundry, dispatch, security, grounds, etc.)   ☐

61. I have been employed by SMHC:

For one year or less	From 1-3 yrs.	From 3-5 yrs.	From 5-10 yrs.	For ten yrs. or more.
☐	☐	☐	☐	☐

Please return in one week. Please do not sign.

their superiors. Cross-tabulations of this type show the correlation between good communication and job satisfaction.

After correlation analysis and interpretation of the survey have been done, the results are presented to the top administrator if the survey originated there. This officer in turn passes them on to all supervisors. In fact, in some organizations the results of attitude surveys are used as discussion material in supervisory training. But aside from this, attitude surveys provide the administrator, department heads, and supervisors with information to guide them in their overall efforts to improve morale. Occasionally, the surveys will reveal certain deficiencies, and the supervisor can do something very specific about them; for example, the questionnaire may show an overwhelming interest in and need for a child care center where young children would be taken care of during the working hours of the parent. This obviously was an area of dissatisfaction, and administration better do something about it. Frequently, however, the results of initial surveys are not so clear. They raise a lot of questions, and sometimes additional surveys are required to probe deeper. Survey techniques are becoming more and more sophisticated, and with their help management should be able to arrive at a solution to almost any morale problem that arises.

Summary

Morale is a state of mind and emotion affecting the attitudes, feelings, and sentiments of groups of employees and individuals toward their work environment, colleagues, supervision, and the enterprise as a whole. It is a composite and not a single feeling. Morale is always present, and it can range from high to low. The level of morale varies considerably from day to day. It is contagious; that is, favorable attitudes spread, and unfavorable attitudes spread even more quickly. High morale is not only the concern of the supervisor—the employees are just as interested in a satisfactory level of morale. Moreover, not only do insiders feel the effect of high or low morale, it is also recognizable to outsiders, such as patients and visitors.

Morale can be influenced by a multitude of factors that can be classified into two broad groups: those factors affecting the employee's activities outside of the enterprise and those factors pertaining to on-the-job situations. There is relatively little the boss can do to directly change the effects of outside factors on the subordinates' morale, but many internal factors, such as incentives, working conditions, and attitudes, are within the supervisor's power to control. These factors can be used to significantly raise the level of subordinates' morale. If the supervisor succeeds in maintaining high morale, it is likely that good teamwork and increased productivity will result. Recent research indicates that this is not always the case.

An astute supervisor can sense changes in the level of morale by keen observation of the subordinates, but often supervisors do not realize that a change has taken place until it is too late. In addition to observation, an attitude survey can be instituted, normally with the help of the personnel department or an outside consultant. This is done primarily by questionnaires submitted to employees. Once a morale survey has been performed, it is absolutely necessary that management do something about those areas of dissatisfaction which appear to contribute to a lowering of morale. In conclusion, good supervisory practices, as advocated throughout this text, are likely to keep morale at a high level.

23

Positive Discipline

Maintaining positive discipline and good influencing go hand in hand. The word discipline is used in many connections and understood in several different ways. To many, discipline carries the disagreeable connotation of punishment. When one hears the word discipline, one is often inclined to think immediately of authority or force. There is a positive way of considering discipline, however, a way that is far more in keeping with good supervisory practices.

Organizational Discipline

For our purposes, discipline can be defined as a state of affairs, as a condition of orderliness, in which the members of the enterprise behave sensibly and conduct themselves according to the standards of acceptable behavior as expressed by the needs of the organization. Discipline is said to be good when the employees willingly follow the rules of the enterprise, live up to or exceed standards, and practice self-discipline. Discipline is said to be poor when subordinates either do this reluctantly or actually refuse to follow regulations, violate the standards of acceptable behavior, and require constant surveillance by their supervisors.

Discipline and Morale

Discipline is not the same as morale. As discussed before, morale is an attitude, a state of mind, whereas discipline is a state of affairs. But the level of morale significantly influences the problems of discipline. Normally, fewer problems of a disciplinary nature can be expected when morale is high. By the same token, low morale brings about increased problems of discipline. It is also conceivable that there could be a high degree of discipline despite a low level of morale. Under these conditions, discipline would probably be controlled by fear and sheer force. On the other hand, however, it is usually not possible to maintain a high level of morale unless there is also a high degree of positive discipline.

Self-Discipline

The best discipline, as stated earlier, is self-discipline. By this we mean the normal human tendency to do what needs to be done and to do one's share and subordinate some of one's own needs and desires to the standards of acceptable behavior set for the enterprise as a whole. From early childhood on, people have been trained to respect rules, accept orders from those legitimately entitled to issue them, and realize that all organized activities set limits on the behavior of their members. Experience shows that most employees want to do the right thing. Even before they start to work, most mature persons accept the idea that following instructions and fair rules of conduct is a normal responsibility that goes with any job. Thus, most employees can be counted on to exercise a considerable degree of self-discipline. They believe in coming to work on time, following the supervisor's instructions, signing the time sheet, and refraining from fights, drinking at work, stealing, and so on. In other words, self-imposed discipline is based on the commitment of employees to conform with the rules, regulations, and orders that are necessary for the proper conduct of the institution.

Once the employees know what is expected of them and believe that the rules by which they are governed are reasonable, they usually will observe them without problems. Of course, from time to time the supervisor must check whether some of these rules and regulations are still reasonable. Times are changing and certain rules that were once reasonable are no longer considered to be so. For example, the dress codes and codes of general appearance have most certainly undergone changes in the past decade. It would be unreasonable to request subordinates to comply with a dress and appearance code set up years ago.

When new rules are introduced, however, the supervisor must show their current reasonableness and need to the employees. For instance, women's fashion may dictate a style such as very short skirts, which is not conducive to a nurse's appearance on the job. But instead of simply outlawing short skirts, a rule giving nurses their choice between wearing a certain length of hemline or uniforms with long pants might be considered a more reasonable dress code for nurses. Another example is that of the operating room supervisor faced with the trend toward long hair and facial hair. Since hair is a danger to asepsis, the supervisor and possibly the chief of surgery, infection committee, and director of nursing might work out rules that will make a hood or helmet-type covering mandatory for operating room personnel. There was no need for such a device previously, but old rules do not provide the necessary protection any longer. In other words, the supervisor must be alert to changing styles and mores and must make certain that the rules and regulations truly respect them; otherwise, many unnecessary disciplinary problems will arise.

Of course, a strong sense of self-imposed discipline on the employees' part will exert group pressure on any possible wrongdoer, thus further reducing the need for disciplinary action on the supervisor's part. Work groups also set standards for conduct and performance; for example, fellow employees are expected by the group to carry their fair share of work, be at work on time, and so on. Group discipline reinforces self-discipline and will exert pressure on those who do not comply with group norms and standards.

Employees must also know that they will have the unqualified support of the supervisor as long as they stay within the ordinary rules of conduct and as long as activities are consistent with what is expected of them. Proper discipline makes it necessary for the supervisor to give positive support to the right action and also criticize and punish the wrong action. The subordinate must know that failure to live up to what is expected will result in "punishment."

The administration cannot expect employees to practice self-discipline unless self-discipline starts at the top. Similar restrictions must be imposed on all managerial personnel to remain within the acceptable patterns of behavior. For example, workers cannot be expected to impose self-discipline if supervisors do not show it. Proper conduct with respect to the needs of the organization requires the supervisor also to comply with the necessity to be on time, observe "no smoking" and "no drinking" rules, and dress and behave in a manner commensurate with the activities.

Maintaining Positive Discipline

Although the vast majority of employees will exercise a considerable degree of self-discipline, a few employees in every large organization occasionally fail to abide by established rules and standards even after having been informed of them. Some employees simply will not accept the responsibility of self-discipline. And a few unruly employees find it difficult to function with policies, rules, and regulations.

Since the job must go on, the supervisor cannot afford to let those few "get away with" violations. Firm action is called for to correct the situation. Unless such action is taken, the morale of the other employees in the work group will be seriously weakened. This is the time when the supervisor has to rely on the authority inherent in the managerial position even though the supervisor may dislike doing so. On such an occasion, the supervisor must clearly realize that he or she is in charge of the department and is therefore responsible for discipline within it. If the supervisor does not correct the situation, some individuals who are merely on the borderline of being undisciplined may follow the bad example. When a defect in discipline becomes apparent, it is the supervisor's responsibility to take proper action firmly and, of course, wisely.

The Purpose of Discipline

Discipline is not for the purpose of punishment or "getting even" with an employee. Rather, its purpose is improvement of the employee's future behavior. It corrects the subordinate's breach of the rules and carries the warning of more serious consequences in the future. Discipline, of course, also serves as a warning for other people in the department. It reminds the disciplined individual's co-workers that rules exist and that violating them does not go unnoticed or without any action from the supervisor. Moreover, discipline reassures all those employees who respect the rules out of their desire to do the right thing. Its primary purpose most certainly is not punishment or retribution.

Indeed, the supervisor should administer discipline so that it motivates rather than demotivates. In other words, the boss must exercise positive discipline. This is not an easy task, since inherently the act of punishing a subordinate for violating a rule always presupposes that the subordinate was caught violating it. Yet many others who may have done the same thing go free, so to speak, because the supervisor did not catch them. This invariably injects a note of unfairness into the disciplinary process. Another reason that it is difficult to administer positive discipline is because any discipline is normally resented, and it places a strain on the relationship between the supervisor and the subordinate. Sometimes all it does is make the subordinate double his or her efforts not to be caught again. Nevertheless, positive discipline will generally be successful and accepted if the supervisor follows a few simple rules when taking disciplinary action.

Taking Disciplinary Action

Taking Responsibility

Normally, a good supervisor will not have too much occasion to take disciplinary action. But when it becomes necessary, it is the supervisor's job to do so.* The supervisor is best qualified to know the employee, alleged violations, and circumstances. By being in charge of the department, the supervisor has the authority and responsibility to take appropriate action. Although it may be expedient for the moment to let the personnel director handle unpleasant problems of this type, the supervisor would be shirking responsibility and abdicating and undermining his or her own position if this were allowed.

The same thing would happen if the supervisor were to ignore or conveniently overlook for any length of time a subordinate's failure to meet the prescribed standards of conduct. If such breaches are condoned, the supervisor is merely communicating to the rest of the employees that he or she does not intend to enforce the rules and regulations. Thus, the supervisor must not procrastinate in administering discipline. On the other hand, the supervisor must take caution against haste or unwarranted action. The first step is to obtain all pertinent facts. Before the supervisor does anything, it is necessary to investigate what has happened and why the employee violated the rule. In ad-

---

*In all of our discussion it is assumed that the employees of the department do not belong to a union, and therefore no contractual obligations restrict the supervisor's authority in the realm of disciplinary action.

dition, the employee's past record should be checked, and all other pertinent information should be obtained before any action is taken.

Maintaining Control of Emotions

Whenever taking disciplinary action, the supervisor must not lose his or her temper. Regardless of the severity of the violation the supervisor must not lose control of the situation, thus running the risk of losing the respect of the employees. This does not mean that the supervisor should face the situation halfheartedly or haphazardly. But if the supervisor is in danger of losing control, action should be avoided, by all means, until tempers have cooled down. Even if the violation is significant, the supervisor cannot afford to lose his or her temper. Moreover, the supervisor should follow the general rule of never laying a hand on an employee in any way. Except for emergencies when an employee has been injured or becomes ill or employees who are fighting need to be separated, such a gesture could easily make matters worse.

Discipline in Private

The supervisor must make certain that all disciplinary action takes place in private. It most certainly should never be done in public. A public reprimand builds up resentment in the employee, and it may permit unrelated factors to enter the situation. For instance, if in the opinion of the other workers, a disciplinary action is too severe for the violation, the disciplined employee would appear as a martyr to the rest of them. A supervisor who is disciplining in public is bound to have his or her performance judged by every other employee in the department. It is possible that the employees may not agree with the facts on which the disciplinary action is based, and the supervisor may end up arguing with the other employees over what happened. It is likely that varying eyewitness reports will only confuse the situation. In addition, of course, public discipline would humiliate the disciplined employee in the eyes of the co-workers and would cause considerable damage to the entire department. Therefore, privacy in taking disciplinary action must be the rule.

Progressive Disciplinary Action

The question of which type of disciplinary action to use is answered differently in different enterprises. But in recent years most enterprises have accepted the idea of progressive discipline that provides for an increase in the penalty with each "offense." First offenders get less severe penalties than repeat offenders; more serious infractions receive more severe penalties than lesser offenses. Unless a serious wrong has been committed, the employee would rarely be discharged for the first offense. Rather, a series of progressive steps of disciplinary action would be taken. The steps presented below are merely suggested; they are not the only means of disciplinary action, nor are they listed necessarily in proper order or are all necessary. But many enterprises have found the progression of these steps to be quite workable: (1) informal talk, (2) oral warning or reprimand, (3) written warning, (4) disciplinary layoff, (5) demotional downgrading, and (6) discharge.

The Informal Talk

If the incident is minor and the employee has no previous record of disciplinary action, an informal friendly talk will clear up the situation in many cases. In such a talk, the supervisor will discuss with the employee his or her behavior in relation to the standards that prevail within the enterprise. The supervisor will try to get to the underlying reason for the undesirable behavior. At the same time, the boss will try to reaffirm the employee's sense of responsibility and reestablish the previous cooperative relationship within the department. It may also be advisable to repeat once more why the action of the employee is undesirable and what it may possibly lead to. If the supervisor later finds that this friendly talk was not sufficient to bring about the desired results, then it will become necessary to take the next step, namely, that of an oral warning.

Oral Warning or Reprimand

In this interview between the employee and the supervisor, it should again be pointed out how undesirable the subordinate's violation is and how it could ultimately lead to more severe disciplinary action. Naturally, such an interview will have emotional overtones, since the subordinate is likely to be resentful for having been caught again and the supervisor may also be angry. The violation should be discussed in a straightforward statement of fact, however, and the supervisor should not begin with a recital of how the fine reputation of the employee has now been "tarnished." Neither should the supervisor be apologetic, but should state the case in specific terms and then give the subordinate a chance to tell his or her side of the story.

The supervisor should stress the preventative purpose of discipline by manners and words, but the employee must be advised that such conduct cannot be tolerated. In some enterprises, a record is made on the employee's papers that this oral warning has taken place. Of course, the purpose of the warning is to help the employee correct the behavior and prevent the need for further disciplinary action. The warning should leave the employee with the confidence that he or she can do better and will improve in the future. Some supervisors believe that such an oral reprimand is not very effective. If it is carried out skillfully, however, many employees will be straightened out at this stage.

Written Warning

A written warning is of a formal nature insofar as it becomes a part of the employee's record. Written warnings are particularly necessary in unionized situations so that the document can serve as evidence in case of grievance procedures. The written warning, of which the employee receives a duplicate, must contain a statement of the violation and the potential consequences. Another duplicate of the warning is sent to the personnel department so that it can be inserted in the permanent record.

Disciplinary Layoff

A disciplinary layoff is the next step when the employee has continued the offense and all previous steps were of no avail. Under such conditions, the supervisor must determine what length of penalty would be appropriate. This, of course, will depend on how serious the offense is and how many times it has been repeated. Usually, disciplinary layoffs extend over several days or weeks. Seldom are they more than a few weeks, however.

Some employees may not be impressed with oral or written warnings, but they will find a disciplinary layoff without pay a rude awakening and probably will be convinced that the institution is really serious. A disciplinary layoff may bring back a sense of compliance with rules and regulations. There are, however, a number of disadvantages to invoking a disciplinary layoff. Some enterprises do not apply this measure at all because it hurts their own productivity, especially in times of labor shortages when the employee cannot be replaced with someone who is just as skilled. It is also believed that the employee might return from the layoff in a much more unpleasant frame of mind than when he or she left. Although most managers consider disciplinary layoff as a serious measure, some employees who frequently violate the rules may not regard it as such; they may even view a few days of disciplinary layoff as a welcome break from their daily routine. Although most institutions use it effectively, quite a few institutions no longer use disciplinary layoffs; instead they move right on to discharge.

Demotional Downgrading

The usefulness of this disciplinary measure is seriously questioned. To demote for disciplinary reasons to a lower level, less desirable, and less paying job is likely to bring about dissatisfaction and discouragement. In fact, over an extended period of time demotional downgrading is a form of constant punishment. The dissatisfaction, humiliation, and ill will that result may easily spread to other employees in the department. Sometimes it can be viewed as an invitation for the employee to quit, rather than be discharged. Many enterprises avoid downgrading as a disciplinary measure just as they avoid layoffs. If so, they will have to use termination of employment as the ultimate penalty.

Discharge

Discharge—corporate capital punishment—is the most drastic form of disciplinary action, and it should be reserved exclusively for the most serious offenses. Supervisors should resort to it infrequently and only after some of the preliminary steps have been taken. Discharge is the ultimate penalty and is costly to the organization and causes real hardships to the person who has been discharged. Of course, when a serious wrong has been committed, discharge should be invoked at once. For instance, when an employee brandishes a loaded gun and threatens to shoot, immediate discharge would be in order. Even for lesser offenses, there are some hospitals where the supervisor goes through the earlier steps of friendly and more formal oral and written reprimands and then points out that the next measure would be discharge without any further discussion. In these institutions there is no intermediate penalty such as a several-day disciplinary layoff, which could hurt the superior-subordinate relationship. Discharge is the only step left in this progression. It is hoped that this severe penalty is invoked infrequently.

For the employee, discharge means hardship because it eliminates the seniority standing, possibly some pension rights, substantial vacation benefits, a high pay scale, and other benefits that the employee has accumulated in many years of service. Discharge also makes it difficult for the worker to obtain new employment. As far as the enterprise is concerned, discharges involve serious losses and waste, including the expense of training a new employee and the disruption caused by changing the makeup of the work team. Discharge may also cause damage to the morale of the group. If the discharged employee is a member of a legally protected group, such as minorities or women, administration has to be concerned about nondiscriminations and quotas. Therefore, because of these possibly serious consequences of discharge, many organizations have removed from the supervisor the right to fire. It has been reserved for higher levels in administration or in some institutions, the supervisor's recommendation to discharge must be reviewed and approved by higher administration and/or by the director of personnel. With unions, management is concerned with possible prolonged arbitration procedures, knowing full well that arbitrators have become increasingly unwilling to permit discharge except for the most severe violations. Of course, there may be cases where there is no other answer but to fire the employee for "just cause." But these cases will be the rare exception and not the rule.

Time Element

In all of the disciplinary steps just discussed, the time element is of significance. It is important to decide how long the violation of a rule should be held against an employee. Current practice is inclined to disregard offenses that have been committed more than a year ago. Therefore, an employee with a poor record because of tardiness would start a new life if he or she maintained a good record for one year or maybe even for six months. This time element will vary, depending on the nature of the violation. The question of elapsed time is of no importance in cases of serious violations. As stated before, if an employee should be brandishing a loaded gun in a heated argument during work, there is no need to worry about any time element of previous offenses. This is enough to warrant immediate discharge!

Documentation

It is essential for the supervisor to keep detailed records of all disciplinary actions, since such actions have the potential of becoming the subject of further discussions, disputes, and even litigation. The written record should cover the time of the event, details of the offense, the supervisor's decision, and action taken. It should also include the reasoning involved. If at some future time the supervisor or the institution is asked to substantiate the action taken, it is not sufficient to depend on memory alone. Presently it is even more important than ever before to keep accurate detailed records because the aggrieved employee may file a claim based on discrimination or for similar reasons. If a union is involved, documentation is a must to justify a disciplinary measure if it is challenged by a formal grievance procedure. Regardless of any potential consequences, written documentation at the time of the event is essential for the institution and the supervisor's own records.

The Supervisor's Dilemma

Throughout this book we have stressed the importance of the relationship of trust, confidence, and help between the supervisor and the employee. Disciplinary action is by nature painful. Therefore, despite all the restraint and wisdom with which the supervisor takes disciplinary action, it still puts a strain on the supervisor-subordinate relationship. It is difficult to impose discipline without generating resentment because disciplinary action is by nature an unpleasant experience and puts a barrier between the supervisor and the employee. The question therefore arises as to how the supervisor can apply the necessary disciplinary action so that it will be the least resented and most acceptable.

The "Red-Hot-Stove" Approach

McGregor* refers to what he calls "the red-hot-stove rule" and draws a comparison between touching a red-hot stove and experiencing discipline. When one touches a hot stove, the resulting discipline has four characteristics: it is *immediate,* with *warning, consistent,* and *impersonal.* First, the burn is immediate, and there is no question of the cause and effect. Second, there was a warning. Everyone knows what happens if one touches a hot stove, especially if the stove is red hot. Third, the discipline is consistent. Every time one touches a hot stove, one is burned. Fourth, the discipline is impersonal. Whoever touches the hot stove is burned. A person is burned for touching the hot stove, not because of who he or she is.

---

*As cited in Leonard R. Sayles and George Strauss, *Managing Human Resources,* 2nd ed. (Englewood Cliffs, N.J.: Prentice-Hall, Inc., 1981), 129; George Strauss and Leonard R. Sayles, *Personnel, The Human Problems of Management,* 4th ed. (Englewood Cliffs, N.J.: Prentice-Hall, Inc., 1980), 221.

This comparison illustrates the fact that the act and the discipline seem almost one. The discipline takes place because the person did something, because he or she committed a particular act. The discipline is directed against the act and not against the person. Following the four basic rules expressed in this "hot-stove" approach will help the supervisor take the sting out of many disciplinary actions. It enables the manager to achieve positive discipline and at the same time generate in the employee the least amount of resentment.

Immediacy

The supervisor must not procrastinate; a prompt beginning of the disciplinary process is necessary as soon as possible after the supervisor notices the violation. The sooner the discipline is invoked, the more automatic it will seem and the closer will be the connection with the offensive act. Of course, as already stated, the supervisor should refrain from taking hasty action, and enough time should elapse for tempers to cool and for assembling all the necessary facts.

There are instances when it is apparent that the employee is guilty of a violation, although the full circumstances may not be known. Here the need for disciplinary action is unquestionable, but there is some doubt as to the amount of penalty. In such cases, the supervisor should tell the employee that he or she realizes what went on, but that some time will be needed to reach a conclusion. There are other cases, however, when the nature of the incident makes it necessary to get the offender off the premises quickly. Some immediate action is required even if there is not yet enough evidence to make a final decision in the case.

Temporary Suspension

To solve this dilemma, many enterprises invoke what is called "temporary suspension." The employee is suspended, pending a final decision in the case. This device of suspension protects management, as well as the employee. It gives management a chance to make the necessary investigation and consult higher levels of administration or the personnel department, and it provides an opportunity for tempers to cool off. In cases of temporary suspension, the employee is told that he or she is "suspended" and will be informed as soon as possible of the disciplinary action that will be taken. The suspension in itself is not a punishment. If the investigation shows that there is no cause for disciplinary action, the employee has no grievance, since he or she is recalled and will not have suffered any loss of pay. If, on the other hand, the penalty is a disciplinary layoff, then the time during which the employee was suspended will constitute part of the layoff assessed. The obvious advantage of this device of temporary suspension is that the supervisor can act promptly without any prejudice to the employee. Nevertheless, temporary suspension should not be used indiscriminately; it should be invoked primarily when the offense is likely to call at least for a layoff.

Advance Warning

To have good discipline and have the employees accept disciplinary action as fair, it is absolutely essential that all employees be clearly informed in advance as to what is expected of them and what the rules are. There must be warning that a certain offense will lead to disciplinary action. Some enterprises rely on bulletin board announcements to make such warnings. But these cannot be as effective as a section in the handbook that all new employees receive when they start working for the institution. Along with the written statements in the handbook, it is advisable to include oral clarification of the rules. During the induction process shortly after new employees are hired, they should be orally informed of what is expected of them and of the consequences of not living up to behavioral expectations.

In addition to the forewarning about general rules, it is essential to let the employees know in advance about the kind of disciplinary action that will be taken. The various steps of disciplinary action should be clarified *before* employees could possibly become involved in an offense. There are considerable doubts, however, as to whether or not a standard penalty should be provided and stated for each offense. In other words, should there be, for example, a clear statement that falsifying attendance records will carry a one-week disciplinary layoff? Those in favor of such a list suggest that it would be an effective warning device and that it would provide greater disciplinary consistency. But such a list would not permit management to take into consideration the various degrees of guilt and mitigating circumstances. In general, it is probably best not to provide a schedule of penalties for specific violations, but merely to state the progressive steps of disciplinary action that will be taken in an orderly sequence. It should be clearly understood that continued violations will bring about more severe penalties. Some enterprises do specify that certain serious offenses will bring the penalty of immediate discharge. But for most violations, it is unwise to spell out a rigid set of disciplinary measures.

The practice of forewarning before taking disciplinary measures also applies to rules that have not been enforced lately. If the supervisor has not disciplined anyone who violated them for a long time, the employees do not expect these rules to be enforced in the future. Suddenly the supervisor may decide that to make a rule valid he or she is going to make "an example of one of the employees" and take disciplinary action. Of course, disciplinary action should not be used in this manner. The fact that a certain rule has not been enforced in the past does not mean that it cannot ever be enforced. What it does mean is that the supervisor must take certain steps before beginning to enforce such a rule. Instead of acting tough suddenly, the supervisor should give the employees some warning that this rule, previous enforcement of which has been lax, will be strictly enforced in the future. In such cases, it is not enough to put the enforcement notice on the bulletin board. It is essential that in addition to a clear written warning, supplemental oral communication be given. The supervisor must explain to the subordinates, perhaps in a departmental meeting, that from the present time on he or she intends to enforce this rule.

Consistency

A further requirement of good discipline is that it must be consistent. The supervisor must be consistent in the enforcement of discipline and in the type of disciplinary action taken. By being consistent, the supervisor sets the limit for acceptable behavior, and every individual wants to know what the limits are. Inconsistency, on the other hand, is one of the fastest ways for a supervisor to lower the morale of the employees and lose their respect. If the supervisor is inconsistent, then the employees find themselves in an environment in which they cannot feel secure. Inconsistency will only lead to anxiety, creating doubts in the employees' minds as to what they can and cannot do. At times, the supervisor may be lenient and overlook an infringement. In reality, however, the supervisor is not doing the employee any favor, but only making it harder for the employee and for the others.

Mason Haire,* a well-known psychologist, compares this situation to the relations between a motorist and a traffic police officer. He says that whenever we are exceeding the speed limit on the highway, we must feel some sort of anxiety, since we are breaking the rule. On the other hand, the rule is often not enforced. We think that perhaps this is a place where the police department does not take the rule seriously, and we can speed a little. But there is always a lurking insecurity because the motorist knows that at any time the police officer may decide to enforce the rule. Most motorists probably feel that it would be easier to operate in an environment where the police would at least be consistent one way or the other. The same holds true for most employees who have to work in an environment where the supervisor is not consistent in disciplinary matters.

Of course, at times extenuating circumstances may make it difficult for the supervisor to exercise consistent discipline. There are occasions when the department is particularly rushed with a large amount of work. The supervisor may be induced to overlook infringements because of the desire not to upset the work force or for fear that if he or she has to suspend someone, a valuable employee will be lost at a critical time. The same kind of consideration may apply whenever it is difficult to get an employee with a certain skill and the offending employee possesses that skill.

In addition, the supervisor faces another problem in trying to be consistent. On one hand, the supervisor has been continuously cautioned to treat all employees alike and to avoid favoritism, whereas on the other hand it has been stated again and again to treat people as individuals in accordance with their special needs and situations. On the surface, these two requirements appear to contradict each other and make it impossible to always apply consistent discipline. But the supervisor must realize that treating people fairly does not mean treating everyone exactly the same. What it does mean is that when an exception is made, it must be considered as a valid exception by the other members of the department. The rest of the employees will regard an excep-

---

*Mason Haire, *Psychology in Management,* 2nd ed. (New York: McGraw-Hill Book Co., 1964), 74.

tion as fair if they know why it was made and if they consider the reason to be justified. Moreover, the rest of the employees must be confident that if any other employee were in the same situation he or she would receive the same treatment. If these conditions are fulfilled, the supervisor has been able to exercise fair play, be consistent in discipline, and still treat people as individuals.

The extent to which a supervisor can be consistent and yet consider the individual's situation is illustrated as follows. Assume that three employees were engaged in horseplay at work. It could very well be that the supervisor will merely have a friendly informal talk with one of the employees, who just started work a few days ago. The second employee may receive a formal or written warning, since he had been warned about horseplay before. And it is conceivable that the third employee would receive a three-day disciplinary layoff, since he had been involved in many previous cases of horseplay. Each case must be considered on its own merit, and each employee must be judged according to background, personal history, length of service, and other factors of this type. Of course, if two of the employees had been in the same situation with the same amount of previous warnings, then their penalties would also have to be identical. In this respect, then, consistency must prevail.

Being Impersonal

Another way that a supervisor can reduce the amount of resentment and keep the damage to the future relations with the subordinates at a minimum is to take disciplinary action on as impersonal a basis as possible. In recalling the "hot-stove" rule, it is worth repeating that whoever touches the stove is burned, regardless of who he or she is. The penalty is connected with the act and not with the person. Looking at disciplinary action in this way reduces the danger to the personal relationship between the supervisor and the employee. It is the specific act that brings about the disciplinary measure, not the personality.

Keeping this in mind, the supervisor will be able to discuss the violation in an objective manner, excluding the personal element as far as possible. The supervisor should take disciplinary action without being apologetic about the rule or what he or she has to do to enforce it and without a sign of anger. Once the disciplinary action has been taken, the supervisor must let bygones be bygones. The supervisor must treat the employee as before and must try to forget about what happened. It is understandable that the person who has been disciplined harbors some resentment; the supervisor who meted out the discipline in all likelihood found doing it distasteful also. Therefore, the supervisor and the employee may feel like avoiding each other for a few days afterwards. Such feelings are understandable, but it would be far more advisable for the boss to lean over backward to find some opportunity to show his or her old friendly feelings toward the disciplined employee as a person. This, of course, is easier said than done. Only the mature person can handle discipline without hostility or guilt. But, as we have said, these feelings can be minimized by following the "hot-stove" approach in practicing positive discipline.

Avenues of Appeal

In every organization, it is always possible that an individual in a position of authority might treat a subordinate unjustly. Thus, there must be a system to right such wrongs. Every enterprise must have a system of corrective justice that is concerned with maintaining a healthy organizational climate. There must be a system for grievances that will enable employees to obtain satisfaction for unjust treatment.

Everyone is familiar with the various steps of the grievance procedure to which each employee has access if he or she belongs to a union. But this right of appeal should also exist in an enterprise that does not have a union. It must be possible for any employee to appeal the supervisor's decision in regard to disciplinary action. Following the chain of command, the immediate supervisor's boss would be the one to whom such an appeal would first be directed. From there, the complaining employee can usually carry the appeal procedure through various levels, ultimately to the administrator or the president of the organization as the final court of appeal. Many health care centers have provided for just this type of appeal procedure.

But great care must be taken that the right of appeal is a real right and not merely a formality. There are supervisors who will gladly tell their subordinates that they can go to the next higher boss, but will never forgive them if they do. Such statements and thinking merely indicate the supervisor's own insecurity in the managerial position. As a superior, he or she must permit the employee to take an appeal to the boss without any resentment. It is management's obligation to provide such an appeal procedure, and the supervisor must not feel slighted in the role as manager or leader of the department when it is used. Indeed, it is likely that management's failure to provide an appeal procedure is one of the chief reasons why employees take recourse to unionization.

There is no doubt, however, that it requires a mature supervisor to not see some threat from appeals which go over his or her head. Such a situation should be handled tactfully by the supervisor's boss. It is possible that in the course of an appeal the disciplinary penalty imposed by the supervisor may be reduced or completely removed. It is understandable that under these circumstances the supervisor may become discouraged and frustrated, since his or her boss has not backed him or her up. This usually happens in situations where doubt remains as to the actual events and where the boss cannot get two stories to coincide. In such cases, the "guilty" employee normally goes free. Although this is unfortunate, it is preferable that in a few instances a guilty employee goes free instead of an innocent employee being punished. In our legal system, the "accused" is assumed innocent until proven guilty, and the burden of proof is on management.

Another reason for the reversal of a decision by higher level management is that the supervisor may have been inconsistent in the exercise of discipline or not all the necessary facts were obtained before disciplinary action was imposed. To avoid such an unpleasant situation, it is necessary for the supervisor to adhere closely to all that has been said in this chapter about the exercise of positive discipline. If a supervisor is a wise disciplinarian, the verdict will normally be upheld by the boss. And even if it should be reversed, this is still not too high a price to pay to guarantee justice for every employee. Without justice, of course, a good organizational climate cannot exist and the influencing function cannot be performed satisfactorily.

Summary

Discipline is a state of affairs. It is likely that if morale is high, discipline will be good, and less need will exist for the supervisor to take disciplinary action. A supervisor is entitled to assume that most of the employees want to do the right thing and that much of the discipline will be self-imposed by the employees. If the occasion should arise, it is essential for the supervisor to know how to take disciplinary action. There is usually a progressive list of disciplinary measures, ranging from an informal talk or an oral warning to "capital punishment," namely, discharge. The supervisor should bear in mind that the purpose of such disciplinary measures is not retribution or humiliation of employees. Rather, the goal of disciplinary action is improvement of the future behavior of the subordinate in question and of the other members of the organization. The idea is to avoid similar violations in the future. Nevertheless, taking disciplinary action is a painful experience for the employee, as well as the supervisor. To do the best possible job, the supervisor must ensure that all disciplinary action fulfills the requirements of immediacy, forewarning, consistency, and impersonality. Moreover, the need for a good organizational climate makes it mandatory that a system of corrective justice exists, whereby any disciplinary action that an employee feels is unfair can be appealed.

Part Seven

Controlling

24

Concepts of Control

Controls play an active part in everyone's life whether they are at work, at home, or anywhere else. Everyone is affected by a multitude of controls, such as thermostats in the home, alarm clocks, coffeemakers, toasters, door openers, fuel gauges in the car, traffic lights, traffic police officers, elevators, timers, bells, and many more. Controls play also an important role in the life of any organization; everyone active in an organized activity depends on controls to make certain that the organization functions effectively.

Controlling is the process that checks performance against standards. It makes sure that the organizational and departmental goals and objectives are achieved. The controlling function is closely related to the other four managerial functions, but it is most closely related to the planning function. When the manager performs the planning function, goals, objectives, and policies are set and become standards against which performance is checked and appraised. If deviations are found, the manager has to take corrective action, and such action may well entail new plans and standards. This is how planning decisions affect controls and how control decisions affect plans, illustrating the circular nature of the entire management process.

The Nature of Controlling

Control and the Other Managerial Functions

Because the discussion of controlling comes last in this book many readers may conclude that controlling is something that the manager does only *after* everything else has been done. In other words, it conveys the general impression that controlling is concerned only with events after the fact. This impression is reinforced by practical considerations, for example, faulty workmanship in a product is usually not discovered until after the mistake was made. Despite such considerations, however, it is much more appropriate to look at controlling as something that goes on *simultaneously* with the other functions. Although the relationship between planning and controlling is particularly close, controlling is interwoven with *all* managerial functions. The better the manager plans, organizes, staffs, and influences, the better the supervisor can perform the controlling function and vice versa.

As stated earlier, there is a circular relationship among all of these functions, and their interrelatedness does not permanently place any one function first or last.

Of course, a supervisor cannot expect to have good control over the department unless sound managerial principles in pursuing the other duties are followed. Well-made plans, workable policies and procedures, a properly planned organization, appropriate delegation of authority, continuous training of employees, good instructions, and good supervision all play a significant role in the department's results. Naturally, the better these requirements are fulfilled, the easier will be the supervisor's function of controlling and there will be less need for taking corrective action.

The Human Aspects of Controls

Another important aspect of control is the *response of people* to it. In previous chapters, we had a great deal to say about work and human satisfaction; we spoke about tight vs. loose supervision, delegation of authority, and on-the-job freedom in connection with motivation. Although controls are an absolute requirement in any organized activity, it must be kept in mind that in behavioral terms control means placing constraints on behavior so that what people do in organizations is more or less predictable. Control systems are designed to regulate behavior, and this implies loss of freedom. Of course, people react negatively to loss of freedom. The amount of control will determine how much freedom of action an individual has in performing the job. Complete absence of control, however, does not maximize an individual's perception of freedom. In fact, some controls are needed to maximize human perception of freedom. The reason for this is that controls not only restrict a person's behavior, but also the behavior of others toward him or her.

A certain amount of control, therefore, is essential for any organizational freedom. But, neither the extremes of tight control or complete lack of control will bring about organizational effectiveness. What is needed is a mixture between the two extremes that will take into consideration the amount of decentralization in the organization, management styles, motivational factors, the situation, the professional competence of the employees, etc. In other words, to arrive at the most desirable mixture of freedom and control, the manager must try to balance the goals of organizational effectiveness and individual satisfaction. These goals must be kept in mind whenever a manager is determining the degree of controls.

The Supervisor and Control

Control is the process of checking to determine whether or not plans and standards are being adhered to, proper progress is being made toward objectives, and, if necessary, correcting any deviations. The essence of control for a supervisor is mainly that action which adjusts performance to predetermined standards if deviations from these standards occur. The supervisor is responsible for the results of the department. The manager must make certain that all functions within the department adhere to the established standards, and, if they do not, corrective action must be taken. At times, the supervisor may enlist experts within the organization for assistance in obtaining control information data and counsel. But it would be out of order for the supervisor to expect anyone else to perform the controlling function for him or her.

Planning, organizing, staffing, and influencing are the preparatory steps for getting the work done. Controlling is concerned with making certain that the work is properly executed. Without controlling, supervisors are not doing a complete job of managing. Control remains necessary whenever supervisors assign duties to subordinates, because the supervisors cannot shift the responsibility they have accepted from their own superiors. A supervisor can and must assign tasks and delegate authority, but, as stated on many occasions, responsibility cannot be delegated. Rather, the supervisor must exercise control to see that the responsibility is properly carried out.

The supervisor knows that the eventual success of the department depends on the degree of difference between what should be done and what is done. Having set up the standards of performance, the supervisor must keep informed of the actual performance through observation, reports, discussion, control charts, and other devices. It is the supervisor's job to use these tools to evaluate the difference between what should be done and what is accomplished. Only then can the corrections necessary to bring about full compliance between the standards and the actual performance be prescribed.

Anticipatory Aspect of Control

To a large degree, controlling is a forward-looking function; it has *anticipatory* aspects. Management is concerned with controls that anticipate potential sources of deviation from standards. Past experience and the study of past events tell the supervisor what has taken place, where, when, and why certain standards were not met. This enables management to make provisions so that future activities will not lead to these deviations. Unfortunately, the anticipatory aspect of controlling is not always sufficiently stressed, and much of the time we are primarily concerned with its *corrective* and *reactive* aspects. Deviations from standards are detected after they have occurred and are corrected at the point of performance, rather than anticipated.

Even if this is the case, however, the corrections will have an effect on the future. There is normally precious little the supervisor can do about the past. For instance, if the work assigned to a subordinate for the day has not been accomplished, the controlling process cannot correct that. Some supervisors are inclined to scold the person responsible and assume that he or she was negligent and deliberate because something went wrong. But there is no use "crying over spilled milk." The wise supervisor will look forward rather than backward. The supervisor must study the past, however, to learn what has taken place and why. This will enable the supervisor to take the proper steps to assure corrective and hopefully preventative action for the future.

Since control is forward looking, it is essential that deviations from the established standards are discovered by the supervisor as quickly as possible.

Therefore, it is the supervisor's duty to minimize the time lag between results and corrective action. For example, instead of waiting until the day is over, it is more advisable for a housekeeping supervisor to check at midday to see whether or not the work is progressing satisfactorily. Even then, the morning is already past and nothing can be done about it any longer. Although this is a painful thought to the supervisor, one cannot alter the fact that sometimes effective control must take place after the event has occurred. Indeed, such control is often unavoidable. But minimizing the time lag between results and doing something about them will enable the supervisor to institute corrective action before the damage has gone too far.

Categories of Control Systems

These considerations are the basis for three different types of control systems in relation to the time factor, namely, controls that are in place before (preliminary), during (concurrent), and after (feedback) the job is being done. Therefore we will distinguish between preventative (anticipatory or preemptive, preliminary or ahead of time), concurrent (or in-process or during the event), and feedback (reactive or after the process, after the event) controls.

Preventative Controls

The supervisor should think through the entire process and task ahead of time and anticipate potential problems. In doing this, forward-looking control mechanisms will be built into the system, and mistakes are likely to be avoided. The purpose of preliminary controls is to anticipate and prevent mistakes by taking care of a possible malfunctioning in advance. For example, the supervisor will plan and arrange for a preventative maintenance program so that the equipment will not break down when needed. Another example of a preventative control is the sign on the curb of the street telling drivers that there is a two-hour parking limit.

Other examples of forward-looking controls are policies, procedures, standard practices, and rules. These are designed so that a predetermined course of action is prescribed to prevent mistakes or malfunctioning. For example, every hospital has established detailed plans and precise procedures in case of an emergency such as a fire. Disciplinary rules dealing with the problem of carrying a weapon on hospital premises constitute a forward-looking control mechanism because it serves as a deterrent. Other examples of preventative control mechanisms are warning signals on a piece of equipment or checklists before starting a test. Just think of the extensive checklist a pilot goes through before takeoff. Using this forward approach to control will enable the supervisor to eliminate many of the daily crises.

Concurrent Controls

Another group of control mechanisms are concurrent controls. The purpose is to apply controls while the operations are going on instead of waiting for the outcome. In these situations the supervisor does not anticipate problems, but monitors operations in process. For example, concurrent control enables the supervisor to keep the quality and quantity of output standardized. There are numerous examples of concurrent control mechanisms all around the supervisor, such as simple numerical counters, automatic switches, warning signals, or even a sophisticated on-line computer system. Whenever the supervisor does not have such aids available, he or she will monitor the activities by observation and instruction and possibly being helped by a number of other employees. Other examples of familiar concurrent control mechanisms are the parking meter and fuel gauge in the car. As stated before, the purpose of concurrent controls covers a middle ground between preventative controls at the one end and feedback controls, after the event, on the other end.

Feedback Controls

A third group of control mechanisms, feedback controls, alerts the supervisor after the event, such as the police officer writing a parking ticket after the time on a meter expires. The feedback control system is the most widely used category. It takes place after the process is finished and the mistake or damage is done. Obviously, it is the least desirable of the three alternatives. The purpose of this type of control is to improve from then on and to prevent any future deviation and recurrence. Examples of feedback controls are quality control, quantity of output, statistical information, accounting reports, etc. The feedback and information should go to the supervisor who is responsible for it and who will have to take action to improve future performances; the supervisor in turn will give as much information to the employees as possible.

Since control after the fact is obviously the least desirable mechanism, the supervisor should make every effort to devise more anticipatory and concurrent control mechanisms. With the help of up-to-date information systems the supervisor should be able to convert many of the after-the-fact controls into on-line, during-the-process mechanisms or even to anticipatory controls.

The Closeness of Control

Knowing how closely to control or follow-up the work of a subordinate is a real test of any supervisor's talents. The closeness of follow-up is based on such factors as the experience, initiative, dependability, and resourcefulness of the employee who is given the assignment. Giving an employee an assignment and allowing that person to do the job is part of the process of delegation. This does not mean, however, that the supervisor should leave the employee completely alone until it is time to inspect the final results. Nor does it mean that the supervisor should be "breathing down the subordinate's neck" and watching every detail. Rather, the supervisor must be familiar enough with the ability of the subordinate to accurately determine how much leeway to give and how closely to follow through with the control measures.

Basic Requirements of a Control System

For any control system to be workable and effective it must fulfill certain basic requirements. Controls should be understandable; register deviations quickly; be timely; provide for appropriate, adequate, and economic control; flexible to a degree; and indicate where corrective action should be applied. These requirements are applicable to all services in all organized activities and to all levels within the management hierarchy. We will discuss them only in a general sense, since it would be impossible to spell out the specific characteristics of controls used in each department or service of a health care center.

Understanding of Controls

The first requirement of a workable control system is that the control mechanisms must be understandable. Both the manager and the subordinates must understand what kind of control is to be exercised. This is necessary on all managerial levels. Of course, the farther down the hierarchy the system is to be applied, the less complicated it should be. Thus, the top administrator may use a complicated system of controls based on mathematical formulas and statistical analysis that is understandable to top administration. The control system for the lower supervisory level, however, should be less sophisticated. It must be designed to the level of the user. If the control system is too complicated, the supervisor will frequently have to devise his or her own control system that for all practical purposes will fulfill the same need and is understood by the employees as well.

Rapid Indication of Deviations

To have a workable control system, controls must indicate deviations without delay. As pointed out, controls are forward looking and the supervisor cannot control the past. The sooner the supervisor is aware of such deviations, however, the sooner he or she can take corrective action. It is more desirable to have deviations reported quickly, even if substantiated only by partial information, approximate figures, and estimates. In other words, it is far better for the supervisor to have prompt approximate information, than highly accurate information that is too late to be of much value. This does not mean that the supervisor should jump to conclusions or take corrective action hastily. The supervisor's familiarity with the job to be done, knowledge, and past experience will come in handy in sensing quickly when something is not progressing the way it should be and that action on the supervisor's part is required.

Appropriateness and Adequacy

Controls must always be appropriate for the activity they are to monitor. Control tools that are suitable for the dietary department are different from those used in nursing. Even within nursing the tools used by the director of nursing services are different from those which the head nurse uses on the floor. The head nurse's controls have to be more specific and precise, whereas the director's have to be more far reaching. Obviously, an elaborate control system that is necessary in a large undertaking would not be needed in a small department; however, the need for control exists just the same. Only the magnitude of the control system will be different. Whatever controls are applied, it is essential that they be appropriate for the job involved. Any mechanism of control should not require more than is necessary.

Economics of Controls

Controls must be worth the expenses involved, that is, they must be economical. At times, however, it may be difficult for management to ascertain how much a particular control system is worth and how much it really costs. One of the important criteria might be the consequences that would follow if the controls did not exist. Thus, the nurses' control of narcotics is stringent and exact, whereas no one is too concerned with close control of bandages or aspirins.

Flexibility

Since all undertakings work in a dynamic situation, unforeseen circumstances could play havoc even with the best-laid plans and standards. The control system must be built so that it will remain flexible. It must be designed to keep pace with the continuously changing pattern of a dynamic setting. It must permit change as soon as the change is required, or else the control system is bound to fail. If the employee seems to run into unexpected conditions early in the assignment—through no fault on the employee's part—it is necessary for the supervisor to recognize this and adjust the plans and standards accordingly. In other words, the supervisor must adjust the criteria by which the employee's job will be checked.

Corrective Action

A final requirement of effective controls is that they must point the way to corrective action. It is not enough to show deviations as they have occured. The system must also indicate *who* is responsible for them and *where* they have occurred. Supervisors must make it their business to know precisely where the standards were not met and who is responsible for not achieving the standard. If successive operations are involved, it may be necessary for the supervisor to check the performance after each and every step has been accomplished and before the work is passed on to the next employee or to another department.

Summary

Controlling is the managerial function in which the manager checks performance against standards and takes corrective action if there are deviations. Control is most closely related to the planning function, but it is interwoven with all the other managerial functions as well. Control is essential in every organized activity, although in behavioral terms control means placing constraints on people. A good control system must be designed so that it will bring about organizational effectiveness without infringing on individual satisfaction.

In relation to the time factor, we can distinguish between preventative, concurrent, and feedback control mechanisms. There are a number of basic requirements for a control system to be effective. The supervisor must make sure that the subordinates fully understand the controls and that the controls established are appropriate for the situation. Since control is anticipatory a control system should be designed to report deviations as quickly as possible. Controls must also be worth the expense involved; in other words, they must be worth the effort put forth. It is likewise imperative that a good control system provide for sufficient flexibility in order to cope with new situations and circumstances in a dynamic setting. Last, but not least, a viable control system must clearly indicate where and why deviations have occurred so that the supervisor can take appropriate corrective action at the proper place.

25

The Control Process

The Feedback Model of Controls

A control system can be viewed as a feedback model. Information on how well the system is doing is obtained by the supervisor; the supervisor, the sensor, then monitors the system by comparing the actual results with the desired performance. Whenever the actual performance deviates from the standards set, the system triggers corrective action in the form of an input. (See Figure 25-1.) This closed-loop feedback system works the same way a thermostat in our home functions. The thermostat is set at the desired degree of temperature. Whenever the room temperature falls below or rises above that temperature, the thermostat, continuously comparing room temperature to the wanted temperature, corrects the variation by turning on or shutting off the furnace or air conditioner. Control systems in organizations work the same way.

In performing the controlling function, the supervisor must follow three basic steps. First, the supervisor sets the standards. Next, the supervisor must check and monitor performance and appraise it against these standards to determine whether the performance meets the expected standards or not. If not, the supervisor must take corrective action, which is the third step in the controlling process. (See Figure 25-2.) This sequence of steps is necessary for effective control. In fact, the supervisor could not possibly check and report on deviations without having set the standards in advance, and corrective action cannot be taken unless deviations from these standards are discovered.

Setting Standards

Standards are criteria against which to judge performance or results. Standards state what should be done. They are closely related to, although more specific than, goals and objectives. In planning, the chief administrator sets the overall objectives and goals that the health care center hopes to achieve. These overall objectives are then broken down into narrower objectives for the individual departments. The supervisor of a department establishes even more specific goals that relate to quality, quantity, costs, time standards, quotas, schedules, budgets, etc. These goals become the criteria, the standards, for exercising control. Of course, the examples just mentioned are tangible; however, many standards are intangible. Although the latter are

346

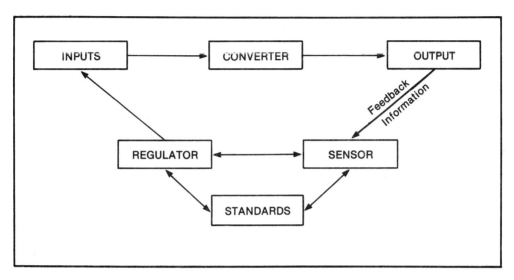

Figure 25-1. Closed-loop system of feedback.

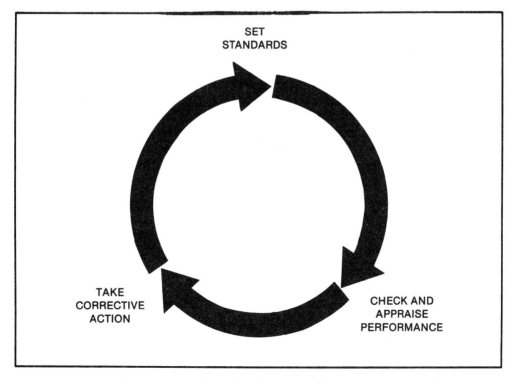

Figure 25-2. Steps in the controlling process.

much more difficult to work with, a health care institution has to consider many intangible standards, especially when it comes to patient care. Let us look at both kinds of standards in more detail.

Tangible Standards

The most common tangible standards are physical standards that pertain to the actual operation of a department in which goods are produced (e.g., the dietary department) or services are rendered (e.g., the nursing service, laboratories, and laundry). Physical standards define the amount of work to be produced within a given time span. Cost standards define direct and indirect labor costs, such as costs of the materials and supplies used and overhead.

These standards are quantitative and qualitative. Not only do they define, for example, how much money can be spent per patient on food, supplies, and materials for three meals a day, but they also state what quality these meals are to be as far as nutritional values, taste, and aesthetic appeal are concerned. Likewise, there are standards on how much one pound of laundry should cost and how many pounds are to be produced in a certain amount of time, taking into consideration the state of mechanization and automation of the laundry. Furthermore, the laundry will have qualitative standards as to sanitation and sterilization, cleanliness of the linens, color, absence of stains, and so forth. In another example, standards specify the number of nursing personnel on a floor in relation to the number of patients to be cared for. Such standards vary depending on the time of day, the nursing unit in question (e.g., an intensive care unit vs. regular floor nursing), and many other factors. There are also standards for the patient's comfort, safety, physical needs, and cleanliness and orderliness of the room.

In setting standards, the supervisor is aided by experience and knowledge of the various jobs to be done within the department. A supervisor has a general idea of how much time it takes to perform a certain job, what resources are required, what constitutes a good quality of performance, and what is a poor job. Job knowledge and experience will be resources the supervisor uses to establish the standards against which to judge the performance and results of the department.

Motion and Time Studies

There are also better, more scientific and systematic ways of establishing objective standards. In some departments, the supervisor can call on industrial engineers who will use work-measurement techniques to help determine the amount of work an average employee should turn out within a given time period. There are many departments in a health care center, for instance, housekeeping, the laundry, the laboratories, the dispatch office, the dietary service, and possibly the nursing service, where this approach is worth the effort and cost. Standards arrived at through work-measurement techniques help the supervisor distribute the work evenly and judge fairly whether an employee is performing satisfactorily.

The supervisor rarely conducts work-measurement techniques, however. They are usually assigned to an industrial engineer or perhaps to an outside consultant trained in doing motion and time studies. *Motion study* involves an analysis of how the job is currently performed with a view to changing, eliminating, or combining certain steps and devising a method that will be quicker and easier. Often flowcharts are drawn up that analyze the steps taken in performing the jobs. After a thorough analysis of the motions and work-flow arrangements, the engineer will come up with what is considered the "best method" for doing the job in question.

Once the best method has been designed, *time studies* are performed to find out the standard time required to do the job using this method. Time studies are done in a scientific and systematic manner by selecting an average employee for observation, measuring the times used for the various elements of the job, applying correction factors, and making allowances for fatigue, personal times, contingencies, and so on. The combined result then leads to a standard time necessary to perform the job. Although this method is rather scientific, it must be kept in mind that considerable judgment and many approximations will be used to arrive at the standard time. There is still the need for decisions involving judgment and discretion.* Standard times, however, are a sound basis on which to determine objective standards. They also enable the supervisor to predict the number of employees required and the probable cost of the job to be done. In many activities outside the health care field standards of this type serve as a basis for incentive plans.

If industrial engineers are not available, the supervisor can perform some of the studies simply by observing and timing the various operations and making the necessary adjustments for fatigue, delay, and so on. If the job to be performed in the department has never been done there before, the supervisor should try to base tentative standards on similar operations. If the new job has no similarity to any previous function, then the best the supervisor can do—unless the help of industrial engineers is available—is to observe the operation while it is being performed for the first few times. The supervisor will have to make approximate time and motion studies to arrive at a standard for the new function. Sometimes, of course, the manufacturer of a new piece of equipment can be helpful to the supervisor in providing standard data, for example, how long it will take a piece of equipment to perform a certain task, etc.

Although they may not be as scientific, standards are more likely to be effective if they are set with the participation of the supervisor and the subordinates instead of being handed down by a staff engineer, a top manager, or an outside consultant. The purpose of any standard is to establish a specific goal for the employees to strive toward, and, as with directives, employees are likely to be more motivated to achieve those standards in which they have had some part.

* For additional information see George Strauss and Leonard R. Sayles, *Personnel: The Human Problems of Management*, 4th ed. (Englewood Cliffs, NJ: Prentice-Hall, Inc., 1980), 622-628.

Intangible Standards

In addition to tangible standards that can be expressed in physical terms, there are also standards of an intangible nature. In a hospital or related health care facility, some of the intangible standards consist of the institution's reputation in the community, the excellence of patient care, or the degree of "tender loving care," including attention to the patients' psychological needs, level of morale of the employees, and so on. It is exceedingly difficult, if not impossible, to express the criteria for such intangible standards in precise and numerical terms. It is much simpler to measure performance against tangible standards, e.g., the number of nursing personnel in relation to number of patients. Nevertheless, a supervisor should not overlook the intangible achievements even if it is difficult to set standards for them and measure their performance. Tools for appraising some of these intangible standards are being developed in the form of attitude surveys, questionnaires, and interviews. Although these tools are not exact, they should be helpful in determining to what extent certain intangible standards are being achieved.

How to Select Standards

Strategic Standards

Obviously, the number of standards that can be used to ascertain the quality and quantity of performance within a department is very large and increases rapidly as the department expands. As the operations within the department become more sophisticated and complex and the functions of the departments increase, it will become more difficult and time consuming for supervisors to check against all the conceivable standards. Therefore, they will need to concentrate on certain standards by selecting some of them as the *strategic* ones. For example, a head nurse making the rounds knows which are the strategic points to check first. She probably checks with the Kardex file and makes certain that the tests and treatments are being done on time, the physical setup of the room is in order, and the patient is comfortable and understands what is being done on that day. She also observes where the other nursing personnel are and what they are doing. Each of these areas constitutes a strategic point of control for the head nurse.

Unfortunately, there are no specific guidelines on how to select these strategic control points. The peculiarities of each departmental function and the makeup of the supervisor and employees will be different in each situation. Thus, only general guidelines can be suggested for selecting strategic standards.

One of the first considerations in choosing one standard as more strategic than another is *timeliness*. Since time is essential in control and controls are anticipatory, the earlier the deviation can be discovered the better. Keeping this in mind, the supervisor can determine at what point in time and the process the work should be checked. For example, in the maintenance department, the strategic control point may be after a crack has been repaired, but before it has been repainted.

Another consideration in choosing strategic control points is that they should permit *economic observations*. In the previous chapter, it was pointed out that a control system must be worth the expense involved, it must be economical. Naturally, the same applies to the strategic control points. A further consideration is that the strategic standards should provide for *comprehensive and balanced control*. The supervisor must be aware that the selection of one strategic control point might have an adverse effect on another. Excessive control on the quantity of achievements often has an adverse effect on the quality. On the other hand, if expenses are selected as a strategic control point, the quality or quantity of the output may suffer. For instance, the executive housekeeper must not sacrifice quality standards that have been designed to prevent infections in order to cut expenses. All of these decisions will depend on the nature of the work within the department, and what serves well as a strategic control point in one activity will not necessarily apply in another.

Standards and Individual Responsibility

For control to have an effective influence on performance, the supervisor must make certain that the goals and standards are known to all the employees within the department. The supervisor must make it clear with whom the responsibility lies for the achievement of standards so that he or she knows who to blame for deviations if the results are not achieved and who to praise if they are. After all, the supervisor is interested in having the standards and objectives reached. Only if each employee knows exactly what is expected as far as his or her own work is concerned can the subordinate try to achieve it. This is why it is necessary to tie the standards in with the individual responsibilities of each employee.

Checking on Performance

The second step in the process of control is to check on performance. Once the standards have been set, it is the supervisor's job to compare the actual performance with these standards. Work is observed, output is measured, and reports are compiled. Such checking activities are usually carried on by the supervisor after the subordinate has completed the function. Since the supervisor does not shift responsibility when assigning a duty to a subordinate and when delegating authority, he or she must make certain that enough controls are available to take corrective action in case the performance does not come up to standards.

There are several ways for a supervisor to check on performance. It can be done either by directly observing the work, personally checking on the employees, or studying various summaries of reports and figures that are submitted to the supervisor. The supervisor compares the information thus obtained with existing standards. Such comparisons are a function of the supervisor that has to be performed daily, weekly, and monthly.

Direct Personal Observation

This is probably the most widely used technique for measurement. There is no better way for a supervisor to check performance than by direct observation and personal contact. Unfortunately, personal observation is time consuming, but every manager should spend a certain part of each day away from the desk inspecting the performance of the employees. For example, regular rounds are not only necessary for the head nurse, they are just as important for the director of nursing. In the latter case, they will be less frequent, but even the director should make some personal observations.

For the supervisor, direct observations are the most effective way of maintaining close contact with employees as a part of their continuous training and development for more efficiency in their jobs. Indeed, this opportunity for close personal observation is one of the great advantages of the supervisor's job; it is something that the top administrator cannot do to any great extent. The farther removed a manager is from the firing line, the less he or she will be able to personally observe and the more he or she will have to depend on reports.

Of course, whenever supervisors observe their employees at work, they must assume a questioning attitude and not necessarily a fault-finding one. Supervisors should not ignore mistakes, but the manner in which they question is essential. They should ask themselves whether or not there is any way in which they could help the employees do the job more easily, safely, or efficiently. They should notice the way the employee is going about the job, whether it is good or bad. Such observations can check specific areas, for instance, inadequate patient care, lack of orderliness, not meeting the physical needs of the patient, sloppy work, poorly performed jobs, etc. At times it may be difficult to convince an employee that his or her work is unsatisfactory; but if reference can be made to concrete cases, it is not easy for the subordinate to deny that they exist. Indeed, it is essential for the supervisor to make specific observations because without being specific one cannot realistically appraise performance and take appropriate corrective action.

As stated above, checking performance through direct personal observation has some shortcomings; for example, it is time consuming and means being away from the desk and office. There are some other limitations. The employee may perform well while the boss is around, but drop back to a lower level performance shortly after the boss is out of sight. Furthermore, it may be difficult to observe some of the activities at the critical time. Also, the supervisor should make an effort to see what is really happening and not only what he or she wants to see. Still, direct observation is practiced widely and is probably the best way of checking performance.

Reports

Written reports—with or without oral presentation—and oral reports are a good means of checking on performance if a department operates twenty-four hours a day, seven days a week, or if it is large or operates in different locations. When a department operates around the clock and one supervisor is responsible for it twenty-four hours each day of the week, this person depends on reports to cover those shifts during which he or she is normally absent. Even with reports, it is wise for the supervisor to get to work a little earlier and stay a little later in the day, so that there is some overlap with the night supervisor in the morning and with the afternoon supervisor later in the day. This gives the supervisors a chance to add some oral explanations to their written reports. Of course, reports should be clear, complete, concise, and correct. They must be brief, but still include all the important aspects.

As the departmental supervisor checks these reports, he or she probably will find many activities that have been performed up to standard. The supervisor should concentrate on the *exceptions*, namely, those areas where the performance significantly deviates from the standard. Only the exceptions require the supervisor's attention. In fact, if the supervisor depends on reports from the various shifts, the subordinates may have been requested not to send data on those activities which have reached the preestablished standards, but to merely report on those items which do not meet the standards or exceed them. In this way, the supervisor can concentrate all efforts on the problem areas. This is known as practicing the *exception principle*. In such situations, however, it is essential that a climate of trust exist between the supervisor and subordinates so that they can freely report the deviations. Subordinates should know that the boss has full confidence in the rest of the employee's activities even though there is no report on them.

If the supervisor does depend on reports for information, it is essential that they are reviewed immediately after they are received and that action is taken without delay when it is needed. It is demoralizing to send reports to a supervisor who does not even read them.

The nature of health care activities calls for reports that are accurate, complete, and correct, especially when patient care is involved. But even in all other areas, most employees will submit truthful reports, even if they are unfavorable to the employee. Much will depend on their relationships and the supervisor's reaction. Of course, the supervisor must check into the matter and correct any shortcomings. As long as the supervisor handles these reports constructively, stressing their honesty, the employees will continue to submit reliable reports instead of "stretching the truth." The supervisor must remember how important upward communications are (Chapter 5), and this is one opportunity to keep the channel open and flowing.

Taking Corrective Action

The third stage in the control model is taking corrective action. Of course, if there are no deviations of performance from the established standards, then the supervisor's process of controlling is fulfilled by the first two steps—setting standards and checking performance. But if there is a discrepancy or a variation, then the controlling function is not fulfilled until and unless the third step, corrective action, is taken. Of course, data must be examined as quickly as possible after the observations are made, so that timely corrective action can be taken to curb undesirable results and bring performance back into line.

It is necessary for the supervisor to first make a careful analysis of the facts and look for the reasons behind the deviations. This must be done before any specific corrective action can be prescribed. The supervisor must bear in mind that the performance standards were based on certain prerequisites, forecasts, and assumptions and that some of these may have been faulty or may not have materialized. A check on the discrepancy may also point out that the trouble was not caused by the employee in whose work it showed up, but in some preceding operation. For instance, a patient's infection might not be caused by the nursing activities or conditions on the nursing floor, but rather by conditions or actions in the recovery room or the surgical suite. In such a situation, of course, the corrective action must be directed toward the real source of the discrepancy. In this instance, the corrective action would emanate from the nursing director's office, assuming that the latter is the common-line superior to all the departments concerned.

The supervisor might also discover that a deviation may be caused by an employee who is not qualified or who has not been given the proper directions and instructions. If the employee is not qualified, additional training and supervision might help, but then again there might be cases where a replacement would be in order. In a situation where directions have not been given properly and the employee was not well enough informed of what was expected of him or her, it is the supervisor's duty to again explain the standards required.

Only after a thorough analysis of the reasons for a deviation has been made will the supervisor be in a position to take appropriate corrective action. It should be stated again that it is not sufficient to merely find the deviation; controlling means to correct the situation. The supervisor must decide what remedial action is necessary to secure improved results in the future. Corrective action may require revising the standards, a simple discussion, an oral reprimand, transferring or even replacing certain employees, or devising better work methods.

But this is not the end of the road. The supervisor must follow up and study the effect of each corrective action on control in the future. With further study and analysis, the supervisor may find that additional or different measures may be required to produce the desired results, keep operations on line, or get them back on the track.

Summary

In performing the controlling function, the manager should follow three basic steps. Standards must be set, performance must be checked, and corrective action must be taken. In setting standards the supervisor must be aware of both intangible and tangible standards. Many of the tangible standards can be established with the help of motion and time studies. It is much more difficult, however, to establish standards for intangible aspects of performance. Moreover, since the number of both types of standards is so large, the supervisor must select certain control points as strategic ones. In each and every department, the supervisor alone can best determine the strategic control points. After establishing the strategic standards, it is the supervisor's function to check and appraise performance against them. In some instances, the supervisor will have to depend on reports, but in most cases direct personal observation is the best means for appraising performance. If discrepancies from standards are revealed, the supervisor must take corrective action to bring matters back into line.

26

Budgetary and Other Controls

Of all available control devices, the budget, especially the expense budget, is probably the one the supervisor is most familiar with and has been coping with for the longest time. A budget is a written plan expressed in numerical terms, primarily in dollars and cents, that extends for a specific period of time; it sets the standards to be met. The budget is the most widely used control device not only in health care centers, but in all other kinds of organized activities. Budgetary control is an extremely effective managerial tool, whether the manager is the executive director of a hospital or the supervisor of a department. For this reason it is essential that every manager learn how to plan budgets, live within their boundaries, and use them properly for control purposes.

As pointed out in Chapter 7, budget making is a planning function, but its administration is part of the controlling function. Budgets are preestablished standards to which operations are compared and, if need be, adjusted by the exercise of control. In other words, a budget is a means of control insofar as it reflects the progress of the actual performance against the plan and in so doing provides information that enables the supervisor to take action, if necessary, to make results conform with the plan.

The Nature of Budgeting and Budgetary Control

Budgetary plans generally include an overall budget for the organization and many subunit budgets for the various divisions and departments. Whereas the overall budget is of great concern to the top administrator and the board of directors, the supervisor is mainly involved with the departmental budget, although overall budget considerations do have their effects on every departmental budget. The term *budgetary control* refers to the use of budgets to control the actual daily operations of the department so that they will conform with the goals and standards set by the budget. Budgetary control goes beyond merely evaluating actual results in relation to established goals. It also means taking corrective action where and when needed.

Numerical Terms

The budget states the anticipated results in specific numerical terms. Although the terms are usually monetary, not all budgets are expressed in dollars and cents to begin with. Many budgets are stated in nonfinancial numerical terms, such as nursing hours, worker hours, quantities of supplies, raw materials, and so forth. Personnel budgets indicate the number of workers needed for each type of skill required, the number of hours allocated to perform certain activities, etc. Although budgets may start out with numerical terms other than monetary values, ultimately every nonfinancial budget must be translated into dollars and cents. This is the common denominator for all activities of an organization, which is why one normally thinks of a budget as a plan expressed in monetary terms.

Improved Planning

Making a budget, whether it is financial or otherwise, leads to improved planning. For budgetary purposes, it is not sufficient just to make a general statement. It is necessary to quantify, date, and state specific plans in a budget. There is a considerable difference between making a general forecast on one hand and attaching numerical values to specific plans on the other. The figures in the budget are the actual plan that will become the standard of achievement. The plans are then no longer merely predictions. Rather, they are the basis for daily operations and are looked on as standards to be met.

Making the Budget

A complete budgetary program requires the involvement of all levels of management; it requires serious and honest consideration. Rigorous budgetary thinking is bound to improve the quality of organizational planning. Indeed, real participation by all the managers and supervisors who will be affected by the various budgets is a prerequisite for their successful administration. Again, this is important because it is natural for people to resent arbitrary orders. Thus, it is imperative that all budget allowances and objectives are determined with the full cooperation of those who are responsible for executing them.

Participation in Budgeting

As stated above, the supervisor responsible for living up to the departmental budget should play a significant role in preparing it. The supervisor should submit a budget and participate in what is commonly known as "grass roots" budgeting. For instance, as the year draws to a close, around the beginning of September, the supervisor of the operating rooms should sit down and gather together those figures which will make up next year's budget. In this

endeavor, the supervisor will need the help and assistance of his or her immediate line superior, in this case most likely, the director of nursing services.
The supervisor must gather all available information as to past performance,
salaries of nursing personnel, other wages, supplies, maintenance, and so
forth. Then the supervisor should think of new developments, for example,
increases in wages, the increased costs of supplies, and additional personnel,
before he or she can prepare an intelligent and achievable budget.

Of course, the full responsibility for preparing the budget does not lie
with the supervisor alone. It is the administrator's and every upper level
manager's duty to work on budgets, and they in turn, together with the controller's and accounting department's printouts, will give the departmental
supervisor a great deal of information on past performance and figures. The
supervisor will use such information to substantiate future estimates and proposals in a free exchange of opinions with the line superior. After both reach a
certain level of agreement, the line boss will carry the overall departmental
budget to higher administration. For example, let us assume that the director
of nursing services supervises three different areas of activities: the regular
floor nursing function, the operating rooms, and the in-service nursing education. After the supervisors of each of these three activities have worked out
their departmental budgets and have discussed and substantiated them fully
with the director of nursing services, he or she will have all these inputs
printed out and come up with a complete budget for the entire nursing services. This budget then will be discussed with the top administration or
whoever is the immediate line superior. Ultimately, the final budget will be
adjusted and set at top administrative levels. Yet its effectiveness is assured,
since true grass roots participation has taken place.

Such participation does not mean, however, that the suggestions of the
supervisors should or will always prevail. A careful and thorough analysis
and study of the figures are necessary. There should be a full discussion between the supervisor and the line superior and the former should have ample
opportunity to be heard and to substantiate his or her case. But the budget
suggestions of subordinate supervisors will not be accepted if the superior
believes the figures are unrealistic, incorrect, or inadequate.

Indeed, some subordinates are inclined to suggest budgets at levels
that they hope to achieve without too much effort. This is obviously done for
self-protection and because the supervisor wants to play it safe. The supervisor rationalizes that by setting the estimates of expenses high enough he or
she can be sure to stay within the allocated amount and will be praised if he or
she stays well below the budget. Of course, this defeats the purpose of grass
roots budgeting. The line superior should remind the supervisor that the purpose of budget participation is to arrive at realistic budgets. It should be
explained that favorable and unfavorable variances will be carefully
scrutinized and that the supervisor's managerial rating will depend among
other factors on how realistic a budget proposal is submitted. Obviously,
many discussions will be needed before the budget is completed and brought
to top administration for final approval.

Zero-Based Budgeting

Conventional budgeting as described above involves projections for the following year based on current expenditures and the previous annual budget. Zero-based budgeting is a fairly new concept of planning and setting a budget; it is not as yet practiced widely. It requires substantiation and justification of each budget item from the ground up, "from scratch." It gives administration an excellent opportunity to reassess all activities, departments, and projects in terms of their benefits and costs to the organization. The great advantage to zero-based budgeting is that each "package" has to be planned anew and costs are calculated from scratch; this avoids the tendency to look only at changes from the previous period. Ongoing programs are reviewed and have to be justified in their entirety. This, of course, involves a great amount of paperwork and is very time consuming.

Budget Director and Budget Committee

Although the authority and responsibility for the budget rest with the line officers and ultimately with the chief executive officer and the board of directors of a health care institution, they will be helped in some cases by a staff unit headed by a budget director or the controller. This staff will provide the line managers with assistance, advice, and data, but should not attempt to prepare the budgets for them. The staff will be particularly helpful, however, in putting the various budget estimates together in final form so that the top administrator can submit it to the board.

Some institutions also have established a budget committee to serve in an advisory capacity in coordinating the various budgets. Clearly, such a committee performs a staff function. It must be distinguished, however, from those budget committees to which the board has delegated the line function of setting rather than just coordinating the budget. In this situation, the budget committee considers all departmental budget estimates and makes the final decisions. The budget committee has ultimate line authority and responsibility for determining the budget instead of the top administrator or executive director of the hospital. The budget is approved by the committee, and nothing can be done without its approval. If budget revisions and changes are requested, it is also up to the budget committee to allow or disallow them. A number of arrangements are possible as to where the final authority for the overall budget rests within these two extremes. Usually it also has to pass the finance committee of the hospital board and eventually the board of directors.

Length of the Budget Period

Although the length of the budget period may vary, most health care centers choose the accounting period of one year. This period is then broken down into quarters, and many hospitals will even divide it by months at the time of the original budget preparation. This is commonly referred to as *periodic budgeting.*

Aside from the annual budgets or without periodic breakdowns, it is common for hospitals also to have budgets extending over a longer term, such as three, five, ten, or even more years. These budgets usually cover such items as capital expenditures, research programs, expansions, and so forth. Long-term budgets of this nature are not direct operating budgets and are of no direct concern to the supervisor. Rather, they are a concern of the chief administrator and the board of directors.

Flexibility of the Budgetary Process

The supervisor should keep in mind that budgets are merely a tool for management and not a substitute for good judgment. Also, care should be taken not to make budgets so detailed that they become cumbersome. Budgets should always allow the supervisor enough freedom to accomplish the best objectives of the department. There must be a reasonable degree of latitude and flexibility. In fact, one of the most serious shortcomings of budgeting is the danger of inflexibility. Although budgets are plans expressed in numerical terms, the supervisor must not be led to believe that these figures are absolutely final and unalterable. Realizing that a budget should not become a straitjacket, enlightened management builds into the budgetary program a degree of flexibility and adaptability.* This is necessary so that the hospital can cope with changing conditions, new developments, and even possible mistakes in the budget because of human errors and miscalculations. Flexibility should not be interpreted to mean, however, that the budget can be changed with every whim, nor that it should be taken lightly.

Nevertheless, if operating conditions have appreciably changed and there are valid indications that the budget cannot be followed in the future, a revision of the budgetary program is in order. Such circumstances may be caused by unexpected events, unexpected wage increases, or large fluctuations in demand. Consider, for instance, the budget of the department of respiratory therapy, in which activities have been and are increasing constantly because of new ideas, technology, applications, and so forth. Naturally, the revenues derived from this service are increasing rapidly at the same time. It would be absurd to expect the supervisor of this department to be able to stay within the budgeted figures for salaries and supplies. If the department is expected to respond and supply the increased demand, this budget must be expanded. In such a case, the old budget has become obsolete, and, unless provisions are available to make the budget flexible, it will lose its usefulness altogether.

Budget Review and Budget Revision

Because of the potential to become obsolete, increasing attention has been given to ways of assuring budget flexibility to avoid the danger of rigid-

---

*Much of this is different in public sector hospitals, e.g., those run by the Veteran's Administration or federal, state, and local governments.

ity. Most health care centers are achieving this by means of periodic budget reviews and revisions. At regular intervals of one, two, or three months the budget is reviewed and, if necessary, changed. Each time the actual performance will be checked and compared with the budgeted figures in meetings between the departmental supervisor and the line superior. At these meetings, the supervisor will be called on to explain the causes for any variations or inadequacies that the line superior finds in the budget. A thorough analysis must be made to discover the reasons for the variances from the budgeted amount. This may then lead to budget revisions or to other corrective measures to prevent further deviations.

Of course, an unfavorable variation by itself does not necessarily require a budget change. But in the example cited above the supervisor of the respiratory therapy department will not have any difficulties in proving the need for an upward budget revision. In some organizations, such a revision can be made on the departmental level, whereas in other institutions, it must be carried up to the chief administrator or even the budget committee. If the deviations are of sufficient magnitude, it is advisable to make the necessary revisions no matter how high up they have to go or how much work they may involve. If the variation is minor, it may be more expedient to let it go, since it is explainable, instead of revising the entire budget.

No matter what decision is made, regular budget reviews and revisions seem to be the best way of ensuring the flexibility of the budgetary process. They prevent the budget from being looked on as a straitjacket and allow the supervisor to consider it a living document and a valuable tool for control purposes.

Budgets and Human Problems

Budgets necessarily represent restrictions, and for this reason subordinates generally resent budgets. Often subordinates have a defensive approach to budgets, an approach they acquire through painful experience. Many times the subordinates become acquainted with budgets only as a barrier to spending, or the budget is blamed for failure to get or give a raise in salary. Moreover, the term budget in the minds of many subordinates has often become associated with penurious behavior rather than with planning and direction.

It is the line manager's job to correct this erroneous impression by pointing out that budgeting is a trained and disciplined approach to many problems and that it is necessary to maintain standards of performance. The budget must be presented to the supervisor as a planning tool and not as a pressure device. Most of the problems, of course, arise at the point of budgetary control. In other words, when deviations from the budget occur, subordinates are often censored for exceeding the budget. Such budget deviations necessitate explanations, discussions, and decisions. As stated before, the budget should not be looked on lightly. The subordinate should also know that in most enterprises enough flexibility is built into the budget system to permit good commonsense departures which are necessary for the best functioning of the institution.

Avoiding unnecessary pressures over the budget, of course, presupposes that a good working relationship exists between the supervisor and the immediate superior. This in turn rests on clear-cut organizational lines and a thorough understanding that the line managers are responsible for control. Staff people are really excluded from the process of controlling; they cannot take operating personnel to task for deviations of the budget; they can merely report the situation to the administrative officer. In the final analysis, effective utilization of budgetary procedures depends on the administration's attitudes toward the entire budgetary process, whether they want it to be an effective planning tool or a pressure device. Only in the first instance will a supervisor believe that whatever can be done without a budget can be done so much more effectively with a budget.

Cost Controls

Cost Containment and Cost Awareness

The providers of health care have been under continuous pressure to keep health care expenditures from spiraling. There has been an unrelenting pressure on everyone in the health care field on this issue. It is safe to predict that the drive to control costs will increase even more because of pressures from government agencies, legislators, insurors, and purchasers of health care, such as large corporations, and even enlightened individuals. In such an environment control of costs is a continuous problem to everyone from the president down to the lowest line supervisor. It is an ongoing problem that will never go away.

Cost control, better referred to as cost awareness, cost consciousness, or cost containment, should be viewed as a significant part of the supervisor's daily job. Supervisors must continuously strive for cost consciousness with even emphasis. Sporadic efforts, crash programs, economy drives, etc., seldom have lasting results. Since cost awareness is a continuous problem, the supervisor must set objectives and make plans for achieving cost containment. The supervisor must set definite numerical objectives to be achieved at a given date. Priorities must be clarified, naturally without infringing on the quality of health care; this is difficult to achieve, especially if there is an escalation of prices and wages all around and more sophistication in patient care.

In order to succeed in cost containment, it is essential to involve the employees of the department in this effort and make them realize that ultimately their action will bring about results. All employees should consider cost consciousness as a part of their job. Most employees will normally try to do the right thing and will help to save costs and reduce waste; most employees are not deliberately wasteful. Many employees can make valuable suggestions and contributions to cost effectiveness. The supervisor should welcome employees' suggestions and not fault them for not having thought of these changes before. Cost awareness should be an ongoing challenge in everyone's daily job.

Allocation of Costs

Every supervisor must see that his or her department contributes effectively to the operation of the institution. In this context of overall controls, we are not referring to the qualitative aspect, but to the financial operation of a department. At times a supervisor is told that the department is operating in the red and that it is losing money each year instead of contributing to a financial surplus. Take, for instance, an operating room supervisor who has been confronted with such a statement. The supervisor may be at a complete loss to understand this. Everyone is working as effectively as possible, the utilization of the operating rooms is high, there is no surplus of employees or waste of materials or supplies, and the supervisor is staying within the expense figures set out in the budget. The charges for using the operating room to the patient have been arrived at by the accounting department in conjunction with the administration. But still the overall figures at the end of the year indicate that the operating rooms are "costing" the hospital a great deal of money because this division ends up as a deficit activity.

The supervisor must realize that in a health care center, just as in all other organized activities, some departments are revenue producing, whereas others are not. Clearly, the operating rooms produce revenues and so does the nursing service. But these patient care departments could not function without the facilities provided by the other departments, for instance, housekeeping, patient food services, medical records, laundry, and administration. Admitting, credit and collections, the executive offices, the personnel department, public relations, purchasing, and the telephone service are additional services without which no other department in the hospital could function. Although these are not revenue-producing departments, their costs must be carried if the hospital is to break even. Indeed, hospitals must allocate such costs to those patient care departments which do produce revenue. The question arises as to *how* the costs of the many non–revenue producing departments are *allocated* to the revenue-producing departments. It is this portion of a department's expenses over which the supervisor has no control whatsoever which can make the difference between ending up with a departmental surplus or with a deficit.

It would be beyond the confines of this text to go into a detailed discussion of the various methods of cost analysis, contribution margin approach, and other bases for allocations. It is a good idea, however, for the supervisor to be informed in a general way of the bases on which a department is being charged for these various expenditures. This is merely for the supervisor's own information, since in reality this person is powerless to influence the costs allocated to the department. The supervisor can readily understand the direct expenses, such as wages, salaries, supplies, and materials, as well as some of the indirect expenses, such as social security, with which the department is charged. It is also understandable that departments are charged with housekeeping based on the hours of service provided, maintenance figures on the basis of work orders, linen based on pounds of laundry, and so forth. But when it comes to the allocation of many other charges, the supervisor should find out what the basis is. Of course, the hospital will try to select a basis of distribution that is fair to all departments and feasible from an accounting point of view.

Obviously, the overall financial performance of a department will be greatly affected by how these allocations are made for other expenditures, for example, administrative expenses, operation of the plant, depreciation, intern and resident service costs, in-service education, interest expenses, and a host of others. Although all of this is determined higher up in the administrative hierarchy, the supervisor is well advised to obtain some information and explanation on how it is done. Then the supervisor will understand how a department operates in the red, despite the effective work of the manager and subordinates.

Additional Controls

It has been stated many times that the supervisor's controlling function is closely related to all other managerial functions and that much of controlling goes on simultaneously with the other functions. Throughout this text many subjects were discussed as part of a particular function at the time, and now their importance also as an aid in the systems of control can be shown.

In Chapter 7 standing plans such as policies, procedures, methods, and rules as basic tools for planning were discussed. But at this time they can be viewed as anticipatory control devices. They are established with the hope and intention that they will be followed and that they work out alright. But if they do not work out or are violated, the supervisor, using feedback control, must take the necessary corrective action to get things back on track; in some cases even disciplinary measures may be necessary.

We discussed positive discipline and disciplinary measures in Chapter 23 as a component of the influencing function. Now this topic can be looked on as a control technique. If a rule has been violated, the supervisor must invoke disciplinary measures, which is synonymous with taking corrective action.

At various occasions management by objectives (MBO) was discussed. This concept includes aspects of controls. After mutually agreed on objectives have been set, results are evaluated in the light of these standards, and, if need be, shortcomings are corrected. This is another example of a control model mechanism.

The discussion of performance appraisal procedures in Chapter 18 can also be viewed as part of the control system. Although performance evaluation measures were presented as a staffing function, they can now be regarded as a feedback control technique in the managerial control system.

These are just a few examples taken from previous discussions of the various managerial functions; they show how closely related controlling is to all the other functions. This confirms the statement that the better the supervisor plans, organizes, staffs, and influences, the better he or she also will perform the controlling function.

Summary

Of all control devices, the budget, and primarily the expense budget, is the one most widely used and hence the one with which most supervisors are familiar. Budget making is planning, whereas living with the budget and budget administration falls into the manager's controlling function. Budgets are plans expressed in numerical terms that ultimately will be reduced to dollars and cents, since this is the common denominator used in the final analysis. Budgets are also preestablished standards to which the operations of the department are compared and, if need be, adjusted by the exercise of control.

The supervisor responsible for living up to the departmental budget must play a significant role in its preparation. Budget making is a line responsibility shared by the supervisor and the direct line superior. Ultimately all budgets are submitted to and approved by top administration, but it is essential that lower level management participate in making their own budgets and have sufficient opportunity to be heard and substantiate their cases.

For a budget to be a live document and not a straitjacket, the budgetary process must provide for flexibility. There must be frequent periodic budget reviews within the normal one-year budgeting period and provisions for budget revision. Such provisions will lessen the human problems that budgetary controls often cause.

In addition to budgetary controls, the supervisor should be aware of other costs that will influence the overall performance of the department. Here the supervisor will be concerned with how the expenditures of the non-revenue producing departments in a health care institution are allocated to those departments which do produce revenues. The bases of these allocations can often make the difference between showing a departmental surplus and operating at a loss. Supervisors also play an important role in cost containment. Cost awareness and cost consciousness should be an ongoing consideration and part of the supervisor's daily activities. Throughout this text we stressed the close relationship between the controlling function and the other managerial functions. Many of the managerial duties and activities discussed now can be viewed also as part of the overall control system.

Part Eight

Labor Relations

27

The Labor Union and The Supervisor

At this time about 20 to 25 percent of the labor force in this country are members of a labor union or some employee association. Collective bargaining gained its major legal basis in 1935 with the enactment of the National Labor Relations Act (also known as the Wagner Act), which guaranteed workers the right to bargain collectively with their employers. In 1947 the Wagner Act was amended by the Labor-Management Relations Act (also known as the Taft-Hartley Act). In 1959 the Labor-Management Reporting and Disclosure Act (sometimes referred to as the Landrum-Griffin Act) was added. In 1974 these laws were extended to cover most health care institutions.

The union movement was primarily a blue-collar movement because there were more blue-collar workers in the United States labor force than white-collar workers. Since the middle 1950s, however, the number of white-collar workers has been on the increase and has surpassed the blue-collar sector. With this change, labor unions have made inroads in representing employees from services, trade, finance, health care, government, and other sectors. A number of unions or employee associations have become the bargaining agents for engineers, teachers, college professors, nurses, airline pilots, and a host of other white-collar workers.*

Union-organizing efforts usually are resisted with vigor by employers and create a period fraught with hostilities. The issues, claims, and counterclaims are on everyone's mind and are present in the workplace, on the parking lot, and even in the local news media. The verbal battle may even accelerate into work slowdowns or stoppages. If the employees vote to join a union, managers are likely to feel that they have lost a battle and that their employees and union representatives have been victorious. It will take time for the ill feelings created during the organizing campaign to disappear.

There is little doubt that the introduction of a union or an employee association into a hospital or related health care facility may be a traumatic experience for the supervisors, as well as for the administrator. It may bring a time of tension during which constructive solutions to problems may be dif-

---

*It is beyond the confines of this text to discuss the details of labor laws or give a history of the union movement in the United States.

ficult. Gradually, however, both the union and the administration must learn to accommodate and live with each other. Every manager must accept the fact that the labor union is a permanent force in our society. Every manager must realize that the union, just as any other organization, has in it the potential for either advancing or disrupting the common effort of the institution. It is in the self-interest of the administration to create a labor-management climate that directs this potential toward constructive ends. But there is no simple or magic formula for overnight cultivation of a favorable climate that will result in cooperation and mutual understanding between the union and management. It takes wisdom and sensitivity from every manager of the organization, from the administrator down to the supervisor, to demonstrate in the day-to-day relations that the union is respected as a responsible part of the institution.

In this effort to create and maintain a constructive pattern of cooperation between the hospital and the union, the most significant factor usually is the supervisor of a department. Supervisors more than anyone else feel the strongest impact of the new situation because they make the most decisions concerning unionized employees. It is the supervisor who in the day-to-day relations with the employees makes the labor agreement a living document for better or for worse. Supervisors are often confused as to how they should behave during an organizing campaign and after the election when the union arrives on the scene. The supervisor should realize that the subordinates decided for a union generally not because they were gullible or naive or because the union used deceit or strong-arm methods; the major reasons lie in the fact that some of the employees' major needs were not satisfied on the job. The supervisor should approach the union professionally and try to build a satisfactory relationship.

It is desirable that the supervisor has been given continuous training in the fundamentals of collective bargaining and in the nature of labor agreements. This is essential for the development of good labor relations. Actually, the supervisor is involved in two distinct phases of labor relations: (1) the inception of unionization and the phase of negotiations and (2) the day-to-day administration of the union agreement, which includes handling complaints and grievances. Although the supervisor is primarily concerned with the second phase of relations with the union, he or she plays a role in the first.

Labor Negotiations

As soon as supervisors learn that union-organizing activities are starting, this information should be passed on to higher administration and/or the personnel director. Often administration has learned of such a campaign through other channels already. This will enable the organization to plan its strategy, usually with the help of legal counsel. Supervisors should be aware of a number of legal restrictions that must be observed during the union-organizing efforts. The following remarks are only of a very general nature; supervisors should receive more detailed instructions from their administrators and lawyers.

Labor laws restrict what managers, including supervisors, are permitted to say and do during this critical period without the danger of their being involved in unfair labor practices. Administration should provide supervisors with information of the dos and don'ts. Generally, supervisors should not make any statements in reference to unionization that could be construed as a promise if the union fails or as a threat if the union is successful. Supervisors should not question their employees privately or publicly about organizing activities. When asked, supervisors can express their opinions about unionization in a neutral manner, if this is possible, without running into the danger of having the answer interpreted as a threat or promise. Finally, supervisors should continue to do the best possible job of supervision during this critical period. These are merely a few guidelines that the supervisor should keep in mind; there certainly are additional guidelines. Usually an election conducted by the National Labor Relations Board will determine the outcome of the organizing campaign. If the union loses the election, the employees will not have a union for some time; if the union wins, management has to recognize the union as the bargaining agent and begin negotiations in good faith.

On the surface, it might not look as if the supervisor is significantly involved in the negotiations of a labor agreement. As stated earlier, the period when a union first enters a department of a health care organization is usually filled with tensions. Emotions run high, and considerable disturbance can result. Under such conditions, it is understandable that the delicate negotiations of a union contract are carried on primarily by members of top administration, probably assisted by legal counsel. There is usually an air of secrecy surrounding the negotiations, which often take place in a hotel room or a lawyer's office.

Since a committee of employees may be participating in these negotiations, there exists a fast line of communication with the other employees of the hospital, but not necessarily with the supervisor. The supervisor often runs the danger of being less well informed about the course of negotiations than the employees are. Therefore, the administrator must see to it that the supervisor is fully advised as to the progress and direction the negotiations are taking. In addition, the supervisor should be given an opportunity to express opinions on matters brought up during the negotiations. In other words, even though top management is representing the institution at the negotiating sessions, supervisors should be able to express their views through them, because ultimately it is the supervisor who bears the major responsibility for fulfilling the contract provisions.

The same necessity exists whenever renegotiations of the labor agreement take place. At that time, top administration should consult with the supervisors as to how specific provisions in the contract have worked out and what changes in the contract the supervisors would like to have made. It is essential for both the administrator and the supervisors to realize that although the supervisors do not actually sit at the negotiating table, they have a great deal to do with the nature of the negotiations. Many of the demands that the union brings up during the negotiations have their origin in the day-to-day operations of the department. Many of the difficult questions to be solved in the bargaining process stem from the relationship that the supervisors have with their employees.

Therefore, it is obvious that there must be a great amount of checking back and forth between the administrator and the supervisor before and during the negotiation of a labor agreement. To supply valuable information, the supervisor must know what has been going on in the department and have facts to substantiate his or her statements. This points to the value of documentation, keeping good records of disciplinary incidents, productivity, leaves, promotions, etc. The supervisor should also be alert to problems that should be called to the administration's attention so that in the next set of negotiations these matters may be worked out more satisfactorily. It is in the interest of both the union and the institution to have as small a number of unresolved problems as possible. But if problems do arise, it is the supervisor's responsibility to see that administration is aware of them at the time of contract negotiations.

Content of the Agreement

Once administration and the union have agreed on a labor contract, this agreement will be the basis on which both parties have to operate. Since the supervisor is now obligated to manage the department within the overall framework of the labor agreement, it is of prime necessity that the supervisor have complete knowledge of its provisions and how they are to be interpreted. The supervisor is the one who can cause disagreements between the union and the hospital by failing to live up to the terms of the agreement. Thus, the content of the union contract must be fully explained to and understood by the supervisor.

A good way to present such explanations is at a meeting arranged for top administration and all the supervisors, which is usually chaired by the personnel or labor relations director. The purpose of the meeting is to brief the supervisors on the content of the labor contract, giving them an opportunity to ask questions about any part they do not understand. Copies of the contract and clarification of the various clauses may be furnished to the supervisors so that they may study them in advance. Since no two contracts are alike, however, it is impossible to pinpoint specific provisions that the supervisor should check into. Normally, all contracts deal with matters such as union recognition, management's rights, union security, wages, bonus rates, conditions and hours of work, overtime, vacations, holidays, leaves of absence, seniority, promotions, and similar matters. Almost certainly there will also be provisions covering complaint and grievance procedures and arbitration. In addition, there are likely to be many other provisions that are peculiar to each institution in question.

It is not only necessary for the administrator to familiarize the supervisors with the exact provisions of the contract, it is just as important to explain to them the philosophy of top administration in reference to general relations with the union. The supervisors should understand that it is the intention of the administration to maintain good working conditions with the union so that organizational objectives can be achieved in a mutually satisfactory fashion. The chief executive officer should clarify the fact that the best way to achieve good union-management relations in a hospital or any other institution is by effective contract administration. Of course, the experts in the personnel department or the labor relations department will have a great deal to do with effective contract administration, but much will still depend on the way in which the supervisor handles the contract on a day-to-day basis.

It is important for the supervisors to bear in mind that the negotiated contract was carefully and thoughtfully debated and finally agreed on by both parties. Thus, it is not in the interest of successful contract administration for the supervisors to try to "beat the contract," even though they may think they are doing the institution a favor. The administrator must make it clear that to achieve satisfactory cooperation, supervisors may not construct their own contractual clauses, nor can they reinterpret clauses in their own way. Once the agreement has been reached, supervisors should not attempt to change or circumvent it.

If the administrator fails to familiarize the supervisors with the provisions and spirit of the agreement, they should insist on briefing sessions and explanations before they apply the clauses of the contract in the daily working situation of the department. The advent of the labor contract does not change the supervisor's job as a manager. The supervisor must still perform the managerial functions of planning, organizing, staffing, influencing, and controlling. There is no change in the authority delegated to the department head by the administrator or in the responsibility that the supervisor has accepted. The significant change is that the supervisor must now perform the managerial duties within the framework of the union agreement. The supervisor still has the right to require the subordinates to carry out orders and the obligation to get the job done within the department. But there are likely to be certain provisions within the union agreement that influence and even limit certain activities, especially within the areas of disciplinary action and dismissal. Undoubtedly, in many instances these provisions of the contract will make it more challenging for the supervisor to be a good manager. But the only way to meet the challenge is for the supervisor to improve his or her own managerial ability, as well as improve his or her knowledge and techniques of good labor relations.

Contract Administration

It is in the daily administration of the labor agreement that the real importance of the supervisor's contribution shows up. The manner in which the day-to-day problems are handled within the framework of the union contract will make the difference between positive labor-management relations and a situation filled with unnecessary tensions and bad feelings. At best, a union contract can only set forth the broad outline of labor-management relations. To make it a positive instrument of constructive relations, the contract must be filled in with appropriate and intelligent supervisory decisions. It is the supervisor who interprets management's intent by everyday actions. In the final analysis, it is the supervisor who, with decisions, actions, and attitudes, really gives the contract meaning and life.

In many instances, it is true that the supervisor "rewrites" or expands on some of the provisions of the contract when interpreting and applying them to specific situations. In so doing, the supervisor sets precedents to which arbitrators pay heed when deciding grievances that come before them. It is impossible for the administrator and the union to draw up a contract that anticipates every possible situation in employee relations and specifies exact directives for dealing with them. Therefore, the individual judgment of the supervisor becomes very important in deciding each particular situation. This again illustrates the vast significance of the supervisor's influence on the interpretation of the labor agreement. As a representative of administration, any error in the supervisor's decisions is the administration's error. It is the immediate supervisor who has the greatest responsibility for seeing that the clauses of the agreement are carried out appropriately. It is therefore necessary for the administrator to realize how significant a role the supervisor plays in the contract administration, and it is just as essential for the supervisor to realize how far reaching his or her decisions can become.

Areas of Difficulty

There are usually two broad areas in which the supervisor is likely to run into difficulties in the administration of a labor agreement. The first covers the vast number of complaints that are concerned with single issues. These would include grievances involving a particular disciplinary action, assignment of work, distribution of overtime, as well as questions of promotion, transfer, downgrading, and so on. In each situation, the personal judgment of the supervisor is of great importance. As long as the contract provisions are met, the supervisor should feel free to deal with grievances as he or she sees fit. Of course, the supervisor must make certain that the actions are consistent and logical even though they are made on the basis of personal judgment rather than hard and fast rules.

The second area of difficulty in contract administration covers those grievances and problems in which the supervisor is called on to interpret a clause of the contract. The supervisor is placed in a situation where an attempt must be made to carry out the generalized statement of the contract but finds that it is subject to varying interpretations. In such instances, it would be wrong for the supervisor to handle the problem without consulting higher management first. Whenever an interpretation of the contract is at issue, any decision is likely to be long lasting. Such a decision may set a precedent that the hospital, union, or even an arbitrator would want to make use of in the future. Therefore, if interpretation of a clause is in doubt, the question should be brought to the attention of higher management, the administrator and possibly the personnel director. Although the supervisor may have been well indoctrinated in the meaning, philosophy, and clauses of the contract, his or her perspective is probably not broad enough to make a potentially precedent-setting interpretation. Since the supervisor did not attend the bargaining meetings, he or she cannot know the intent of the parties nor the background of this provision. For these and other reasons the supervisor should consult with superiors.

The Supervisor's Right to Decision Making

In non–precedent-setting situations and in the daily administration of the labor agreement, the supervisor must bear in mind that as a member of management, he or she has the right and even the duty to make a decision. The supervisor must realize that the union contract does not abrogate management's right to decide; it is still management's prerogative to do so. The union has a right to protest the decision, however.

For instance, it is the supervisor's job to maintain discipline and if disciplinary action is necessary, the supervisor should take action without discussing it with the union's representative. The supervisor should understand that usually there is no co-determination clause and should not set any precedent of determining together with the union what the supervisor's rights are in a particular disciplinary case. Of course, before any disciplinary measures are taken, a prudent supervisor will examine all the facts in the case, fulfill the preliminary steps, and think through the appropriateness of the action.

In a few cases, the union contract will call for consultation or advance notice before the supervisor can proceed. Advance notice or consultation does not mean agreement on the final decision, however. Repercussions or protests from the union can still occur, although prior communication on anticipated action can avoid some of them. In any event, the right to decide on day-to-day issues of contract administration still rests with the supervisor and not with the union.

The Supervisor and the Shop Steward

The supervisor will probably have the most union contact with the shop steward who is the first-line official of the union and is sometimes referred to as shop committeeman, committeewoman, or departmental chairperson. The shop steward* normally remains an employee of the hospital or related health care facility and is expected to put in a full day's work for the employer, regardless of the fact that this person has been selected by the fellow workers to be their official spokesperson both with the institution and with the union. This obviously is a difficult position, since the steward has to serve two masters. As an employee, he or she has to follow the supervisor's orders and directives; as a union official, he or she has responsibilities to fellow co-workers.

Just as individuals vary in their approach to their jobs, so stewards vary in their approach to their position. Some are unassuming; others are overbearing. Some are helpful and courteous, whereas others are difficult. But unless there are special provisions, the steward's rights are merely those of any other union member. Moreover, the steward is subject to the same

---

*The shop steward is not the same as a union business agent or business representative; these are normally full-time union officials who are paid and employed by the local or national union. At times the supervisor will also have to deal with them.

regulations regarding quality of work and conduct as every other employee of the department. Certain privileges may be specified in the union contract, however, such as how much hospital or "company" time the steward can devote to union business or other matters, whether or not solicitation of membership or collection of dues may be carried on during working hours, and other questions of this type.

As stated above, the role of the shop steward will depend considerably on the makeup of the individual. There are those who will take advantage of their position to do as little work as possible, whereas others will perform a good day's work. The supervisor should always remember that the steward is an employee of the hospital and should be treated as such. But it should also be remembered that the steward is the representative of the other employees and in this capacity the shop steward learns quickly what the other employees are thinking and what is going on in the grapevine. Thus, the supervisor will come to understand and take advantage of the fact that the dual role can make the steward a good link between management and employees.

Although stewards perform a number of union functions, such as collecting dues, soliciting membership, and promoting political causes, the supervisor should understand that the most important responsibility of the steward is probably in relation to complaints and grievances coming from the employees. It is the steward's job to bring such complaints and grievances before the supervisor, and it is the supervisor's job to settle them to the best of his or her ability, using the grievance procedures that are described in great detail in every union contract. Naturally, throughout these procedures, which we shall discuss more fully in the next chapter, the supervisor represents management, and the steward represents the employees for the union. In most cases, the steward is sincerely trying to redress the aggrieved employee by winning a favorable ruling. At times, however, the supervisor may be under the impression that the steward is out looking for grievances merely to stay busy. This may be partly true, since the steward does have a political assignment, and it is necessary to assure the employees that the union is working in their behalf. Indeed, the steward must be able to convince the employees that they can rely on him or her, and therefore on the union, to protect them. On the other hand, an experienced steward knows that there is normally a sufficient number of real grievances to be settled and that there is no need to look for complaints which do not have a valid background and would rightfully be turned down by the supervisor.

Most unions will see to it that the shop steward is well trained to present the complaints and grievances so that they can be carried to a successful conclusion. The steward is usually well versed in understanding the content of the contract, management's obligations, and employees' rights. Before presenting a grievance, the steward should determine such matters as whether or not the contract has been violated, the employer acted unfairly, the employee's health or safety has been put in jeopardy, etc. In grievance matters, the union is usually on the offensive and the supervisor is on the defensive. The shop steward will challenge the management decision or action, and the supervisor must justify what he or she has done.

Because the shop steward's main interest is in the union, at times this may antagonize the supervisor. In some instances, it will be difficult for the supervisor to keep a sense of humor and remain calm. Often it is also difficult for the supervisor to discuss a grievance with a shop steward on an equal footing, since the steward is a subordinate within the normal working situation. But when playing the role of a shop steward, the position as representative of the union members gives him or her equal standing. The supervisor should always bear in mind that the steward's job is a political one and as such it carries certain weight. At the same time, the supervisor should understand that a good shop steward will keep any supervisor on the alert and force him or her to be a better manager.

Summary

About 20 to 25 percent of the labor force in this country are members of an employee association or a labor union. Since unions are representing more and more white-collar workers, it is essential that supervisors in health care undertakings are familiar with some basic aspects of labor relations.

The supervisor's role in the union relations of a hospital or related health care facility cannot be minimized. Although the supervisor is not normally a member of the management team that sits down with union negotiators to settle the terms of the labor contract, he or she does play an important indirect role in this meeting. Many of the difficulties and problems discussed at a negotiating meeting can be traced back to the daily activities of the supervisor. But at best the union contract resulting from the negotiations can set forth only the broad outline of labor-management relationships. It is the day-to-day application and administration of the agreement that will make the difference between harmonious labor relations and a situation filled with unnecessary tensions and bad feelings. The supervisor is the person who, through daily decisions and actions, gives the contract real meaning. The supervisor must therefore be thoroughly familiar with the contents of the contract and with the general philosophy of the hospital administration toward the union. There must be an understanding of the difficult and important political role of the union steward, who serves in a dual capacity as one of the regular employees and as the representative of the union members. In grievance cases, the supervisor must learn to regard the steward as an equal, as one who is trained to present the complaints of union members as effectively as possible. The shop steward will challenge management's decision, and the supervisor must justify it. Although at times it may be difficult to keep a balanced perspective, the supervisor should always remember that a good shop steward can serve to make him or her a better manager.

28

Handling
Grievances

A grievance is a complaint that usually results from a misunderstanding, misinterpretation, or violation of a provision of the labor agreement. Almost all union contracts contain provisions for a grievance procedure. This first step of the procedure begins at the departmental level, with the supervisor or the foreman or forelady and the shop steward. If the grievance is not settled there, it can be appealed to the next higher level of management; at this point usually a chief steward or a business agent of the union will enter into the picture. At times the contract may provide for an appeal to an even higher level of management. The procedure usually sets a time limit for each of these steps to be finished. If the dispute cannot be settled by the first two or three steps to the mutual satisfaction of both parties, the agreement usually has an arbitration provision; this means that the issue may be submitted to an impartial outsider, an arbitrator, who, after hearing testimony and evidence, will render a final decision that is binding on both parties.

This points to the necessity for the supervisor to be well qualified in handling complaints and settling grievances. Indeed, in a unionized setting one of the supervisor's most important duties is to make certain that the majority of complaints and grievances are properly disposed of during the first step of the grievance procedure. Most organizations require that supervisors check and consult with a labor relations specialist in the personnel department when handling complaints. This is important because many complaints could have hospital-wide or organization-wide implications. Grievances that refer to discrimination and equal employment opportunities could have legal implications for the entire organization. And there are many additional reasons why the human resources department should be involved. The supervisor is not shirking responsibility or admitting ignorance by consulting and checking with these specialists. In some organizations management even has conferred on the members of the labor relations department the final authority to adjust grievances by conferring on them functional authority as discussed in Chapter 12.

The following discussion is based on an organizational setup in which the personnel and labor relations experts are in a staff position, and the initial formal authority and responsibility to handle grievances rest with the line supervisor. In every unionized organization, line supervisors know that handling grievances is part of their job and that it takes judgment, tact, and often more patience than comes naturally. Supervisors should not feel threatened by them. Supervisors frequently may feel that too much of their time is taken up in discussing complaints and grievances instead of getting the job done in the department. Or they may feel that they have to be more of a labor lawyer than a supervisor. But they should also realize that higher management regards the skill in handling grievances to be an important index of supervisory ability, and the number of grievances that come up within a department is considered a good indication of the state of employee-management relations.

It should be pointed out that although a fine distinction can be made between the terms complaint and grievance, from the supervisor's point of view a grievance simply means a complaint that has been formally presented either to the supervisor as a management representative or to the shop steward or any other union official. Normally, a grievance is a complaint resulting from a misunderstanding, misinterpretation, or violation of the provisions of the labor agreement. The supervisor must learn to distinguish, however, between those grievances which are admissible and those which are gripes and merely indicate that the employee is unhappy or dissatisfied. In the latter case, the supervisor should by all means listen to what the employee has to say in order to decide what action can be taken to correct the situation other than the grievance procedure. The grievance procedure, for the purposes of this chapter, means that there is a process to resolve a misunderstanding, misinterpretation, or violation of the union contract.

The Steward's Role

The steward is usually the spokesperson for the employee in a grievance procedure. He or she is familiar with the labor agreement and has been well indoctrinated as to how to present the employee's side of the grievance. A good shop steward is eager to get the credit for settling a grievance. Therefore, the question arises as to what the supervisor should do if an employee approaches him or her without the shop steward or without having consulted the shop steward. In such a case, it is appropriate for the supervisor to listen to the employee's story to see whether or not the case is of interest to the union or involves the union. If the indications are that the contract or the union are involved, then the supervisor by all means should call in the shop steward to listen to the employee's presentation. Although it is unlikely that a union member would present a grievance without the shop steward, the supervisor will do well to notify the steward if this should happen.

Similarly, if the steward submits a grievance by himself or herself, the supervisor should also listen carefully and with understanding. It is always best to listen to complaints when both the steward and the complaining employee are present, however. But if the steward does not bring the employee along, it still is necessary to listen to what the steward has to say. There is nothing to keep the supervisor from speaking directly to the employee later on, either with or without the steward. If the steward is not present, the supervisor should take great care not to give the impression that he or she is undermining the steward's authority or relationship with the union members. There should always be free and open communication between the supervisor and the shop steward despite the fact that it is the steward's job to represent employees and to fight hard to win their cases.

The Supervisor's Role

It is one of the supervisor's prime functions to dispose of all grievances at the first step of the grievance procedure. This means that it is part of the supervisor's job, usually with help from staff people in the personnel department, to fully explore the details of the grievance, deal with the problems brought out, and try to settle them. The supervisor will quickly learn that it pays to settle grievances early, before they grow from molehills into mountains. There occasionally will be some grievances that go beyond the first step and have to be referred to higher levels of management. But normally if many grievances go beyond this step, it may indicate that the supervisor is not carrying out the supervisory duties properly. Unless circumstances are beyond the supervisor's control, every effort should be made to handle grievances brought to his or her attention within reasonable time limits and to bring them to a successful conclusion. To achieve prompt and satisfactory adjustments of grievances at this early stage, the supervisor will do well to observe the following checklist.

Availability

The supervisor must be readily available to the shop steward and to the aggrieved employee. Availability does not only mean being physically around. It also means being approachable and ready to listen with an open mind. The supervisor must not make it difficult for a complaining employee to see him or her and sound off. This does not mean that the supervisor must stop immediately what he or she is doing, but every effort must be made to set a time as quickly as possible for the first hearing.

Listening Skills

Everything stated in the chapters on communication and interviewing (Chapters 5 and 17) is applicable to this situation also. When a complaint is brought to the supervisor, the steward and the employee should be given the opportunity to present their case fully. Sympathetic listening by the supervisor is likely to minimize hostilities and tensions during the settlement of the case. The supervisor must know how to listen well. He or she must give the steward and the employees a chance to say whatever they have on their minds. If they believe that the supervisor is truly listentling to them and that fair treatment will be given, the complaint will not loom as large to them as it did. It may even happen that halfway through the story the complaining employee realizes that he or she does not have a true complaint at all. Indeed, sympathetic listening can often produce this result. Or sometimes the more a person talks, the more likely he or she is to make contradictory and inconsistent remarks, thus weakening the argument. But only an effective listener will be able to catch these inconsistencies and use them to help resolve the case.

Emotional Control

The supervisor must take great caution not to get angry at the shop steward or the employee. It is the steward's job to represent the employee even when the steward knows that the grievance is not valid. In such a situation, it is the supervisor's job to objectively point out that there are no merits in the grievance. The supervisor cannot expect the shop steward to do this, because he or she must serve as the employee's spokesperson at all times.

Sometimes a union deliberately creates grievances to keep things stirred up. But even this type of situation must not arouse the anger of the supervisor. If the supervisor does not know how to handle such occurrences successfully, he or she should discuss the matter with higher management and experts in the labor relations or personnel department. But by no means must the supervisor get upset, even if a grievance is phony.

If arguments, tempers, and emotional outbursts run high and make good communications difficult, the supervisor may want to terminate the meeting and reschedule it. The supervisor must use caution not to participate in a shouting match. It is hoped that at the next meeting tempers have cooled down and a good discussion will be possible.

Defining the Problem

To determine whether a grievance is valid under the contract, it is necessary to precisely define the employee's complaint and the extent of the problem. Often the shop steward and the employee are not sufficiently clear in their presentations. It is then the supervisor's job to clearly summarize what has been presented and make certain that everyone understands the problem the complaint is trying to solve. Sometimes the complaint merely deals with the symptoms of the problem. The supervisor must know how deeply to delve in order to get at the root of the situation. Once the real problem is clarified and dealt with properly, it is not likely that grievances of the same type will come up again.

Obtaining the Facts

To arrive at a solution of the problem and a successful adjustment of the grievance, it is necessary to get all the facts as quickly as possible. The supervisor can get the facts by asking the complaining employee pertinent questions that may bring out inconsistencies. In so doing, the supervisor should be objective and should try not to confuse either the shop steward or the employee. The supervisor must ascertain who, what, when, where, and why. In other words, the supervisor must find out who or what caused the grievance, where and when it happened, and whether there was unfair treatment, intentionally or deliberately. He or she must also determine whether there is any connection between the current grievance and other grievances. Although it sometimes may be tempting to hide behind the excuse of searching for more facts, the supervisor must not do so. He or she must make a decision on the basis of those facts which are available and which can be obtained without undue delay.

Sometimes, however, it is impossible to gather all the information at once, and therefore it will not be possible to settle the grievance right away. Under those conditions, it is necessary to inform the aggrieved employee and the shop steward. If they see that the supervisor is working on the problem, they are likely to be reasonable and wait for an answer.

Familiarity With the Contract and Consultation

After having determined the facts, it is now essential for the supervisor to ascertain whether or not this is a legitimate grievance in the context of the contract. As mentioned earlier, a grievance is usually not a grievance in the legal sense unless provisions of the labor contract have been violated or administered inconsistently. Therefore, it is necessary to check the provisions in the contract when any reference to a violation of it is made. If the supervisor has any question about this, it would be wise to consult with someone in the personnel or labor relations department or higher management. Provisions in the labor agreement may not be clearly stated, and there may be a question as to whether a certain provision in the contract is applicable at all. It may be that changes have been made in the contract, and the supervisor must become acquainted with their intent and meaning and how they are to be interpreted.

Time Limits

Usually the grievance procedure sets a time limit within which the grievance must be answered. The supervisor must see that all grievances are settled as promptly and justly as possible. Postponing an adjustment in the hope that the complaint may disappear is courting trouble and more grievances. Moreover, an unnecessary postponement is unfair because the employee and the steward are entitled to know the supervisor's position as quickly as the facts can be obtained.

Speed is definitely important in the settlement of grievances, but not if it will result in unsound decisions. If it is impossible for the supervisor to obtain the necessary facts at once, the aggrieved parties must be informed, instead of leaving them under the impression that they are getting the runaround. Waiting for a decision is bothersome to everybody concerned; if a delay cannot be avoided, the grievance should be reduced to writing and signed by the steward and the employee so they do not forget what is involved.

Adjustment of Grievances as a Supervisory Function

It is part of the supervisor's job to see that all grievances are properly adjusted at the first step of the grievance procedure. As already pointed out, this is part of the managerial aspects of the supervisory function. It is far better to settle a minor issue at this stage before it escalates into a major case. The only cases that should be referred to higher levels of management are those which are of an unusual nature, require additional interpretation of the meaning of the union contract, contain problems that have not shown up before, or involve broad policy considerations.

Consistency of Action

In the adjustment of grievances, the supervisor must make certain that the rights of the administration are protected and that the policies and precedents of the hospital are followed. If the supervisor must deviate from previous adjustments, it is necessary to explain the reason to the employee and the shop steward. The supervisor must make certain that both of them understand that this exception does not set a precedent. In such cases, of course, it is always necessary for the supervisor to have this checked out with higher levels of administration and/or the personnel department.

The Consequences of the Settlement

The supervisor should not come up with a decision that is not consistent with previous decisions. It is necessary for the supervisor to check previous settlements and make certain that the current intended decision is consistent with past decisions, the institution's policy, and the labor agreement. The supervisor should avoid making an exception because this decision is likely to become a precedent; in adjusting grievances the supervisor must consider not only what effect the adjustment will have in this particular instance, but also its implications for the future. Whenever the supervisor settles a grievance, there is the possibility that this settlement will show up as part of the labor contract in following years. Also, if the case goes to arbitration, the arbitrator is likely to look for precedents and use them as a valid basis for the final decision.

Providing a Clear Answer

The supervisor must answer the grievance in a straightforward reasonable manner that is perfectly clear to the aggrieved parties. The answer must not be phrased in language that the aggrieved parties cannot understand, regardless of whether or not the adjustment is in favor of the employee. If the supervisor rules against the employee, the employee is that much more entitled to a clear and straightforward reply. Although the employee may disagree with such a reply, at least it will be understood.

Clarity is even more necessary if the supervisor has to reply to the grievance in writing. In that case, the answer must be restricted to the specific complaints involved, the words used must be appropriate, and any reference to a particular provision of the labor agreement or to plant rules must be clearly cited. Unless required, a written reply should not be rendered. But if such a reply is required by the labor agreement, then it is appropriate for the supervisor to discuss all the implications with higher management or with the personnel department so that a properly worded reply is available.

Record Keeping

It is essential for the supervisor to keep records whenever a decision is made. If the employee's request is satisfied, this decision will probably become a precedent. If the complaint cannot be settled in the first step, it is likely that this grievance will go farther, possibly to arbitration. It will certainly go to higher levels of management, and it is not wise for the supervisor to defend the action by depending on memory. Diligent records of the facts, reasoning, and decisions should be available. With this documentation at hand, the supervisor will be able to substantiate the actions whenever asked. Indeed, good records are an absolute necessity because the burden of proof is usually on the supervisor. It is correct to state that management has the right to decide, but that the union has the right to grieve. Whenever the employee or the union maintains that the supervisor has violated the agreement or has administered its provisions in an unfair or inconsistent manner, the supervisor must defend the action, and without good records this will often be difficult, if not impossible.

• • •

Supervisors should familiarize themselves with all of the twelve foregoing points as aids in handling grievances. No doubt the supervisors' decisions and actions will have a heavy impact on employee-union relations at the hospital or related health care facility. For this impact to be favorable, supervisors must not only be familiar with the above-mentioned points, but must also apply them during honest face-to-face discussions with employees and the shop steward whenever grievances do arise.

Summary

The labor agreement sets forth a broad, general outline of labor-management relationships. This outline must be filled in with intelligent supervisory decisions. Occasions to make such decisions arise mainly in the settlement of complaints and grievances. Indeed, the proper adjustment of grievances is one of the important components of the supervisory position. Whenever the supervisor settles grievances, the labor contract is referred to and interpreted, and the settlements have far-reaching implications because they set precedents. Much of what the union will discuss at the next contract negotiations has its origin in day-to-day supervisory decisions. And if a grievance should go to arbitration, the impartial arbitrator will also attach great importance to precedents set by the supervisor. Often it is not so much what the contract says that counts, but how it has been interpreted by management's front-line representative, namely, the supervisor. This shows how important a role the supervisor actually plays in the adjustment of grievances and how necessary it is to gain considerable skill in the use of adjustment techniques. In most organizations specialists in labor relations will be involved in arriving at the appropriate settlement.

To apply adjustment techniques appropriately, the supervisor will do well to always be available and listen, without losing his or her temper, even if the grievance is a "phony" one. The supervisor must learn to define the problem, get the facts, and then draw on a thorough knowledge of the clauses of the contract. It is also important to avoid unnecessary delays and settle grievances at an early stage. Moreover, the supervisor must be fair in all decisions, protecting the rights of the institution and respecting the content and spirit of the agreement; the supervisor, furthermore, must keep good records, give clear replies, and above all remain consistent.

APPENDIX B

Job Descriptions

Executive Department
Personnel Department
Nursing Service Department
Clinical Laboratories Department
Dietetic Department
Housekeeping Department
Laundry Department
Radiology—Nuclear Medicine Department

Job Descriptions

The purpose of this appendix is to provide the reader with sample job descriptions and organization charts illustrating many of the positions found in hospitals. The material is taken from *Job Descriptions and Organizational Analysis for Hospitals and Related Health Services,* U.S. Department of Labor, revised edition 1971, 1978 printing, published by the U.S. Government Printing Office.* The information in this document was compiled from a number of different sources and the results therefore show a composite picture. Naturally, the job descriptions "cannot be expected to coincide exactly with any single position in a specific institution. Therefore, usually it will be necessary to adapt descriptions to fit individual organization patterns and jobs before they can be used with complete accuracy."† In other words, the following information must be adjusted to accommodate specific local needs and peculiarities of a particular organization.

In deciding which of the many activities of a hospital to illustrate, the author wanted to cite some examples that are directly involved in patient care and some that support patient care. As examples of the first, the reader will find information on the nursing service, the clinical laboratories, and the dietary department. Housekeeping and laundry were chosen as examples of supportive activities. In addition, some information is given for a few overall administrative activities; the executive job of the administrator and the activities of the personnel department are examples. Of course, the choice of these activities at the exclusion of many others is not an indication that they are more important. In a hospital no activity can exist alone. All are needed and vital.

For each of the above-specified activities, the reader will find a short description of the functions, goals, and objectives of the department, followed by an organization chart. These charts are merely for illustrative purposes and should not necessarily be considered a

*For a more recent government publication see *Health Careers Guidebook*, 4th ed. (Washington DC: U.S. Department of Labor, Employment, and Training Administration and U.S. Department of Health, Education, and Welfare, Health Resources Administration, U.S. Government Printing Office, 1979). This publication contains information on the multitude of careers in the health care field and describes the duties, functions, job requirements, opportunities, education, etc., but does not contain job descriptions in the proper meaning of the term as used in our book.

†*Health Careers Guidebook*, 2.

recommended pattern of organization. Again, they are only a composite picture of what is often found. In addition, there are examples of job descriptions of supervisory positions in each department. The author has chosen the nursing service to show descriptions of all the jobs in at least one department. Again, this was not done to indicate that this department has greater importance over the others. They were chosen simply because more of all hospital employees usually work in this service than in the others.

Throughout this book the author has spoken about supervisors and department heads without referring to them as women or men. This was accomplished by using nouns or plural pronouns or the phrase "he or she." Occasionally these job descriptions refer to an individual, and the original government material may still refer to the individual by gender; this is not the author's choice but is in the quoted original source.

The author once more would like to point out that the material in this appendix should not be taken as "gospel." It must be adjusted to the idiosyncrasies of a particular job in a particular hospital. In some instances more up-to-date titles might be applicable; for example, the administrator might be referred to as the president, the personnel director as the director of human resources, the executive housekeeper as director of environmental services, etc. But the content of the job is essentially the same. This appendix is added with the hope that it will provide many additional examples and greater clarification of the material discussed in the text and will serve as a good start in writing specific job descriptions whenever the need arises.

EXECUTIVE DEPARTMENT

PURPOSE: Direct all functions of the hospital in keeping with over-all policies established by the governing board, in order that objectives of health care, advancement of knowledge, and over-all contribution to community welfare may be achieved most effectively, economically, and to the satisfaction of patients, employees, and medical staff.

RESPONSIBILITY: Interpreting and administering policies of governing board, and acting as technical advisor and liaison officer in matters involving formulation of these policies. To execute these functions properly, the department is responsible for management and supervision of all aspects of hospital activities, including planning and direction, public relations, budget and finance, personnel administration, volunteer services, purchase and supply, plant maintenance, housekeeping, general administrative services, and coordination of medical staff activities into the patient care program.

More specifically, responsibilities of the Executive Department include:

1. Transmitting, interpreting, and implementing policies, rules, and regulations affecting all hospital activities and personnel; establishing procedures for systematic performance of hospital duties; and coordinating activities of all departments.

2. Acting as liaison among governing board, medical staff, and hospital personnel, and encouraging maintenance of professional and medical standards through insistence on an organized medical staff prepared to adhere to prescribed quality standards. The ADMINISTRATOR is the chief executive officer of the board. In cooperation with medical staff and governing board, the Executive Department contracts for services of members of medical staff who are licensed to practice in the State.

3. Providing for equipment and facilities consistent with community needs and goals of the hospital, and insuring that high professional standards are maintained for health care. The Executive Department has primary responsibility for the safety and protection of hospital patients.

4. Formulating and maintaining an effective program of public relations. This involves explaining hospital costs and functions to the public, interpreting purpose and importance of the hospital in relation to community welfare, and participating in community affairs.

5. Maintaining sound financial structure, including establishing fee schedules, providing for careful, economical, and safe administration of funds, and maintaining accurate records of hospital finances. In cooperation with all departments, the Executive Department prepares a budget for approval by the board and drafts recommendations covering future operations of the hospital.

6. Formulating sound personnel policies and disseminating these policies to all hospital employees, developing an organizational structure with clearly defined lines of authority and areas of responsibility which will enable the employees to work together toward common objectives, selecting and training qualified department heads, coordinating all department activities, and establishing lines of communication between administrative and line employees.

7. Supervising maintenance and protection of buildings and grounds, giving final approval on equipment and supplies, and contracting for new construction.

8. Keeping up to date with advances in management techniques and business methods, technological changes, and economic and political trends, and broadening the perspective and scope of hospital services to meet expanding needs of the community.

9. Preparing periodic reports to the governing board covering progress and programs, as well as the activities of, and projected plans for, the hospital.

10. Maintaining liaison with local, State, and regional hospital and government health councils and planning agencies.

AUTHORITY: The ADMINISTRATOR reports directly to the governing authority, known as the Board of Directors, Board of Governors, or Trustees, and responsibility is delegated to him for carrying out established rules and regulations of the board. The guiding and directing force for administration comes from the governing authority as the primary policymaking body, and it specifically expresses the aims and goals to be achieved. The ADMINISTRATOR assists the governing authority in policy determination and initiates action on many matters which require an expressed policy. He develops statements of policy for consideration and approval by the governing authority. At the same time, constant review and periodic modification of policies are essential. After policies are adopted, the ADMINISTRATOR is delegated full authority to conduct activities of the hospital to achieve desired results. The ADMINISTRATOR, in turn, delegates to department heads authority over their respective departments.

INTERRELATIONSHIPS AND INTRARELATIONSHIPS: Ultimate responsibility for all hospital activities rests with the ADMINISTRATOR. Coordination of various sections or departments is a major function of the Executive Department. To accomplish this the Executive Department maintains effective communication with all departments of the hospital.

The personal contacts between the ADMINISTRATOR and governing authority, medical staff, department heads, auxiliaries, patients, public health officials, civic organizations, and numerous other groups and individuals typify interrelationships in activities of the Executive Department.

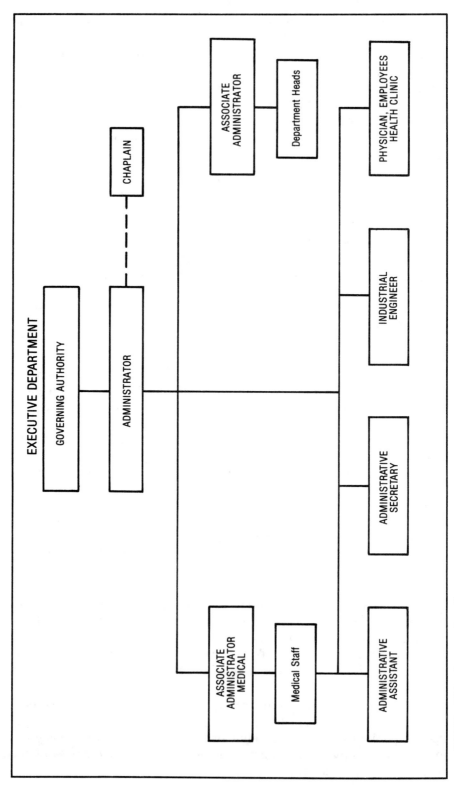

NOTE: This chart is for illustrative purposes and should not be considered a recommended pattern of organization.

The education and training functions of the hospital require careful organization and followup of all programs to insure that standards are achieved and maintained.

STANDARDS: Certain minimum standards for medical and professional care established by the Joint Commission on Accreditation of Hospitals, the American College of Surgeons, American Medical Association, American Hospital Association, American Osteopathic Hospital Association, and other accrediting and licensing agencies are obligatory for the hospital. All standards must be thoroughly understood to insure conformance.

In addition, the American College of Hospital Administrators promotes increasing efficiency of hospital administration by encouraging programs for the continuing education of hospital administrators.

STAFFING: Staffing of the Executive Department will vary in accordance with size, type, and activities of the hospital. In the large hospital, the ADMINISTRATOR may have one or more assistants in several primary administrative areas. In a small institution the ADMINISTRATOR may attend to details in many functional areas.

Executive Department   Superintendent, Hospital 187.118

ADMINISTRATOR

executice director
executive vice president
hospital administrator

JOB DUTIES

Administers, directs, and coordinates all activities of the hospital to carry out its objectives in the provision of health care, furtherance of education and research, and participation in community health programs:

Is responsible for the operation of the hospital, for the application and implementation of established policies, and for liaison among the governing authority, the medical staff, and the departments of the hospital.

Organizes the functions of the hospital through appropriate departmentalization and the delegation of duties. Establishes formal means of accountability from those to whom he has assigned duties. Regularly schedules interdepartmental and departmental meetings, where appropriate, to maintain liaison between the medical staff and other departments. Names appropriate departmental representatives to the multidisciplinary committee of the hospital.

Prepares reports for, and attends meetings with, the governing body regarding the total activities of the institution as well as governmental developments which affect health care. Provides for personnel policies and practices that adequately support sound patient care and maintain accurate and complete personnel records.

Reviews and acts upon the reports of authorized inspecting agencies.

Implements the control and effective utilization of the physical and financial resources of the hospital. Employs a system of responsible accounting, including budget and internal controls.

Participates, or is represented, in community, State, and national hospital associations and professional activities which define the delivery of health care services and aid in short- and long-range planning of health services and facilities. Provides an acceptable public relations program.

Pursues a continuing program of formal and informal education in health care, administrative, and management areas to maintain, strengthen, and broaden his concepts, philosophy, and ability as a health care administrator.

Delegates administrative responsibilities to ASSOCIATE ADMINISTRATORS and to department heads.

MACHINES, TOOLS, EQUIPMENT, AND WORK AIDS
None.

EDUCATION, TRAINING, AND EXPERIENCE

Graduation from an accredited college or university, with graduate work in an accredited program in hospital administration.

Education and experience requirements may vary according to individual background, size of hospital, and section of the country. However, a minimum of 3 years of serving in subordinate administrative positions is required by most hospitals. Larger hospitals may require 1 year of resident or administrative internship experience.

WORKER TRAITS

Aptitudes: Verbal ability is required to express ideas and views effectively when speaking to groups, hospital directors, and personnel. Must be able to gather and analyze data contained in reports.

Numerical ability required to evaluate statistical data and to make various computations in planning hospital operations and budget.

Clerical ability is necessary to read reports and utilize data accurately for other purposes.

Interests: A preference for activities involving esteem of others is required to lead professional and nonprofessional workers and to participate in community activities.

Temperaments: Organizational ability to plan and control the total activity of the hospital and the activities of all its personnel.

Ability to relate to people in a manner so as to win confidence and establish support.

Ability to evaluate reports, research studies, and other data against both judgmental and verifiable criteria.

Flexibility to adjust to changing conditions and the various details of the job.

Physical Demands and Working Conditions: This is light work. Sits and walks throughout the working day.

Talking and hearing to converse with individual members of hospital staff and to address various groups.

Handling office equipment and supplies.

Works inside. Usually has own office.

Visual acuity to prepare and read reports.

Hours of duty may be long and irregular.

JOB RELATIONSHIPS

Workers supervised: All employees of hospital through ASSOCIATE ADMINISTRATORS and department heads.

Supervised by: Governing authority of hospital.

Promotion from: ASSOCIATE ADMINISTRATOR.

Promotion to: No formal line of promotion. This is the highest occupation level in the hospital.

PROFESSIONAL AFFILIATIONS

American College of Hospital
Administrators
840 North Lake Shore Drive
Chicago, Illinois 60611

Association of University Programs
in Hospital Administration
1642 East 56th Street
Chicago, Ill. 60637

Local, state, and national hospital
associations.
Local and State civic and services
organizations.

PERSONNEL DEPARTMENT

PURPOSE: To coordinate the needs and interests of the institution with those of the employees in a manner so as to provide the community with efficient, economical hospital service, and to staff the hospital with qualified, productive employees.

RESPONSIBILITY: Personnel administration is characterized by the philosophy, motives, and methods of organizing and treating people so that they will consistently perform at the highest levels of which they are capable, while obtaining the greatest degree of satisfaction.

The number and kinds of functions assigned the Personnel Department will vary greatly depending upon the needs, size, and goals of the hospital.

The department is responsible within delegated authority, for planning and administering a comprehensive personnel program, including participation in development of an overall personnel policy. It is responsible for developing techniques and procedures to assist line supervisors in improving the personnel aspects of their jobs. It serves as advisor to the ADMINISTRATOR on personnel problems, proposes changes in established personnel policies, and consults with and assists supervisors on a continuing basis. The major functions of this department may be classified as (1) developing sources of qualified employees, (2) recruiting and retaining competent personnel, and (3) increasing employee productivity and job stability.

Specifically, the Personnel Department performs some or all of the following functions: Recruits and screens job applicants; inducts and orients new employees; advises on methods of training and may plan and conduct training programs; develops procedures and policies to promote employee stabilization; develops procedures for position control through job analyses and job evaluations; establishes and maintains programs of wage and salary administration, and employee benefits; assists in planning and establishing lines of communication; may take part in collective bargaining procedures; establishes health and safety programs; advises the administration on legal problems relating to employment; does research to determine causes of and solution to personnel problems; advises on hospital organization and helps establish employee budgetary controls; maintains complete personnel files on all employees; and maintains organization charts and staffing patterns.

AUTHORITY: Final authority for applying sound personnel policies rests with the ADMINISTRATOR. The PERSONNEL DIRECTOR exercises line authority only over employees in the Personnel Department. Personnel administration is a staff function. As such, it has no direct authority over operating or line supervision.

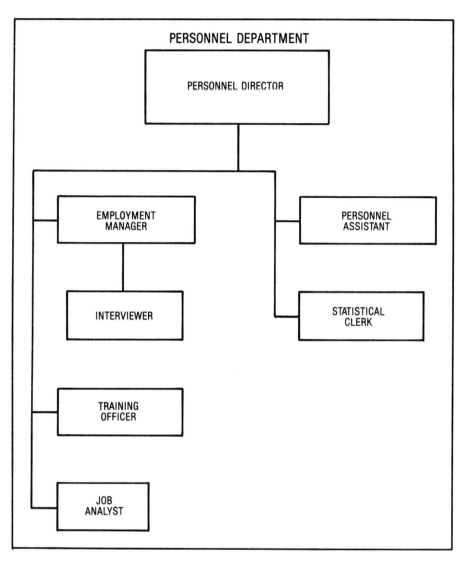

NOTE: This chart is for illustrative purposes only and should not be considered a recommended pattern of organization.

INTERRELATIONSHIPS AND INTRARELATIONSHIPS: Because administrative officials recognize the need for specialized knowledge and careful planning to insure sound personnel relations, personnel administration has become a separate department. Since the PERSONNEL DIRECTOR, as a specialist, is chief advisor to the ADMINISTRATOR on all matters involving employee relations, he should report directly to the ADMINISTRATOR. As a staff officer, he works in cooperation with each department head to secure the maximum in employee efficiency and morale within the hospital.

Sound employee relations tend to be reflected in employee contacts with the public; therefore, the Personnel Department is a key to good public relations. Through direct contacts with other departments, job applicants, employment agencies, social agencies, schools, public officials, and many other groups and individuals, the Personnel Department is in a unique position to create a favorable impression of the hospital and promote progressive public relations.

PHYSICAL FACILITIES AND STAFFING: The personnel offices should be easily accessible to job applicants and hospital personnel. They should be attractive and impress visitors favorably. Provision should be made for privacy in employment interviews and discussions with employees.

The Personnel Department is normally under the supervision of a PERSONNEL DIRECTOR, who has mature judgment, leadership, and specialized knowledge of personnel administration. No exact ratio has been established between numbers of employees in the Personnel Department and total personnel in the organization. The needs of the institution and functions assigned to the Personnel Department will affect the number of employees required. In smaller hospitals, personnel functions are often combined with other administrative responsibilities. With such combinations, there should be a clear division of time and responsibility, so that the personnel function is not subordinated to another function.

Both the professional and clerical staffs of this department are subject to combinations of job duties. Depending upon the size and organizational makeup of the particular hospital, each job shown on the organization chart may merit standing alone as described in the JOB DUTIES, or be broken into additional job titles (not shown), or be combined into any one of the job titles listed.

Personnel Department   Manager, Personnel 166.118

PERSONNEL DIRECTOR

JOB DUTIES

Plans, coordinates, and administers policies relating to all phases of hospital personnel activities:

Plans and develops a personnel program and establishes methods for its installation and operation. Develops the techniques and procedures for and directs the activities of recruitment, induction, placement, orientation and training. He may also be responsible for the safety and security programs. Interprets hospital policies and regulations to new employees, arranges for their physical examinations, and conducts or advises on training programs. Establishes uniform employment policies and confers with department heads and supervisors to discuss improvement of working relationships and conditions. Assists in development of plans and policies related to personnel and advises supervisors and administrative officials regarding specific personnel problems. Initiates and recommends policies and procedures necessary to achieve objectives of the hospital and insure maximum utilization and stability of personnel. Initiates and directs surveys related to turnover, wages, benefits, morale, and other personnel considerations. Prepares training manuals and directs job analysis program, including preparation of job descriptions and specifications. Acts as liaison between employees and administrative staff. Investigates causes of disputes and grievances and recommends corrective action. Supervises workers engaged in carrying out personnel department functions.

Plans and sets up system of recordkeeping. Devises forms relative to the personnel functions. Organizes system for maintenance of central personnel files that will provide ready analysis of all personnel management functions.

Administers benefit services and other employer-employee programs, including recreation, pension and hospitalization plans, credit union, vacation and leave policies, and others. Initiates and implements employee suggestions and performance evaluation systems.

Informs employees of hospital activities and administrative policies by means of handbooks, house organs, bulletin boards, and other media. Performs research as a basis for recommending changes in procedures and policies. Interviews all terminating employees to determine causes of termination. Represents hospital at conferences relative to personnel activities. Prepares budgets.

MACHINES, TOOLS, EQUIPMENT, AND WORK AIDS
Office supplies and equipment.

EDUCATION, TRAINING, AND EXPERIENCE
Graduation from a recognized college or university with a degree in personnel management, industrial relations, or business administration.

Courses should include tests and measurements, statistics, applied psychology, personnel and business administration, economics, labor relations, and cost accounting.

Experience as Assistant Personnel Director is recommended. Receives inservice indoctrination in hospital policies and regulations.

WORKER TRAITS
Aptitudes: Verbal ability is required to discuss personnel programs with administrative staff and employees of varying levels of verbal ability, to effectively promote the personnel program, and to explain hospital policy to individuals and groups. Capability also required to prepare manuals.

Numerical ability is required to evaluate personnel statistical data, to make various computations of departmental operations, and to prepare budgets.

Clerical ability is required to avoid and detect errors in verbal and tabular material prepared for submission to administrative personnel.

Interests: A preference for technical activities in order to develop and administer personnel policies.

A preference for activities that involve working with people in order to make the personnel policy effective and satisfactory to all hospital employees and to administrators.

Temperaments: Ability to direct and plan the activities of the entire Personnel Department.

Ability to communicate with hospital staff and outsiders as well as workers within his department, in making and carrying out personnel policies and regulations.

Must be able to make decisions.

Physical Demands and Working Conditions: Work is sedentary, requiring lifting and handling personnel records and files, seldom exceeding 10 pounds.

Frequent talking and hearing when conferring on personnel matters, interviewing, or assigning work to subordinates.

Works inside. Usually has own office.

JOB RELATIONSHIPS

Workers supervised: EMPLOYMENT MANAGER; INTERVIEWER; TRAINING OFFICER; JOB ANALYST; and clerical staff.

Supervised by: ADMINISTRATOR.

Promotion from: Assistant Personnel Director or EMPLOYMENT MANAGER.

Promotion to: No formal line of promotion. May be promoted to an ASSOCIATE ADMINISTRATOR.

PROFESSIONAL AFFILIATIONS

American Society for Personnel
   Administration
52 East Bridge Street
Berea, Ohio 44017

American Personnel and Guidance
   Association
1605 New Hampshire Avenue, NW.
Washington, D.C. 20009

Public Personnel Association
1313 East 60th Street
Chicago, Ill. 60637

American Society for Hospital
   Personnel Directors
840 North Lake Shore Drive
Chicago, Ill. 60611

State and local personnel associations and societies.

NURSING SERVICE DEPARTMENT

PURPOSE: To provide safe, efficient, and therapeutically effective nursing care.

RESPONSIBILITY: To care for the patient. The Nursing Service Department carries out its functions according to the philosophy, objectives, and policies of the hospital established by the governing authority. Within this framework the department's functions are:

1. To provide and evaluate nursing service for patients and their families in support of medical care as directed by the medical staff.

2. To define and carry out the philosophy, objectives, policies, and standards for nursing care of patients and related nursing services.

3. To provide and implement a departmental plan of administrative authority which clearly delineates responsibilities and duties of each category of nursing personnel.

4. To coordinate the department's functions with the functions of all other hospital departments and services.

5. To estimate the department's requirements and to recommend policies and procedures to maintain an adequate and competent nursing staff.

6. To provide the means and methods by which the nursing personnel can work with other groups in interpreting the objectives of the hospital and nursing service to the patient and community.

7. To participate in the formulation of personnel policies, interpret established policies, and evaluate their effectiveness.

8. To develop and maintain an effective system of clinical and administrative nursing records and reports.

9. To estimate needs for facilities, supplies, and equipment, and to establish an evaluation and control system.

10. To participate in and adhere to the financial plan of operation of the hospital.

11. To initiate, utilize, and/or participate in studies or research projects for improving patient care and other administrative and hospital services.

12. To provide and execute a program of continuing education for all nursing personnel.

13. To participate in and/or facilitate all educational programs which include student experiences in the Nursing Service Department.

The special nursing units in the Nursing Service Department usually include medical, surgical, pediatric, obstetric, and psychiatric. In addition to the overall responsibilities and functions of nursing service, the units also carry more specific responsibilities and functions of patient care, varying with each nursing unit. The establishment and execution of educational programs for staff and student nurses are functions of these special nursing units.

Medical and Surgical: Nursing care is provided in medical and surgical units in accordance with physician's instructions and recognized techniques and procedures. While medical conditions are not easily divided into distinct categories, medical nursing is considered a specialty in that normal and abnormal reactions or symptoms of diagnosed diseases must be recognized and reported. The patient with a stroke or a cardiac condition requires a much different type of nursing from that given the patient with an ulcer or diabetes. Surgical patients also require special preoperative and postoperative care.

Pediatrics: This service embraces the care of children. Care of the newborn is usually in a separate unit located in the obstetric unit. The activities of the pediatric unit require understanding of the unique needs, fears, and behavior of children, which is reflected in the type and degree of nursing care given. Where illnesses require protracted convalescence, educational and occupational therapy become concerns of the nursing service. Relationships with parents pose further important responsibilities.

Obstetrics: Prenatal care, observation, and comfort of patients in labor, delivery room assistance, and care of mother after delivery, as well as nursing care of newborn, are important responsibilities of this unit. Obstetric nurses assist in instructing new mothers in postnatal care and care of the newborn. Care of the newborn, particularly the premature, requires special nursing skills dictated by their unique requirements.

Psychiatric: While most emotionally disturbed patients are treated in specialized hospitals, the general hospital also recognizes a responsibility and provides facilities for the mentally ill. Nursing care of the mentally ill requires a knowledge of their various behavior patterns and how to cope with them. Techniques must be learned for dealing with all types of problem behavior, so that skilled, therapeutic care is given to such patients. Family and community education is also an important function of the psychiatric unit.

Other special units within the Nursing Service Department are Operating Room, Recovery Room, Emergency Room, and an Intensive Care Unit.

Operating Room: This unit has primary responsibility for comforting patients in the O. R.; maintaining aseptic techniques; scheduling all operations in cooperation with surgeons; and determining that adequate personnel, space, and equipment are available. Nursing personnel assist the surgeon during operations and are part of the surgical team. Preparation for operations includes sterilization of instruments and equipment; cleaning up after operations is also part of the unit's responsibility.

Recovery Room: In many hospitals, the Recovery Room unit is an adjunct responsibility of the Operating Room unit. Special nursing attention must be given patients after an operation until they have completely recovered from the effects of anesthesia.

Emergency Room: This unit is responsible for emergency care, and for arrangements to admit the patient to the hospital, if necessary. The unit completes required records; makes reports to police and safety and health agencies; handles matters of payment, and notification of relatives; and refers patients to other services within the hospital or community, as needed.

Intensive Care: Many hospitals have an Intensive Care unit; some hospitals have several. These units usually accommodate a limited number of patients whose conditions are very critical or require specialized care and equipment such as electronic instruments for observation, signaling, recording, and measuring physiological functions. In addition to providing continuous recording of cardiac function, bedside systems may monitor temperature, blood pressure, respiration rate, and other measurements. More nurses are assigned per number of patients and they are continuously in the room or within sight of the patient under care. This makes it possible to give close attention to the critically ill or postoperative patient requiring intensive care, and to concentrate special equipment where it is most likely to be needed. An increasing number of specialized "teams" consists of one or more physicians and other medical specialists, nurses, and ancillary personnel who respond to emergency situations. They are known by the specialized function they perform such as "cardiac team" or "kidney failure team."

AUTHORITY: At the head of the department is a DIRECTOR, NURSING SERVICE, who reports to the ADMINISTRATOR, and as a part of top management, is delegated authority to provide a nursing service in accordance with overall hospital policies. Although professional nursing practices are developed cooperatively with the medical and other professional staffs, the DIRECTOR, NURSING SERVICE retains authority over nursing practice.

The ASSISTANT DIRECTOR, NURSING SERVICE, assists in planning and directing all hospital nursing service activities.

Each of the special units described earlier is usually headed by a nurse supervisor who reports to the ASSISTANT DIRECTOR, NURSING SERVICE. Nurses and ancillary workers assigned to each unit are supervised by the unit supervisor, who is delegated authority for accomplishing the unit's functions.

A single composite job description has been prepared for NURSE, SUPERVISOR, one for NURSE, HEAD, and one for NURSE, STAFF. Nurses within each of these three categories perform essentially the same duties and have the same responsibilities.

The variations and additional duties depend upon the specialized nursing unit to which the nurse is assigned or in which she has specialized. Nursing positions have been treated in this manner to eliminate repetition and simplify presentation of the jobs in the Nursing Service Department.

INTERRELATIONSHIPS AND INTRARELATIONSHIPS: The relationships between the Nursing Service Department and other hospital departments are complex and numerous.

Smooth operation of hospital services and patient care and treatment depend upon coordinated activities of all hospital departments. The Nursing Service Department is the hub around which many of the activities of direct patient care are centered. The department should participate in the development of administrative policies and procedures affecting nursing as well as other hospital services. Relationships with other departments such as dietary, housekeeping, laundry, laboratories, and medical records and the importance of each in the care of a patient should be mutually understood and appreciated. A definite program of conferences to work out common problems helps in developing more effective work relationships. Manuals of standard techniques, procedures, and policies to accomplish this objective should be written and periodically reviewed, discussed, and revised.

Nursing personnel have closer contact with patients over longer periods of time than any other group of hospital personnel. The nurses' attitudes are vitally important to the emotional and physical well-being of patients. The nurse-patient relationship cannot be given too much emphasis. The Nursing Service Department plays an important role in the development of good public relations for hospitals.

STANDARDS: Standards for this department have been defined by the American Nurses' Association, National League for Nursing, and the Joint Commission for Accreditation of Hospitals. Registered Nurses must be licensed by their State; most States also require the licensing of practical nursing personnel.

PHYSICAL FACILITIES AND STAFFING: The physical facilities of the Nursing Service Department will depend upon, among other factors, the size and type of hospital. Certain special facilities have already been mentioned. In addition to patient care facilities, the department will need administrative offices, conference rooms, and dressing rooms for personnel.

Ancillary workers, such as NURSING AIDES, ORDERLIES, clerical workers, and others, assume many of the nonprofessional responsibilities associated with care of the patient.

An inservice training program should be set up for both professional and nonprofessional workers. All members of the Nursing Service Department should be included in order to develop and main-

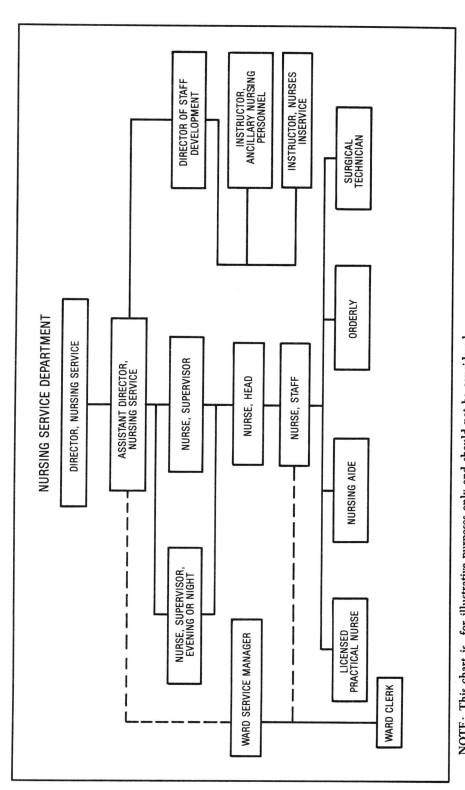

NURSING SERVICE DEPARTMENT

NOTE: This chart is for illustrative purposes only and should not be considered a recommended pattern of organization.

tain an esprit de corps, foster new ideas, improve technical and professional skills of the individual, and provide a means of group expression.

Certain special demands on nursing service personnel exist because of their relationship with the patients they care for. They must be able to work with the realization that incompetence and errors may have serious consequences for the patient. Understanding, patience, and tact enhance the emotional well-being of patients. These qualities are needed, also, in dealing with patients' visitors and relatives. Nursing service personnel must be alert in recognizing symptoms and skillful in applying techniques and procedures in which they have been trained, in treating unusual, unfavorable, and often unpleasant conditions. Resourcefulness and the ability to think clearly in emergencies are also needed.

GENERAL WORKING CONDITIONS: Although nursing service personnel may be subject to various physical strains in caring for patients who are wholly or partially unable to move themselves, this hazard, as well as danger to the patient, can be minimized by following proper lifting techniques and using various devices and equipment designed for this purpose.

There is also the possibility of exposure to communicable disease or infections. When these conditions are suspected or become known, special isolation and asepsis procedures are followed to prevent spreading of the condition to self and others.

Some patients undergo radiological treatments which require the presence of nursing personnel or may bear radiological materials as a result of certain treatments. Where the possibility of exposure to dangerous amounts of radioactivity exists, personnel wear film badges which are periodically analyzed, as well as following specified procedures in caring for such patients.

Traditionally, nursing service personnel wear distinctive clothing on duty. In special units, such as operating room, nursery, or in rooms isolated due to presence of communicable disease, special (often sterile) clothing is usually required. Special clothing is worn to prevent the spread of disease or other contamination. In the operating room, clothing is sterile to prevent contamination.

Nursing Service Department   Director, Nursing Service 075.118

DIRECTOR, NURSING SERVICE

JOB DUTIES

Organizes and administers the department of nursing:

Establishes objectives for the department of nursing and the organizational structure for achieving these objectives. Interprets and puts into effect administrative policies established by the governing authority. Assists in preparing and administering budget for the department. Selects and recommends appointment of nursing staff.

Directs and delegates management of professional and ancillary nursing personnel. Plans and conducts conferences and discussions with administrative and professional nursing staff to encourage participation in formulating departmental policies and procedures, promote initiative, solve problems, and interpret new policies and procedures. Coordinates activities of various nursing units, promoting and maintaining harmonious relationships among nursing personnel and with medical staff, patients, and public. Plans and directs orientation and inservice training programs for professional and nonprofessional nursing staff. Analyzes and evaluates nursing and related services rendered to improve quality of patient care and plan better utilization of staff time and activities. Participates in community educational health programs.

MACHINES, TOOLS, EQUIPMENT, AND WORK AIDS
Office equipment.

EDUCATION, TRAINING, AND EXPERIENCE
Graduation from an accredited school of nursing with a bachelor's degree preferred, and a master's degree desirable. Current licensure by State Board of Nursing required, and demonstrated administrative ability.

Five to 10 years' nursing experience, including satisfactory experience as instructor or supervisor, or as assistant director in a school of nursing.

WORKER TRAITS
Aptitudes: Verbal ability is required to express ideas and views effectively when speaking to groups, hospital directors, and personnel, and to gather and analyze data and prepare reports.

Numerical ability is required to evaluate statistical data and to make various computations in planning departmental operations and budget.

Interests: A preference for contacts with people, such as organizing and planning programs, developing staff, and assigning personnel.

Temperaments: Organizational ability to plan and control the entire activities of the Nursing Service Department and personnel activities.

Ability to relate to people to win their confidence and establish support for programs.

Ability to evaluate reports, programs, and other data against both judgmental and verifiable criteria.

Physical Demands and Working Conditions: Work is sedentary. Occasional walking about office and to and from various hospital areas.

Talking and hearing when supervising and conferring with others.

Works inside.

JOB RELATIONSHIPS
Workers supervised: General supervision of all nursing personnel in the hospital.
Supervised by: ADMINISTRATOR.
Promotion from: ASSISTANT DIRECTOR, NURSING SERVICE.
Promotion to: No formal line of promotion.

PROFESSIONAL AFFILIATIONS

American Nurses' Association
10 Columbus Circle
New York, N.Y. 10019

American Society for Nursing
Service Administrators
840 North Lake Shore Drive
Chicago, Ill. 60611

National League for Nursing
10 Columbus Circle
New York, N.Y. 10019
State and local nursing associations.

Nursing Service Department   Director, Nursing Service 075.118

ASSISTANT DIRECTOR, NURSING SERVICE

JOB DUTIES

Assists in organizing and administering the department of nursing; assumes responsibilities delegated by DIRECTOR, NURSING SERVICE:

Conducts conferences and discussions with personnel to encourage participation in formulating departmental policies, promote initiative, solve problems, and present new policies and procedures.

Analyzes nursing and auxiliary services to improve quality of patient care and to obtain maximum utilization of staff time and abilities. Coordinates activities of the nursing service units to achieve and maintain efficient and competent nursing service and to promote and maintain harmonious relationships among personnel supervised, medical staff, patients, and others. Assists in establishing lines of authority and responsibility, and defining the duties of nursing service personnel, consistent with good administrative techniques, to assure that department objectives are accomplished.

Assists in review and evaluation of budget requests against current and projected needs of nursing service.

Interviews applicants and recommends appointment of staff personnel, outlining their duties, scope of authority, and responsibilities. Participates in establishing and administering orientation and inservice training programs for both professional and nonprofessional personnel. Insures proper and economical use of equipment, supplies, and facilities for maintaining patient care. Maintains personnel and other records, and directs maintenance of patient care records.

Cooperates with medical staff performing research projects or studies as they affect nursing. Works with other agencies and groups in the community to promote the growth and broaden knowledges and skills of professional staff, and improve quality of hospital services.

MACHINES, TOOLS, EQUIPMENT, AND WORK AIDS

Office equipment.

EDUCATION, TRAINING, AND EXPERIENCE

Graduation from an accredited school of nursing with bachelor's degree preferred, and master's degree desirable. Current licensure by State Board of Nursing required, and demonstrated administrative ability.

Experience in a supervisory capacity with demonstrated executive ability and leadership.

WORKER TRAITS

Aptitudes: Verbal ability is necessary to understand and present oral and written material in communicating with superiors and subordinates.

Numerical ability is required to evaluate statistical data and to make various computations in planning departmental operations and budget.

Clerical ability is necessary to read reports and utilize data accurately for other purposes.

Interests: A preference for contacts with people, implemented in organizing and planning programs and assigning personnel to provide nursing service for patients.

Temperaments: Ability to plan and direct hospital nursing service program, coordinating it with activities of other departments.

Ability to confer and cooperate with other department heads, personnel of outside agencies, and supervisors.

Physical Demands and Working Conditions: Work is sedentary; occasional walking about office and to and from various hospital areas.

Talking and hearing are involved in supervising and conferring with others.

Works inside.

JOB RELATIONSHIPS

Workers supervised: Direct supervision of NURSE, SUPERVISORS and indirect supervision of all professional and ancillary nursing staff in the department.

Supervised by: DIRECTOR, NURSING SERVICE.

Promotion from: May be promoted from a nursing position in which administrative ability has been demonstrated.

Promotion to: DIRECTOR, NURSING SERVICE.

PROFESSIONAL AFFILIATIONS

American Nurses' Association
10 Columbus Circle
New York, N.Y. 10019
State and local nursing associations.

National League for Nursing
10 Columbus Circle
New York, N.Y. 10019

Nursing Service Department   **Nurse, Supervisor 075.128**

NURSE, SUPERVISOR

JOB DUTIES

Supervises and coordinates activities of nursing personnel engaged in specific nursing services, such as obstetrics, pediatrics, or surgery, or for two or more patient care units:

Supervises Head Nurses in carrying out their responsibilities in the management of nursing care. Evaluates performance of Head Nurse and nursing care as a whole and suggests modifications. Inspects unit areas to verify that patient needs are met.

Participates in planning work of own units and coordinates activities with other patient care units and with those of related departments.

Consults with NURSE, HEAD, on specific nursing problems and interpretation of hospital policies. Supervises maintenance of personnel and nursing records.

Plans and organizes orientation and inservice training for unit staff members and participates in guidance and educational programs. Interviews prescreened applicants and makes recommendations for employing or for terminating personnel. Assists

DIRECTOR, NURSING SERVICE in formulating unit budget. Engages in studies and investigations related to improved nursing care.

NURSE, SUPERVISOR is usually known by name of nursing section to which assigned or in which she has specialized, such as NURSE, SUPERVISOR, MEDICAL AND SURGICAL or NURSE, SUPERVISOR, PEDIATRICS. Specialized duties will be required by the specialized section.

MACHINES, TOOLS, EQUIPMENT, AND WORK AIDS

Manuals, patient charts, nursing care plans, records, and work schedules.

EDUCATION, TRAINING, AND EXPERIENCE

Graduation from an accredited school of nursing and current licensure by State Board of Nursing. Advanced education desirable. Experience as NURSE, HEAD in which administrative, supervisory, and teaching abilities have been demonstrated.

WORKER TRAITS

Aptitudes: Verbal ability is necessary to present information and ideas essential to supervisory duties, to understand advanced nursing theory and practice, and to maintain good working relationships with staff and medical personnel.

Clerical perception is necessary to prepare records and charts and to organize training programs.

Interests: A preference for contacts with people, as in supervising and instructing nursing personnel.

A preference for scientific and technical activities for understanding and responding to medical problems and concepts.

Temperaments: Ability to plan, supervise, and coordinate activities.

Ability to interpret operating policies and procedures and to review work performance in determining conformance to recognized standards.

Able to make decisions regarding performance methods.

Physical Demands and Working Conditions: Work is of medium demand; walking and standing most of the time on duty.

Frequent reaching, handling, and fingering of instruments, equipment, records, and reports.

Talking and hearing essential to instruct and supervise nursing personnel.

Near-visual acuity required to detect changes in patients' condition.

Color vision for perceiving changes in patients' skin color and colors of medicines and solutions.

Works inside.

JOB RELATIONSHIPS

Workers supervised: NURSES, HEAD directly, and indirectly other professional and nursing personnel.

Supervised by: ASSISTANT DIRECTOR, NURSING SERVICE.

Promotion from: NURSE, HEAD.

Promotion to: ASSISTANT DIRECTOR, NURSING SERVICE.

PROFESSIONAL AFFILIATIONS

American Nurses' Association
10 Columbus Circle
New York, N.Y. 10019

National League for Nursing
10 Columbus Circle
New York, N.Y. 10019

State and local nursing associations.

Nursing Service Department   Nurse, Supervisor 075.128

NURSE, SUPERVISOR, EVENING OR NIGHT
assistant director of nursing, evening or night

JOB DUTIES

Supervises and coordinates activities of nursing personnel on evening or night tour to maintain continuity for around-the-clock nursing care:

Visits nursing units to oversee nursing care and to ascertain condition of patients. Advises and assists nurses in administering new or unusual treatments. Gives advice for treatments, medications, and narcotics, in accordance with medical staff policies, in absence of physician. Arranges for emergency operations and reallocates personnel during emergencies. Admits or delegates admissions of new patients. Arranges for services of private-duty nurses. Determines necessity of calling physician. May perform some bedside nursing services.

Delegates preparation of reports covering such items as critically ill patients, new admissions, discharges or deaths, emergency situations encountered, and private-duty nurses employed. Informs supervisory personnel on ensuing tour of duty of patients' condition and hospital services rendered during work period.

Interprets hospital policies and regulations to staff members, patients, and visitors, and insures conformance. Evaluates work performance and assists in preparing performance reports for nursing staff. Participates in staff education and conferences for formulating policies and program plans and for integration of various nursing services.

MACHINES, TOOLS, EQUIPMENT, AND WORK AIDS

Manuals, patient charts, nursing care plans, records, and work schedules.

EDUCATION, TRAINING, AND EXPERIENCE

Graduation from an accredited school of nursing and current licensure by State Board of Nursing. Experience desirable as NURSE, SUPERVISOR, during which executive ability has been demonstrated.

WORKER TRAITS

Aptitudes: Verbal ability is necessary to present information and ideas essential to supervisory duties.

Numerical ability is required to evaluate statistical data and to make various computations in planning operations and budgets for units.

Clerical perception is necessary for the preparation of records and charts.

Interests: A preference for business contacts with people, for supervising and instructing nursing personnel.

A preference for scientific and technical activities, for understanding and responding to medical problems and concepts.

Temperaments: Ability to plan, supervise, and coordinate activities of nursing personnel on night duty.

Ability to interpret operating policies and procedures and to review work performance in determining conformance to recognized standards.

Ability to make decisions regarding work performance of nursing personnel.

Physical Demands and Working Conditions: Work is of medium demand; walking and standing most of the time on duty.

Frequent reaching, handling, and fingering of instruments, equipment, records, and reports, and in caring for patients' needs.

Talking and hearing essential to instruct and supervise nursing personnel.

Near-visual acuity required to detect changes in patients' condition.

Color vision for perceiving changes in patients' skin color and colors of medicines and solutions.

Works inside.

JOB RELATIONSHIPS

Workers supervised: Professional and ancillary nursing personnel assigned to evening or night service.

Supervised by: DIRECTOR, NURSING SERVICE or ASSISTANT DIRECTOR, NURSING SERVICE.

Promotion from: NURSE, SUPERVISOR.

Promotion to: DIRECTOR, NURSING SERVICE.

PROFESSIONAL AFFILIATIONS

American Nurses' Association
10 Columbus Circle
New York, N.Y. 10019
State and local nursing associations.

National League for Nursing
10 Columbus Circle
New York, N.Y. 10019

Nursing Service Department   Nurse Head 075.128

NURSE, HEAD

JOB DUTIES

Directs nursing service activities including the preparation of nursing care plans, and instructs nurses in an organized hospital patient care unit:

Assigns duties to professional and ancillary nursing personnel based on patients' needs, available staff, and unit needs. Supervises and evaluates work performance in terms of patient care, staff relations, and efficiency of service. Provides for nursing care in unit and cooperates with other members of medical care team in coordinating patients' total needs. Identifies and studies nursing service problems and assists in their solution. Observes nursing care and visits patient to insure that nursing care is carried out as directed and treatment is administered in accordance with physicians' instructions and to ascertain need for additional or modified services. Maintains a safe environment for patients. Operates or supervises operation of specialized equipment assigned to unit and provides assistance and guidance to nursing team as required.

Accompanies physician on rounds to answer questions, receive instructions, and note patients' care requirements. Reports to replacement on next tour on condition of patients or of any unusual actions taken. May render professional nursing care and instruct patients and members of their families in techniques and methods of home care after discharge.

Directs preparation and maintenance of patients' clinical records, including nursing and medical treatments and related services provided by NURSE, STAFF. Compiles daily reports on staff hours worked and care and condition of patients. Investigates and adjusts complaints or refers them to supervisor.

Insures established inventory standards for medicines, solutions, supplies, and equipment. Accounts for narcotics. Provides orientation for new personnel to job requirements, equipment, and unit personnel. Instructs unit personnel in new nursing care techniques, procedures, and equipment. Presides over unit personnel meetings to discuss patient care needs. Evaluates individual work performance through observation, spot-checking work completed, and conferences. Promotes individual staff development.

Attends meetings of supervisory and administrative staff to discuss unit operation and staff training needs and to formulate programs to improve these areas. May assist in developing and administering budget for nursing unit to which assigned. Assists with studies related to improvement of nursing care.

NURSE, HEAD is usually known by the nursing unit to which assigned or in which she has specialized, such as NURSE, HEAD, MEDICAL AND SURGICAL or NURSE, HEAD, PEDIATRICS. Specialized duties will be required by the specialized unit.

In smaller hospitals, duties and responsibilities of this job may be combined with those of NURSE, SUPERVISOR.

MACHINES, TOOLS, EQUIPMENT, AND WORK AIDS

Medical equipment, patient charts, nursing care plans, records and reports, and work schedules.

EDUCATION, TRAINING, AND EXPERIENCE

Graduation from an accredited school of nursing and current licensure by State Board of Nursing. Advanced preparation in the clinical specialty, ward management, principles of supervision, and teaching is preferred.

Experience as a professional nurse in which potential administrative and supervisory competence has been demonstrated.

WORKER TRAITS

Aptitudes: Verbal ability is necessary to present information and ideas essential to supervisory duties and to understand general nursing theory and practice.

Motor coordination and manual dexterity are required to coordinate hands, eyes, and fingers in administering medications and treatments, using clinical instruments, and handling patients.

Some clerical ability is necessary to prepare and review records and charts.

Interests: A preference for business contacts with people, for supervising and instructing nursing personnel.

A preference for performing services that will benefit and help people. A preference for scientific and technical activities to understand and work with medical concepts while performing nursing duties.

Temperaments: Ability to direct activities of a single nursing unit.

Capable of dealing with people in actual job duties. Works intimately with patients, family members, and medical staff.

A sense of discipline to work in accordance with accepted nursing and medical standards.

Physical Demands and Working Conditions: Work is of medium demand; walking and standing most of time on duty.

Reaches for, handles, and fingers reports and charts, instruments, and equipment.

Talking and hearing essential in instructing and supervising nursing personnel and in receiving doctors' orders and patients' requests.

Near-visual acuity required to work with charts and records and to observe patients.

Color vision to perceive changes in patients' skin color and colors of medicines and solutions.

Works inside.

JOB RELATIONSHIPS

Workers supervised: NURSES, STAFF and ancillary nursing personnel assigned to the unit.

Supervised by: NURSE, SUPERVISOR, assigned unit.

Promotion from: NURSE, STAFF.

Promotion to: NURSE, SUPERVISOR.

PROFESSIONAL AFFILIATIONS

American Nurses' Association   National League for Nursing
10 Columbus Circle   10 Columbus Circle
New York, N.Y. 10019   New York, N.Y. 10019
State and local nursing associations.

Nursing Service Department   Nurse, General Duty 075.378

NURSE, STAFF

JOB DUTIES

Renders professional nursing care to patients within an assigned unit of a hospital, in support of medical care as directed by medical staff and pursuant to objectives and policies of the hospital:

Performs nursing techniques for the comfort and well-being of the patient. Prepares equipment and assists physician during treatments and examinations of patients. Administers prescribed medications, orally and by injections; provides treatments using therapeutic equipment; observes patients' reactions to medications and treatments; observes progress of intravenous infusions and subcutaneous infiltrations; changes or assists physician in changing dressing and cleaning wounds or incisions; takes temperature, pulse, respiration rate, blood pressure, and heart beat to detect deviations from normal and gage progress of patient, following physician's orders and approved nursing care plan. Observes, records, and reports to supervisor or physician patients' condition and reaction to drugs, treatments, and significant incidents.

Maintains patients' medical records on nursing observations and actions taken such as medications and treatments given, reactions, tests, intake and emission of liquids and solids, temperature, pulse, and respiration rate. Records nursing needs of patients on nursing care plan to assure continuity of care.

Observes emotional stability of patients, expresses interest in their progress, and prepares them for continuing care after discharge. Explains procedures and treatments ordered to gain patients' cooperation and allay apprehension.

Rotates on day, evening, and night tours of duty and may be asked to rotate among various clinical and nursing services of institution. Each service will have sepcialized duties and NURSE, STAFF may be known by the section to which assigned such as NURSE, STAFF, OBSTETRICS or NURSE, STAFF, PEDIATRICS. May serve as a team leader for a group of personnel rendering nursing care to a number of patients.

Assists in planning, supervising, and instructing LICENSED PRACTICAL NURSES, NURSING AIDES, ORDERLIES, and students. Demonstrates nursing techniques and procedures, and assists nonprofessional nursing care personnel in rendering nursing care in unit.

May assist with operations and deliveries by preparing rooms; sterilizing instruments, equipment, and supplies; and handing them, in order of use, to surgeon or other medical specialist.

MACHINES, TOOLS, EQUIPMENT, AND WORK AIDS

Medical and nursing equipment and supplies.

EDUCATION, TRAINING, AND EXPERIENCE

Graduation from an accredited school of nursing and current licensure by State Board of Nursing.

Orientation training in specific unit only; no experience required beyond that obtained in school of nursing.

WORKER TRAITS

Aptitudes: Verbal ability is necessary to understand patients' charts, doctors' orders, nursing care plan, and medication orders and to communicate with patients and staff.

Motor coordination and manual dexterity are necessary to coordinate hands, eyes, and fingers in administering medications and treatments, using clinical instruments, and handling patients.

Some clerical perception is required to prepare records and charts.

Interests: A preference for performing services of benefit and help.

A preference for scientific and technical activities, for understanding and responding to medical problems and concepts.

Temperaments: Ability to perform of variety of duties characterized by frequent change as work schedules will change on a daily basis.

Able to work intimately with patients, doctors, nursing staff, and families of patients.

Capable of working to prescribed hospital and nursing standards.

Physical Demands and Working Conditions: Work is of medium demand; walking and standing most of time on duty.

Occasional lifting of patients with assistance.

Frequent reaching, handling, and fingering of instruments and equipment, and caring for patients' needs.

Hearing to distinguish differences in heartbeat and breathing of patient.

Near-visual acuity to read gages and dials on equipment.

Color vision for perceiving changes in patients' skin color and colors of medicines and solutions.

Works inside.

JOB RELATIONSHIPS

Workers supervised: May supervise ancillary nursing personnel of unit.
Supervised by: NURSE, HEAD.
Promotion from: No formal line of promotion.
Promotion to: NURSE, HEAD.

PROFESSIONAL AFFILIATIONS

American Nurses' Association
10 Columbus Circle
New York, N.Y. 10019
State and local nursing associations.

National League for Nursing
10 Columbus Circle
New York, N.Y. 10019

Nursing Service Department   Nurse, Licensed, Practical 079.378

LICENSED PRACTICAL NURSE
licensed vocational nurse
JOB DUTIES

Performs a wide variety of patient care activities and accommodative services for assigned hospital patients, as directed by the Head Nurse and/or team leader:

Performs assigned nursing procedures for the comfort and well-being of patients such as assisting in admission of new patients, bathing and feeding patients, making beds, helping patients into and out of bed. Takes patients' temperature, blood pressure, pulse, and respiration, and records results on patients' charts. Collects specimens, such as sputum and urine, in containers, labels containers, and sends to laboratory for analysis. Dresses wounds, administers prescribed procedures, such as enemas, douches, alcohol rubs, and massages. Applies compresses, ice bags, and hot water bottles. Observes patients for reaction to drugs, treatment, cyanosis, weak pulse, excessive respiratory rate, or any other unusual condition, and reports adverse reactions to NURSE, HEAD or NURSE, STAFF. Administers specified medication, and notes time and amount on patients' charts. Assembles and uses such equipment as catheters, tracheotomy tubes, and oxygen supplies. Drapes or gowns patients for various types of examinations. Assists patients to walk about unit as permitted, or transports patient by wheelchair to various departments. Records food and fluid intake and emission. Sterilizes equipment and supplies, using germicides, sterilizer, or autoclave. Answers patients' call signals, and assists NURSE, STAFF or physician in advanced medical treatments. Assists in the care of deceased persons.

May specialize in work of a particular patient care unit and be known by the name of that unit, such as LICENSED PRACTICAL NURSE, RECOVERY ROOM or LICENSED PRACTICAL NURSE, PSYCHIATRICS.

May be required to work rotating shifts.

MACHINES, TOOLS, EQUIPMENT, AND WORK AIDS

Nursing supplies and equipment such as blood-pressure device, thermometer, and surgical dressings.

EDUCATION, TRAINING, AND EXPERIENCE

High school graduation plus graduation from a recognized 1-year practical nurse program. Must pass State Board of Nursing licensing examination.

WORKER TRAITS

Aptitudes: Verbal ability is necessary to understand instructions, limited medical terminology, and concepts; to communicate with patients and hospital staff; and to keep accurate records.

Form perception is necessary to observe pertinent detail when reading thermometers and blood-pressure devices and to observe patients' condition.

Manual dexterity is necessary for easy and skillful use of the hands when working with patients or equipment.

Interests: A preference for performing services of benefit and help.

A preference for people and communication of ideas in caring for patients.

Temperaments: Ability to perform a variety of activities characterized by change and short duration in caring for patients.

Adapted to working with ill people who may be difficult in carrying out job duties.

Physical Demands and Working Conditions: Work is of medium demand. Standing and walking most of time on duty.

Occasionally lifts patients with assistance.

Frequent reaching and handling of instruments and equipment when attending to patients' needs.

Fingering when changing dressings and bandages.

Talking and hearing for discussions with patients and supervisors.

Near-visual acuity for accurate reading of gages and thermometers and for recording on patients' charts.

Works inside.

JOB RELATIONSHIPS

Workers supervised: None

Supervised by: A member of professional nursing staff, depending upon organization of the hospital and nursing unit to which assigned.

Promotion from: No formal line of promotion.

Promotion to: No formal line of promotion.

PROFESSIONAL AFFILIATIONS

National Federation of Licensed
    Practical Nurses
250 West 57th Street
New York, N.Y. 10019

National Association for Practical
    Nurse Education and Service, Inc.
535 Fifth Avenue
New York, N.Y. 10017

Nursing Service Department   Surgical Technician 079.378

SURGICAL TECHNICIAN

scrub technician

JOB DUTIES

Performs a variety of duties in an operating room to assist the surgical team:

Assists surgical team during operative procedure. Changes into operative clothing, scrubs hands and arms, puts on sterile gown and gloves. Arranges sterile setup for operation. Passes instruments, sponges, and sutures to surgeon and surgical assistants. Assists circulating nurse to prepare patient for surgery. May assist in positioning patient in prescribed position for type of surgery to be performed. May assist in preparation of operative area of patient. May assist the ANESTHESIOLOGIST during administration of anesthetic. Adjusts light and other equipment as directed. Assists other team members, upon completion of surgery, in moving patient onto wheeled stretcher for delivery to the recovery room. Assists in cleanup of operating theater following operation including disposal of used linen, gloves, instruments, utensils, equipment, and waste.

May count sponges, needles, and instruments used during operation. May prepare operative specimens, place in preservative solution, and deliver to laboratory for analysis. May record data on patients' record data sheets.

May be required to work rotating shifts.

MACHINES, TOOLS, EQUIPMENT, AND WORK AIDS

Instruments and operating room equipment.

EDUCATION, TRAINING, AND EXPERIENCE

High school graduation or equivalent. Some employers prefer graduation from a recognized 1-year practical nurse program.

Hospital-conducted on-the-job training in operating room techniques.

WORKER TRAITS

Aptitudes: Verbal ability is required to use and understand medical terminology to fulfill quickly and accurately surgeons' and nurses' instructions.

Motor coordination is required for rapid and accurate movements of body and hands in response to visual and audio stimuli.

Interests: A preference for performing services of benefit and help.

A preference for working with scientific objects used to aid people.

Temperaments: Ability to perform a variety of duties in the operating room under supervision.

Capable of attaining set standards of asepsis and antisepsis techniques.

Physical Demands and Working Conditions: Work is of medium demand. Standing and walking during tour of duty.

Assists in lifting patients onto operating table and carrying instruments and supplies.

Reaching, handling, and fingering instruments during surgery and in sterilizing equipment.

Hearing to understand verbal instructions.

Near-visual acuity to distinguish between different instruments.

Works inside. While certain anesthetics are explosive, they are not critical because of safety measures taken.

JOB RELATIONSHIPS

Workers supervised: None.
Supervised by: NURSE,STAFF.
Promotion from: No formal line of promotion.
Promotion to: No formal line of promotion.

PROFESSIONAL AFFILIATIONS

None.

Nursing Service Department   Nurse Aid 355.878

NURSING AIDE

nurse aide
nursing assistant

JOB DUTIES

Performs various patient care activities and related nonprofessional services necessary in caring for the personal needs and comfort of patients:

Answers signal lights and bells to determine patients' needs. Bathes, dresses, and undresses patients and assists with personal hygiene to increase their comfort and well-being. May serve and collect food trays, feed patients requiring help, and provide between-meal nourishment and fresh drinking water, when indicated. Transports patients to treatment units, using wheelchair or wheeled carriage, or assists them to walk. Drapes patients for examinations and treatments; remains with patients, performing such duties as holding instruments and adjusting lights. Takes and records temperatures, pulse, respiration rates, and food intake and output, as directed. May apply ice bags and hot water bottles. Gives alcohol rubs. Reports all unusual conditions or reactions to nurse in charge. May assemble equipment and supplies in preparation for various diagnostic or treatment procedures performed by physicians or nurses.

Tidies patients' rooms and cares for flowers. Changes bed linen, runs errands, directs visitors, and answers telephone. Collects charts, records, and reports, delivers them to authorized personnel. Collects and bags soiled linen and stores clean linen. May clean, sterilize, store, and prepare treatment trays and other supplies used in the unit. May be known by unit or section of hospital to which assigned, such as NURSING AIDE, PSYCHIATRIC or NURSING AIDE, NURSERY, where special duties required by patients are performed.

May be required to work rotating shifts.

MACHINES, TOOLS, EQUIPMENT, AND WORK AIDS

Nursing supplies and equipment.

EDUCATION, TRAINING, AND EXPERIENCE

High school graduation preferred.

Hospital-conducted on-the-job training programs. To work in some departments, additional training is given.

WORKER TRAITS

Aptitudes: Verbal ability is required to communicate with patients and to understand instructions received from nursing staff.

Manual dexterity is required to move and use hands easily and skillfully while aiding patients and giving treatments.

Interests: A preference for performing services of benefit and help.

Temperaments: Able to perform a variety of activities characterized by change and short duration in caring for patients.

Adapted to working with ill people in carrying out job duties.

Physical Demands and Working Conditions: Work is of medium demand. Standing and walking most of time on duty.

Lifting and pushing patients, carts, and wheelchairs.

Handling, reaching, and feeling when distributing supplies and equipment and checking patients.

Talking and hearing to converse with patients and staff members.

Near-visual acuity for accurate reading of gages and thermometers and for recordings on patients' charts.

Works inside.

JOB RELATIONSHIPS

Workers supervised: None.

Supervised by: A member of nursing staff, depending on organization of hospital and unit to which assigned.

Promotion from: This is an entry job in the department of nursing.

Promotion to: No formal line of promotion.

PROFESSIONAL AFFILIATIONS

None.

Nursing Service Department Orderly 355.878

ORDERLY

nursing assistant, male

JOB DUTIES

Assists nursing service personnel by performing a variety of duties for patients (usually male) and certain heavy duties in the care of the physically or mentally ill and the mentally retarded:

Performs same job duties as NURSING AIDE.

MACHINES, TOOLS, EQUIPMENT, AND WORK AIDS

Nursing supplies and equipment.

EDUCATION, TRAINING, AND EXPERIENCE

High school graduation preferred.

Hospital-conducted on-the-job training programs. For work in some departments, additional training is given.

WORKER TRAITS

Aptitudes: Verbal ability is required to communicate with patients and to understand instructions received from nurse.

Manual dexterity is necessary to move hands easily and rapidly when working with small equipment and in aiding patient with personal care.

Interests: A preference for performing services of benefit and help.

A preference for routine and organized activities and working under direct supervision to aid and assist patients.

Temperaments: Ability to perform a variety of repetitive duties involving aid to patients.

Adapted to working with ill people in performing job duties.
Physical Demands and Working Conditions: Work is heavy.
Standing and walking most of time on duty.
Lifting and carrying equipment, supplies, and patients.
Pushing and pulling wheelchairs, wheeled bed, or stretcher.
Reaching, handling, and fingering equipment and supplies when assisting patient.
Talking and hearing for conversing with patients and supervisors.
Works inside. May be member of a team. Care must be exercised when lifting or assisting patients.

JOB RELATIONSHIPS

Workers supervised: None.
Supervised by: A member of nursing staff, depending on organization of hospital and unit to which assigned.
Promotion from: This is usually an entry job in the department of nursing.
Promotion to: No formal line of promotion.

PROFESSIONAL AFFILIATIONS

None.

Nursing Service Department   Ward Service Manager 187.—T

WARD SERVICE MANAGER

unit manager
ward supervisor

JOB DUTIES

Supervises and coordinates administrative management functions for one or more patient care units:

Supervises clerical staff and assures accomplishment of administrative functions on a 24-hour basis by scheduling working hours and arranging for coverage of nursing care unit by nonnursing personnel. Performs personnel-management tasks by orienting and training new personnel. Evaluates performance of assigned workers by checking for quality and quantity.

Inventories and stores patients' personal effects either within the unit or in the hospital vault.

Establishes and maintains an adequate inventory of drugs and supplies for the unit.

Coordinates with other departments such as housekeeping and maintenance to maintain a unit that is hygenically safe and functional. Checks for cleanliness of the units and reports discrepancies to the appropriate supervisor. Performs daily maintenance inspection, and through proper channels initiates minor facility improvement projects.

Maintains close contact with medical and surgical reservations in regard to admissions, transfers, discharges, and other services. Serves as liaison between the specific patient care unit and other departments. Reviews special tests at the end of shift.

Insures that the medical record is completed in accordance with the standards of the Joint Commission on Accreditation of Hospitals. Insures hospital compliance with Medicare requirements insofar as certification and related administrative matters are concerned. Checks charts of patients scheduled for surgery or other special procedures to verify completeness of orders of consents, preparation orders, and lab results, and for necessary signatures.

Greets, directs, and gives nonprofessional factual information to patients, visitors, and personnel from other departments.

Participates in projects, surveys, and other information-gathering activities approved by hospital management.

MACHINES, TOOLS, EQUIPMENT, AND WORK AIDS

Nursing Service supplies, medications, and records.

EDUCATION, TRAINING, AND EXPERIENCE

One year of college or equivalent.

A minimum of 1 year's supervisory experience.

On-the-job training in coordinating nonnursing services for the assigned nursing units.

WORKER TRAITS

Aptitudes: Verbal ability is required to schedule, assign, and supervise workers and to communicate with personnel from other departments.

Numerical ability is required to verify quantities of incoming items and prepare reports of stock on hand.

Interests: A preference for activities involving contact with subordinates and other hospital employees.

Temperaments: Ability to perform a wide variety of duties when supervising the nonnursing personnel of the units.

Able to plan, control, and direct the work activities of the nonnursing personnel of one or more nursing units.

Capable of dealing with subordinates, department heads,, and nursing personnel.

Physical Demands and Working Conditions: Work is light. Lifts and carries supplies weighing from 5 to 10 pounds.

Reaches for and handles supplies, records, and equipment.

Talking and hearing for communicating with other personnel of the department and other departments.

Near-visual acuity for reading reports and records.

Works inside.

JOB RELATIONSHIPS

Workers supervised: WARD CLERK and other nonnursing personnel assigned to the unit.

Supervised by: ASSISTANT DIRECTOR, NURSING SERVICE or ADMINISTRATOR.

Promotion from: No formal line of promotion.

Promotion to: No formal line of promotion.

PROFESSIONAL AFFILIATIONS

None.

Nursing Service Department   Ward Clerk 219.388

WARD CLERK

floor clerk
nursing station assistant

JOB DUTIES

Performs general clerical duties by preparing, compiling, and maintaining records in a hospital nursing unit:

Records name of patient, address, and name of attending physician on medical record forms. Copies information, such as patients' temperature, pulse rate, and blood pressure, from nurses' records. Writes requisitions for laboratory tests and procedures such as basal metabolism, X-ray, EKG, blood examinations, and urinalysis. Under supervision, plots temperature, pulse rate, and other data on appropriate graph charts. Copies and computes other data, as directed, and enters on patients' charts. May record diet instructions. Keeps file of medical records on patients in unit. Routes charts when patients are transferred or dismissed, following specified procedures. May compile census of patients.

Keeps record of absences and hours worked by unit personnel. Types various records, schedules, and reports and delivers them to appropriate office. May maintain records of special monetary charges to patient and forward them to the business office. May verify stock supplies on unit and prepare requisitions to maintain established inventories. Dispatches messages to other departments or to persons in other departments and makes appointments for patients' services in other departments as requested by nursing staff. Makes posthospitalization appointments with patients' physicians. Delivers mail, newspapers, and flowers to patients.

MACHINES, TOOLS, EQUIPMENT, AND WORK AIDS

Office supplies and equipment.

EDUCATION, TRAINING, AND EXPERIENCE

High school graduation or equivalent, including courses in English, typing, spelling, and arithmetic, or high school graduation supplemented by commercial school course in subjects indicated.

No previous experience is required.

On-the-job training in practices and procedures of the hospital and certain medical terminology.

WORKER TRAITS

Aptitudes: Verbal ability is necessary for understanding procedure routines and instructions.

Numerical ability is needed to make accurate computations of patients' and other data.

Clerical perception is necessary to perceive and maintain detail in entering data on patients' charts and to avoid errors in arithmetic.

Interests: A preference for established routine in keeping patients' charts, preparing schedules, and verifying supplies.

Temperaments: Ability to carry out repetitive operations, under specific instructions and in accordance with established procedures.

Physical Demands and Working Conditions: Work is sedentary. Occasionally walks about ward and to and from other departments.

Reaching for and handling charts, reports, and other office supplies.

Talking and hearing when receiving instructions and conversing on telephone.

Near-visual acuity to record information accurately.

Works inside.

JOB RELATIONSHIPS

Workers supervised: None.

Supervised by: WARD SERVICE MANAGER or nurse in charge of unit or ward in which work is performed.

Promotion from: This is usually an entry job.

Promotion to: No formal line of promotion. May be promoted to higher grade clerical job for which ability is demonstrated.

PROFESSIONAL AFFILIATIONS

None.

Nursing Service Department   Director of Staff Development 075.118

DIRECTOR OF STAFF DEVELOPMENT
inservice-education coordinator

JOB DUTIES

Plans, develops, and directs program of education for all hospital nursing service personnel, and coordinates staff development with nursing service program:

Develops, schedules, and directs orientation program for professional and auxiliary nursing service personnel. Develops instructional materials to assist new personnel in becoming oriented to hospital operational techniques. If not scheduled by Personnel Department, schedules hospital tours and addresses by administrative staff to acquaint new personnel with over-all operation and interrelationship of hospital services. Determines effectiveness of orientation materials and procedures through practice sessions. Sets up demonstrations of nursing service equipment to acquaint hospital staff with new equipment and make them more familiar with established equipment.

Plans, coordinates, and conducts regular and special inservice training sessions for hospital nursing staff to acquaint them with new procedures and policies and new trends and developments in patient care techniques; and to provide opportunity for individual members to develop to their full potential.

Keeps current on latest developments by attending professional seminars, institutes, and reading professional journals. Assists Supervisors and Head Nurses in planning and implementing staff development programs in their units. Keeps bulletin boards current by listing information on seminars and institutes and promotes appropriate staff attendance at these professional meetings. Plans training sessions for supervisory staff members.

May participate with committees in writing and maintaining policies and procedures manuals and nursing service forms. Reviews suggestions submitted by nursing service staff for changes or clarification in policies and procedures.

Writes annual reports on activities and prepares plans for future activities. Prepares budget requests.

MACHINES, TOOLS, EQUIPMENT, AND WORK AIDS

Nursing supplies and equipment for demonstration purposes, manuals and clerical forms, and audiovisual equipment.

EDUCATION, TRAINING, AND EXPERIENCE

Graduation from an accredited school of nursing and current licensure by State Board of Nursing; graduation from a recognized college or university with specialization in education; bachelor's degree required. Experience as NURSE, HEAD; NURSE, SUPERVISOR; or Nurse, Educator.

WORKER TRAITS

Aptitudes: Verbal ability is necessary in communicating and in compiling written reports; must be able to understand and use medical terminology.

Clerical perception is necessary to organize materials for program and to proofread technical materials.

Interests: A preference for activities dealing with scientific and technical materials.

A preference for activities dealing with the communication of technical ideas and concepts.

Temperaments: Ability to plan and direct a nursing development program.

Capable of dealing with people in actual job duties in developing nursing policies and procedures.

Physical Demands and Working Conditions: Work is sedentary.
Reaching for and handling reports, forms, and equipment.
Talking and hearing while discussing procedures and instructing nursing staff.
Near-visual acuity for demonstrating techniques and reviewing manuals.
Works inside.

JOB RELATIONSHIPS

Workers supervised: Supervises other training personnel in Nursing Service Department.
Supervised by: ASSISTANT DIRECTOR, NURSING SERVICE or Head of Training Department.
Promotion from: NURSE, SUPERVISOR or NURSE, HEAD.
Promotion to: No formal line of promotion.

PROFESSIONAL AFFILIATIONS

American Nurses' Association
10 Columbus Circle
New York, N.Y. 10019
State and local nursing associations.

National League for Nursing
10 Columbus Circle
New York, N.Y. 10019

Nursing Service Department   Nurse Instructor 075.128

INSTRUCTOR, ANCILLARY NURSING PERSONNEL

JOB DUTIES

Plans, coordinates, and carries out educational programs (theoretical and practical aspects of nursing) to train ancillary nursing personnel:

Prepares and issues trainee manuals (which describe duties and responsibilities of nursing assistants) to be used as training guides. Familiarizes new employees with physical layout of hospital and hospital policies and procedures, organizational structure, hospital etiquette, and employee benefits. Plans educational program and schedules classes in basic patient care procedures, such as bedmaking, blood-pressure and temperature taking, and feeding of patients. Teaches NURSING AIDES and ORDERLIES nursing procedures by demonstration in classrooms and clinical units and by lectures in classrooms, using such aids as motion pictures, charts, and slides. Observes trainees in practical application of procedures. Secures cooperation of Supervisors and Head Nurses to assist in teaching their specialty; coordinates training with all nursing service units to maintain consistency in practice and establish relationships, to give scope to program, and to point out variations of duties required by different units and on different shifts.

Prepares, administers, and scores examinations to determine trainees' suitability for the job. Makes recommendations to nursing service regarding placement of trainees according to test scores and practical application performance. Evaluates trainees' progress following training period and submits report to nursing service for further processing. Conducts meetings with trainees and with supervisors to discuss problems and ideas for improving nursing service training program.

MACHINES, TOOLS, EQUIPMENT, AND WORK AIDS

Teaching aids such as movies and charts, nursing supplies, and equipment for demonstration purposes.

EDUCATION, TRAINING, AND EXPERIENCE

Graduation from an accredited school of nursing and current licensure by State Board of Nursing; advanced training in teaching methods and supervision.
One year's experience as NURSE, HEAD or NURSE, SUPERVISOR.

WORKER TRAITS

Aptitudes: Verbal ability is necessary to present ideas and subject matter to trainees, to express clearly new ideas and techniques, to understand medical terminology, and to prepare manuals.

Some clerical ability is necessary to prepare, administer, and score performance tests, and to prepare course content.

Interests: A preference for scientific and technical materials and a desire to teach these to others.

A preference for people and communication of ideas to instruct trainees and to communicate with fellow staff members.

Temperaments: Ability to organize and direct course content and classroom and clinical instruction for a class of nonprofessional nursing personnel.

Able to deal with people in actual job duties in training new employees.

Equipped to make decisions when evaluating trainees' achievement and potential.

Physical Demands and Working Conditions: Work is light. Considerable walking and standing while instructing and observing students.

Reaching, handling, and fingering instruments, supplies, and teaching aids.

Talking and hearing when conducting classes.

Near-visual acuity to demonstrate techniques and keep records.

Works inside.

JOB RELATIONSHIPS

Workers supervised: Trainees during training period.
Supervised by: DIRECTOR OF STAFF DEVELOPMENT.
Promotion from: NURSE, HEAD or NURSE, SUPERVISOR.
Promotion to: DIRECTOR OF STAFF DEVELOPMENT.

PROFESSIONAL AFFILIATIONS

American Nurses' Association
10 Columbus Circle
New York, N.Y. 10019
State and local nursing associations.

National League for Nursing
10 Columbus Circle
New York, N.Y. 10019

Nursing Service Department   Nurse, Instructor 075.128

INSTRUCTOR, NURSES, INSERVICE

JOB DUTIES

Plans, directs, and coordinates inservice orientation and educational program for professional nursing personnel:

Assists DIRECTOR OF STAFF DEVELOPMENT in planning and carrying out program of staff development. Confers with DIRECTOR OF STAFF DEVELOPMENT to schedule training programs for professional nurses already on the staff, according to departmental work requirements. Lectures to nurses and demonstrates improved methods of nursing service. Lectures and demonstrates procedures, using motion pictures, charts, and slides.

Orients new staff members and provides inservice refresher training for professional nurses returning to hospital nursing service.

Instructs volunteer workers in routine procedures such as aseptic practices and blood-pressure and temperature taking.

MACHINES, TOOLS, EQUIPMENT, AND WORK AIDS

Teaching aids such as movies and charts, nursing supplies, and equipment for demonstration purposes.

EDUCATION, TRAINING, AND EXPERIENCE

Graduation from an accredited school of nursing and current licensure by State Board of Nursing; advanced training in teaching methods and supervision.

One year's experience as NURSE, HEAD or NURSE, SUPERVISOR.

WORKER TRAITS

Aptitudes: Verbal ability is necessary to present ideas and subject matter to trainees, express clearly new ideas and techniques, and understand medical terminology.

Some clerical ability is necessary to prepare, administer, and score performance tests and to prepare course content.

Interests: A preference for scientific and technical materials and a desire to teach and explain these to others.

A preference for people and communication of ideas to instruct nurses and to communicate with fellow staff members.

Temperaments: Ability to organize and direct course content and classroom and clinical instruction for professional nursing personnel.

Able to deal with people in actual job duties in training nursing personnel.

Ability to make decisions when evaluating nurses' achievements and potentials.

Physical Demands and Working Conditions: Work is light. Considerable walking and standing while instructing and observing nurses' performance.

Reaching, handling, and fingering instruments, supplies, and teaching aids.

Talking and hearing when conducting classes.

Near-visual acuity to demonstrate techniques and keep records.

Works inside.

JOB RELATIONSHIPS

Workers supervised: None.

Supervised by: DIRECTOR OF STAFF DEVELOPMENT.

Promotion from: NURSE, HEAD or NURSE, SUPERVISOR.

Promotion to: DIRECTOR OF STAFF DEVELOPMENT.

PROFESSIONAL AFFILIATIONS

American Nurses' Association
10 Columbus Circle
New York, N.Y. 10019
State and local nursing associations.

National League for Nursing
10 Columbus Circle
New York, N.Y. 10019

CLINICAL LABORATORIES DEPARTMENT

PURPOSE: To perform laboratory tests necessary for diagnosis and treatment of hospital patients, and engage in research essential to medical advancement.

RESPONSIBILITY: To perform laboratory tests in the six main fields of bacteriology, biochemistry, histology, serology, hematology, and cytology in order to assist medical staff in making or confirming diagnoses. In addition to specialized tests, clinical laboratories in all general hospitals are responsible for making routine tests that are agreed upon by medical staff and hospital administration. These usually include urinalyses for all patients on admission, blood cell and hemoglobin count, and gross and microscopic examination of all tissues removed at operations. The laboratories also determine causes of communicable diseases and, upon request, render bacteriological service as a control and continual check on all apparatus used for sterilization. In larger hospitals, the clinical laboratories will be divided into a number of specialized units:

Histopathology: Prepare and examine tissue to provide data on cause and progress of disease, make microscopic examinations of tissue pathology, engage in research to develop new histopathological methods and new stains to produce greater clarity during examination of special tissue structures or chemical components, perform autopsies and interpret gross and microscopic autopsy findings in conferences with medical staff and technologists for future diagnoses and treatment of patients.

Biochemistry: Perform chemical tests of body fluids and exudates to provide information for diagnosis and treatment of disease, investigate chemical processes involved in functioning and malfunctioning of the human body, and study effects of chemical compounds upon physiological and biochemical functions of the body to provide information on optimum methods of treating pathological conditions.

Hematology: Analyze and test blood specimens and interpret test results to provide a basis for treatment of diseases and engage in research related to hematological methods and diagnosis.

The blood bank, in a hospital having these special units, is usually a part of hematology. The bank provides for storage and preservation of blood plasma. Blood may be procured either directly from donors or from other blood banks. When obtained from donors, this unit extracts blood and makes necessary laboratory tests.

Microbiology: Cultivate, classify, and identify microorganisms found in body fluids, exudates, skin scrapings, or autopsy and surgical specimens to provide data on cause, cure, and prevention of disease; engage in research to develop new or improved bacteriological methods for discovering and identifying pathogenic organisms; and investigate biology, distribution, and mode of transmission of bacteria and nature and efficiency of chemotherapeutic treatment.

Serology: Prepare serums used to treat and diagnose infectious diseases and immunize against these diseases, and identify diseases based on characteristic reactions of various serums; investigate safety of new commercial antibiotic products and accuracy of therapeutic claims; direct immunology tests and injections; investigate problems of allergy; and conduct tests to determine therapeutic and toxic dosages and most effective methods of administering serums, vaccines, antibiotics, anti-toxins, antigens, and related drugs.

Cytology: Examine human cells to detect evidence of cancer in its early stages and other diseased conditions; engage in research to develop new cytological methods, and new stains to produce greater clarity during examination of cell structures.

The clinical laboratories may be responsible for a number of other functions, such as basal metabolism tests; activities of clinical photographic laboratory, medical illustration unit, and morgue; and care and treatment of animals used in research. Teaching programs for student nurses, interns, residents, and MEDICAL TECHNOLOGISTS and other laboratory personnel may also be a function of this department.

AUTHORITY: The PATHOLOGIST is assigned authority and responsibility for organization and operation of all pathological services. He is director of the clinical laboratories and is also the hospital PATHOLOGIST. He reports to the ASSOCIATE ADMINISTRATOR on administrative functions and supervises all personnel assigned to the laboratories. For professional standards, the PATHOLOGIST is respon-sible to the chief of the medical staff. He may delegate certain administrative duties to the MEDICAL TECHNOLOGIST, CHIEF.

INTERRELATIONSHIPS AND INTRARELATIONSHIPS: Laboratory services must be coordinated with all other diagnostic functions of the hospital, which requires consultation with members of the medical staff, the ASSOCIATE ADMINISTRATOR or the ADMINISTRATOR, and other department heads. A system should be established for performing all routine tests within a specified period of time after admission of a patient. Emergency laboratory service must be available on a 24-hour basis.

Laboratory services are important to the work of the Outpatient Department, and close cooperation is necessary between these services. Personnel in the laboratory have occasional contact with patients; medical, admitting, and nursing staff; and with other employees. The PATHOLOGIST may lecture to students, professional societies, and medical organizations. There is cooperation with other department heads, private physicians, and personnel in other laboratories and related activities in radiology and technical services.

STANDARDS: All regularly employed laboratory technologists and technicians should be on the registry sponsored by the American Society of Clinical Pathologists. They must have completed instruction in a school for technologists or technicians approved by the Council on Medical Education and Hospitals of the American Medical Association. Many hospitals, particularly those connected with schools of medicine or osteopathy, offer courses in medical technology. These school must also meet the standards formulated by the Council on Medical Education and Hospitals of the American Medical Association or their equivalent.

PHYSICAL FACILITIES AND STAFFING: The physical facilities of this department will depend on its workload. The very small hospital, which performs only routine examination in its laboratory, requires a minimum of space and equipment. In the large hospital, the laboratory space may be divided into a number of divisions, including an office for the PATHOLOGIST and a central workroom for facilities that may be utilized in common by all laboratory units. Where a great deal of outpatient work is performed, a small branch laboratory may be set up in the Outpatient Department or Clinic for routine tests.

The director of this department is a doctor of medicine or osteopathy with qualifications in pathology acceptable to the Council on Education and Hospitals of the American Medical Association or the Committee on Hospitals of the Bureau of Professional Education of the American Osteopathic Association. Where it is not possible to secure the full-time services of a PATHOLOGIST, arrangements should be made for the services of a PATHOLOGIST for tissue and postmortem examinations and for the interpretation of tests and examinations.

Depending upon the hospital, requirements for a clinical laboratory director can be met by: (1) A full-time clinical PATHOLOGIST, (2) a part-time clinical PATHOLOGIST (frequently, arrangements can be made for a PATHOLOGIST to serve two or more hospitals within a given area), (3) a consulting PATHOLOGIST to whom materials can be sent for diagnosis and who will come to the laboratory periodically to supervise the services and meet with the medical staff, or (4) a member of the medical staff who has had training in clinical pathology and will direct the laboratory in those cases where the volume of work is insufficient to warrant the full-time services of a specialist. In the latter instance, tissue examinations requiring extensive equipment and skill can be sent to the nearest clinical laboratory which is headed by a qualified PATHOLOGIST.

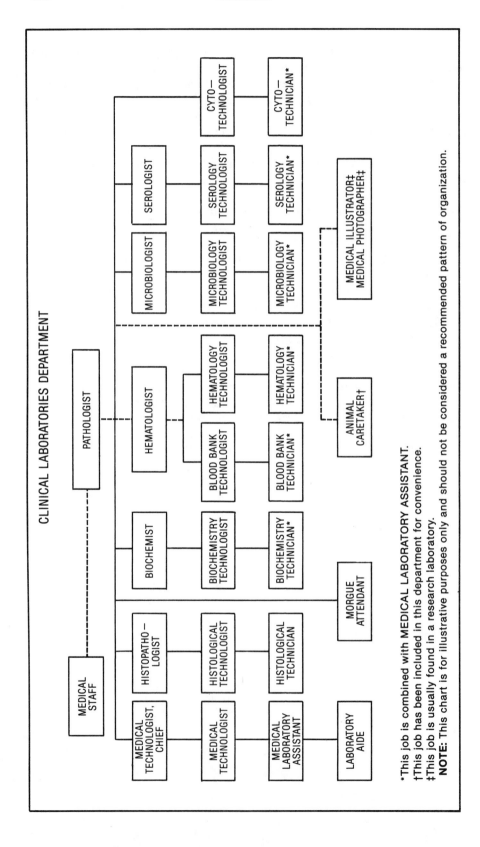

CLINICAL LABORATORIES DEPARTMENT

*This job is combined with MEDICAL LABORATORY ASSISTANT.
†This job has been included in this department for convenience.
‡This job is usually found in a research laboratory.
NOTE: This chart is for illustrative purposes only and should not be considered a recommended pattern of organization.

Clinical Laboratories Department   Pathologist   070.081

PATHOLOGIST

JOB DUTIES

Supervises and directs activities of the clinical laboratories in accordance with accepted national standards and administrative policies of the hospital:

Establishes department procedures and methods. Assigns and supervises activities of department personnel. Directs training of resident physicians, interns, technologists, and technicians assigned to the department. Requisitions supplies and equipment. Serves as consultant to other department heads and visiting physicians, to interpret laboratory findings and assist in determining appropriate method and extent of treatment necessary. Participates, along with personnel of other departments, in planning joint administrative and technical programs and recommends methods and procedures for coordination of pathological services with related patient care services. May engage in research projects and prepare scientific papers on the nature, cause, and behavior of diseases. Investigates and studies trends and developments in pathological practices and techniques and evaluates their adaptability to specific needs of the pathological program. Lectures to students, professional societies, and organizations in the medical field. Prepares budget for the fiscal year and submits to administrative officials for approval.

Provides pathological services to aid in the diagnosis of diseases and the treatment of patients and to assist in postmortem diagnoses.

Supervises all laboratory work, demonstrating new techniques to staff and performing difficult tasks demanded by complex or unusual situations. Conducts macroscopic and microscopic examinations of specimens of body tissues, fluids, and secretions, and diagnoses nature of pathological condition. Prepares report on each case, incorporating recommendations for treatment, such as surgery, chemotherapy, or roentgen-ray therapy. Prepares vaccines and immune serums. Conducts autopsies, performing macroscopic anatomical examinations and microscopic studies of all tissues or fluids showing evidence of pathological conditions. Prepares complete report on postmortem study, including description of pathology performed, postmortem diagnosis conditions, and statement of cause of death.

MACHINES, TOOLS, EQUIPMENT, AND WORK AIDS

Budget forms, laboratory slips, laboratory supplies, microscope, specimens, surgical tools, reference texts, and work schedules.

EDUCATION, TRAINING, AND EXPERIENCE

Graduation from a medical school approved by the Council on Medical Education and Hospitals of the American Medical Association or the Committee on Hospitals of the Bureau of Professional Education of the American Osteopathic Association. Must have a state license to practice medicine or osteopathy and/or a certificate of National Board of Medical Examiners or National Board of Osteopathic Examiners.

Certification by American Board of Pathology requires: (1) 5 years' experience, 4 years of which shall have been in institutions approved by council on Medical Education and Hospitals of the American Medical Association or by the board; or (2) 11 years' experience if none has been in institutions that have been approved by the board. Must have successfully completed written, oral, and practical examinations. For certification in pathological anatomy, applicant must successfully complete a written and oral examination in gross pathology and a practical examination in microscopic pathology. For certification in clinical pathology, applicant must successfully complete a written, oral, and practical examination in bacteriology, hematology, clinical chemistry, parasitology, serology, and clinical microscopy. Applicants may be certified in one or both specialities.

WORKER TRAITS

Aptitudes: Verbal ability required to advise physicians and nursing staff on the diagnosis and treatment of diseases, confer with laboratory personnel, lecture at conferences, and write reports on pathological studies and tests.

Numerical ability required to determine validity and reliability of testing procedures, establish quality controls, and prepare budget estimates.

Spatial ability required to visualize the various functions of the human body in performing pathological studies and tests.

Form perception required to make visual comparisons of body cells and microorganisms.

Manual and finger dexterity required to perform microscopic tests and to conduct autopsies.

Color discrimination required to detect color variations of specimens under study.

Interests: A preference for scientific and technical activities to diagnose diseases based on test results and assist in determining appropriate method and extent of treatment necessary.

A preference for activities carried out according to specified processes and techniques is required to conduct difficult and complex laboratory tests and to perform autopsies.

Temperaments: Capability to direct, control, and plan the entire activities of the clinical laboratory.

The evaluation of information against sensory or judgmental criteria is involved when making diagnoses based on typical test results and in conducting postmortem examinations.

Responsibility for maintenance of exact standards by all clinical laboratory personnel when conducting tests.

Physical Demands and Working Conditions: Work is light. Lifts and carries a variety of relatively light objects such as specimens, test manuals, textbooks, and reports.

Reaches for, handles, and fingers surgical instruments, specimens, microscopes, textbooks, and case records.

Talking and hearing essential to confer with laboratory personnel, lecture in educational conferences, and consult with staff physicians.

Near-visual acuity required to read technical and scientific textbooks, technical manuals, and reports.

Color vision required to perform autopsies and other diagnostic tests.

Works inside. Exposed to danger from disease-bearing specimens. Exposed to odorous chemicals and specimens.

JOB RELATIONSHIPS

Workers supervised: All personnel assigned to the clinical laboratories.

Supervised by: ASSOCIATE ADMINISTRATOR in administrative activities, and Chief of Medical Staff in professional activities.

Promotion from: No formal line of promotion. May be promoted from Assistant Pathologist.

Promotion to: ASSOCIATE ADMINISTRATOR.

PROFESSIONAL AFFILIATIONS

American Association of
Pathologists and Bacteriologists
University of Rochester School of
Medicine and Dentistry
Department of Pathology
Rochester, N.Y. 14620

American Board of Pathology
University of Michigan
Department of Pathology
1335 East Catherine Street
Ann Arbor, Mich. 48104

American Medical Association
535 North Dearborn Street
Chicago, Ill 60610

American Osteopathic Association
212 East Ohio Street
Chicago, Ill. 60611

American Osteopathic Board of
Pathology
212 East Ohio Street
Chicago, Ill. 60611

American Osteopathic College of
Pathologists
3921 Beecher Road
Flint, Mich. 48504

American Society of Clinical
Pathologists
445 North Lake Shore Drive
Chicago, Ill. 60611

American Society of Experimental
    Pathology
9550 Rockville Pike
Bethesda, Md. 20014

College of American Pathologists
230 North Michigan Avenue
Chicago, Ill. 60601

State and local organizations.

Clinical Laboratories Department   Biochemist   041.081

BIOCHEMIST

chemist, biological

JOB DUTIES

Directs and supervises chemical tests of body fluids and exudates of hospital patients to provide information for diagnosis and treatment of disease:

Trains and supervises BIOCHEMISTRY TECHNOLOGISTS and biochemistry technicians in collecting specimens from hospital patients and in conducting tests to identify chemical composition of body fluids. Assists technologists with more difficult analyses, interprets results, and performs unusual or complicated tests. Submits diagnostic reports for approval by PATHOLOGIST. Studies, refines, and modifies established techniques to produce more accurate qualitative and quantitative analyses and improved methods for identifying changes of a chemical nature caused by disease.

Devises methods of testing toxic or therapeutic effect of new experimental drugs, toxins, or poisons on humans and on microorganisms or parasites. Determines which elements of a mixture are responsible for toxic effects. Conducts tests to identify chemical processes involved in functioning of living tissues and organs, and studies metabolism, utilization, and oxidation of foodstuffs in body, using experimental animals as needed. Isolates, identifies, synthesizes, and studies characteristics of natural organic products, such as enzymes, hormones, and vitamins. Investigates chemical aspects of allergies, allergens, antigens and antibodies, and serums, and studies related problems of immunology and serology.

May conduct biochemical research in highly specialized areas, such as metabolism of steroid hormones or origins of cancer. May lecture to lay and professional students.

Prepares budget for laboratory supplies and equipment. Writes reports recording number of tests performed, kinds of tests, amount of supplies used, and progress made on research projects. May interview and hire new laboratory workers and conduct on-the-job training.

The duties of BIOCHEMISTRY TECHNOLOGIST may be combined with this job.

MACHINES, TOOLS, EQUIPMENT, AND WORK AIDS

Chemicals, laboratory equipment, microscopes, reports, testing machines, work schedules.

EDUCATION, TRAINING, AND EXPERIENCE

Bachelor's degree in chemistry and biochemistry is essential. Master's or doctor's degree is desirable and frequently is required.

At least 3 years' experience in biochemistry in a medical laboratory is usually required.

WORKER TRAITS

Aptitudes: Verbal ability required to supervise laboratory personnel, to understand technical terminology, and to write diagnostic and research reports.

Numerical ability required to compute results of automated tests.

Form perception required to recognize pertinent details of specimens under microscope.

Color discrimination required to detect minute differences or similarities of specimens under microscopic study.

Interests: A preference for scientific and technical activities to conduct chemical experiments under controlled conditions in studying chemical reactions and interactions in living organisms.

A preference for activities carried on in relation to processes and techniques, used in conducting tests to determine the nature and extent of disease conditions.

Temperaments: Capability to plan, control, and direct the activities of all personnel in the biochemistry section of the clinical laboratories.

Equipped to evaluate information against verifiable criteria, required when conducting research to develop new drugs and vaccines for the prevention, arresting, or treatment of disease, and investigating effects of new drugs on living tissues.

Responsible to insure that tests and experiments are conducted within established standards.

Physical Demands and Working Conditions: Work is light. Lifts and carries laboratory equipment and supplies around the laboratory.

Reaches for, handles, and fingers laboratory supplies, equipment, and specimens.

Talking and hearing essential to converse with assistants and other clinical laboratory personnel.

Near-visual acuity required to examine specimens during tests and to read printed materials.

Color vision to detect color variations of specimens under microscopic study.

Works inside. Works with specimens capable of transmitting disease. Exposed to odorous chemicals and specimens.

JOB RELATIONSHIPS

Workers supervised: BIOCHEMISTRY TECHNOLOGIST.
Supervised by: PATHOLOGIST.
Promotion from: No formal line of promotion.
Promotion to: No formal line of promotion. Promotion is through increased administrative and supervisory duties.

PROFESSIONAL AFFILIATIONS

American Society of Biological Chemists
9650 Wisconsin Avenue, NW.
Washington, D.C. 20014

Clinical Laboratories Department   Biochemistry Technologist   078.281

BIOCHEMISTRY TECHNOLOGIST

medical technologist, biochemistry
urinalysis technician

JOB DUTIES

Performs chemical tests on body fluids and exudates from hospital patients to provide information for diagnosing and combating infectious diseases:

Receives patient specimens, such as urine, blood, spinal fluid, and gastric juices, or collects specimens directly from patient. Centrifuges specimen to separate cells and sediment from serum or supernatant fluids. Adds specific quantities of reagents or solutions to body specimens and heats, filters, or shakes solutions according to prescribed procedures. Notes appearance, change of color, or resulting precipitate or examines results by means of photometer, spectograph, colorimeter, and microscope to identify chemical composition and concentrations and to observe processes of change. Titrates specimen samples against standard reagents to make quantitative determinations. Calculates and tabulates results, and makes reports of observations.

Performs other qualitative and quantitative tests using titration apparatus, centrifuge, incinerator-furnace, filters, shakers, pH meter, and microgasometer. Notes readings of machine registers on work sheets and logs. Examines graph tracings made by machine analyzers to locate or plot test values. Calculates test findings, using mathematical formulas, conversion tables, and slide rule. Posts test findings to laboratory tickets, logbooks, and quality control records.

Performs a number of specific tests: Tests urine for determination of sugar and albumin content, alkalinity, and presence of acetone bodies, blood, bile derivatives, Bence-Jones protein, sulfonamides, uric acids, and various drugs and poisons. Adds specific reagents to urine samples which act as indicators, and notes change of color or appearance of precipitates. Makes quantitative determinations by comparing resultant colors against standards, or by making simple calculations based on quantity of reagent or sample used to obtain specific color. May detect presence of blood by means of a spectroscope. Centrifuges urine and examines resultant sediments under a microscope to detect presence of various types of cell bodies. Determines specific gravity of urine, using a urinometer, and notes general odor, color, and turbidity of sample. Tests blood to determine urea nitrogen, carbon dioxide, sulfonamides, calcium, iron, chlorides, creatinine, uric acid, phosphorous content, and glucose tolerance. Tests gastric contents for free and total acidity and occult blood; spinal fluid for chlorides, globulin, and total proteins; and feces for bile, occult blood, and urobilinogen. Tests for presence of vitamins and hormones, using established chemical procedures or by observing their effect on test animals under experimental conditions. May test purity, alkalinity, and total solid contents of water, milk, and food products.

The duties of biochemistry technician may be combined with this job; it is also frequently combined with that of BIOCHEMIST.

MACHINES, TOOLS, EQUIPMENT, AND WORK AIDS

Centrifuge, chemical glassware, colorimeter, logbook, laboratory equipment, microgasometer, photometer, reports, spectrograph, and urinometer.

EDUCATION, TRAINING, AND EXPERIENCE

Three years of college with courses in biology, chemistry, and mathematics, plus 1 year of training in a school of medical technology approved by the American Society of Clinical Pathologists.

Must be registered as a Medical Technologist by the Registry Board of the American Society of Clinical Pathologists.

Some states require a license issued by the state board of health in order to practice.

Worker will usually receive 3 to 6 months' on-the-job training by the BIOCHEMIST to become familiar with procedures and practices of hospital.

WORKER TRAITS

Aptitudes: Verbal ability required to use and understand medical terminology and to prepare written reports in technical language.

Numerical ability required to calculate by formula the strength of unknown samples, convert machine readings to reportable data, and use slide rule to calculate test results.

Form perception required to examine specimens for changes in appearance and to observe precipitates.

Finger dexterity required to manipulate test tubes, pipettes, and similar small objects during performance of tests.

Interests: A preference for scientific and technical activities to perform qualitative and quantitative analyses of specimens for use in diagnosing and combating infectious diseases.

A preference for activities carried on in relation to processes and techniques to perform tests.

Temperaments: Performance of tests involves the capability to evaluate information against measurable criteria.

Worker must adhere to rigid medical standards in performing tests.

Physical Demands and Working Conditions: Work is light. Lifts and carries laboratory equipment and supplies.

Reaches for, handles, and fingers test equipment.

Near-visual acuity necessary to read test instruments and to plot and calculate test results.

Color vision required to detect color changes when testing specimens.

Works inside. Subject to danger of infection from disease-bearing specimens. Exposed to odorous chemicals and specimens.

JOB RELATIONSHIPS

Workers supervised: MEDICAL LABORATORY ASSISTANT specializing in biochemistry, may be designated as Biochemistry Technician.
Supervised by: BIOCHEMIST or MEDICAL TECHNOLOGIST, CHIEF.
Promotion from: No formal line of promotion.
Promotion to: No formal line of promotion.

PROFESSIONAL AFFILIATIONS

American Society of Medical Technologists
Suite 25, Hermann Professional Building
Houston, Tex. 77025

Clinical Laboratories Department   Blood Bank Technologist   078.281

BLOOD BANK TECHNOLOGIST

medical technologist, blood bank

JOB DUTIES

Collects, tests, and stores blood, administers transfusions, and maintains records of blood donations or transfusions. Supervises or performs the following procedures of a blood bank:

Schedules donor's appointments to maintain adequate supply of various types of blood. Confers with donor to obtain medical history data required as safeguard against collecting diseased or otherwise unusable blood. Takes donor's temperature, blood pressure, and pulse, following specified procedures and records data. Cleans area of puncture site with disinfectants and distends vein, using rubber tourniquet. Inserts needle on one of disposable siphon tube into patient's medial-cubital vein, following strict procedures of asepsis and antisepsis to avoid infection of patient and contamination of blood being obtained. Inverts bottle and opens clamp on tube to allow siphoning process to begin. Shakes bottle to assure that blood mixes with anticoagulant mixture placed in bottle, or turns switch of electric-powered shaking device. Observes donor during entire procedure to detect signs of reaction. Notifies physician or nursing personnel if complications arise. Fills blood bottle and test tubes used for performance of blood tests. Unhooks donor and observes him throughout his immediate convalescence to verify his strength and color. Posts data to record donation of blood into log. May take blood samples from patients by piercing finger or earlobe.

Groups or types blood by mixing red cells of person to be typed with typing serums, noting whether clumping of cells occurs. Prepared and examines microscopic test slides to determine the blood group of donor or patient, using pipette and microscope. Verifies the blood group of patient or donor by back-typing the blood samples, using microscope. Cross-matches blood to determine compatibility. Identifies antibodies in donors' or patients' blood that could react adversely during transfusion and cause harm to the person receiving the transfusion. Performs tests for syphilis and sterility. Records all tests results in log. Files transfusion slips and enters data pertaining to the transfusion into the log.

Processes blood plasma for future use in blood transfusion. Separates plasma from red blood cells, using centrifuge machine and separating devices.

Prepares solutions and reagents in accordance with standard formulas. Maintains written records of tests performed and keeps inventory of blood bank. Inspects stored blood to detect signs of spoilage, and removes spoiled blood for discard. Retests donor and recipient blood after adverse transfusion reaction to determine and record for study by PATHOLOGIST the possible causes for this reaction.

MACHINES, TOOLS, EQUIPMENT, AND WORK AIDS

Centrifuge, glass slides, indicator solutions, labels, logbook, microscope, reagents, test equipment, tourniquet, transfusion equipment.

EDUCATION, TRAINING, AND EXPERIENCE

Three years of college with a major in biology, chemistry, and mathematics; 1 year of training and study in a school approved by the American Society of Clinical Pathologists; plus 1 additional year of study and training in a school approved by the American Association of Blood Banks.

Must be registered as a Medical Technologist by the Registry Board of the American Society of Clinical Pathologists.

Some states require a license issued by the state board of health in order to practice.

WORKER TRAITS

Aptitudes: Verbal ability required to use and understand medical terminology for preparing written reports in technical langauge and for periodic review of test instructions and literature.

Numerical ability required to calculate by formula the strength of unknown serum samples.

Form perception required to recognize details in cell structure under microscope and to make visual comparisons and color discriminations in performing blood tests and microscopic examinations.

Interests: A preference for working with things in a technical context is required, to collect, test, store, and administer blood as prescribed.

A preference for activities that are carried on in relation to processes and techniques, such as conducting blood tests and transfusions.

Temperaments: The worker must be accurate to evaluate the test samples against known criteria to determine the exact nature of the sample.

Capable of precise attainment of set standards in conducting tests and transfusions. Accuracy of testing and recording test results is of vital importance. Must have stamina when faced with numerous emergency situations.

Physical Demands and Working Conditions: Work is light. Worker stands for greater part of working day.

Lifts and carries laboratory equipment weighing up to 10 pounds.

Reaches for, handles, and fingers blood bank apparatus and laboratory equipment.

Talking and hearing essential to receive instructions from supervisor and to give instructions to blood donors.

Near-visual acuity required to perceive minute particles and details in blood when testing.

Color discrimination required to detect reactions during tests and for daily examination of stored blood.

Works inside. Worker is frequently exposed to diseases from handling diseased blood specimens. Exposed to odorous chemicals.

JOB RELATIONSHIPS

Workers supervised: MEDICAL LABORATORY ASSISTANT specializing in hematology, may be designated as Blood Bank Technician.

Supervised by: HEMATOLOGIST or MEDICAL TECHNOLOGIST, CHIEF.

Promotion from: No formal line of promotion.

Promotion to: No formal line of promotion.

PROFESSIONAL AFFILIATIONS

American Society of Medical Technologists
Suite 25, Hermann Professional Building
Houston, Tex. 77025

CYTOTECHNOLOGIST

medical technologist, cytology

JOB DUTIES

Stains, mounts, and studies cells of human body to detect evidence of cancer and other pathological conditions:

Receives body materials and fluids such as blood, exudates, and scrapings, or collects specimens directly from patients. Centrifuges fluid specimens on separate sediment and cells from supernatant fluids. Places specimen on microscope slide, using pipette, spatula, or swab. Draws blank microscope slide over specimen slide. Immerses slides in fixative solution to preserve specimen and prevent cellular distortion. Immerses into a series of staining solutions to dehydrate, clear, and stain slides, and to render specific parts of the cell more visible under microscopic study.

Mounts slide on microscope and examines cells to detect evidence of cancer or other diseased condition. Classifies slides according to established classifications ranging from normal to cancerous cells, applying knowledge gained through study and experience of typical and atypical cell structures. Records classifications on slides and presents slides with unusual cell structures to PATHOLOGIST for further examination and decision as to whether biopsy or further cytological study is necessary. Compiles listing of patients from whom PATHOLOGIST has requested follow-up specimens and be analyzed within specific periods of time. Prepares new specimen for examination and studies cells of specimen to determine if cell abnormalities have remained the same, been eliminated, or intensified. Reports findings to PATHOLOGIST.

Maintains records of all work performed in cytology section. Catalogues and files all slides to be used as part of patients' medical records. May take periodic inventory of supplies and equipment. Prepares chemical reagents and stains used in performing tests.

MACHINES, TOOLS, EQUIPMENT, AND WORK AIDS

Centrifuge, chemical reagents, logbook, microscope, pipettes, reagents, swabs.

EDUCATION, TRAINING, AND EXPERIENCE

Two years of college with courses in biology and chemistry, plus 1 year of training in a school of cytology approved by the American Medical Association.

Worker must be certified by the Registry Board of Medical Technologists of the American Society of Clinical Pathologists.

Some states require a license issued by the state board of health in order to practice.

WORKER TRAITS

Aptitudes: Verbal ability required to use and understand medical terminology and for periodic review of test instructions and literature.

Form perception required to perceive minute details of cellular structures of varying size, symmetry, and color.

Color discrimination required to perceive colors, shades, and hues for accurate staining of slides.

Interests: A preference for scientific and technical activities, to examine cells to detect evidence of diseased conditions.

A preference for activities carried on according to processes and techniques, required in order to prepare slides and to master the techniques of cellular examinations.

Temperaments: Ability to evaluate cellular components against established and measurable criteria when conducting tests.

Disciplined to adhere to rigid medical standards when conducting laboratory tests.

Physical Demands and Working Conditions: Work is light. Lifts and carries trays of prepared slides and relatively light laboratory equipment about the laboratory.

Occasionally walks about the institution to obtain specimens from patients.

Reaches for, handles, and fingers microscopic slides and other small pieces of laboratory equipment.

Near-visual acuity required to observe specimens under microscope.

Color vision required to examine suitability of stains on specimens used in study.

Works inside. Exposed to specimens that are capable of transmitting disease and to odorous chemicals and specimens.

JOB RELATIONSHIPS

Workers supervised: MEDICAL LABORATORY ASSISTANT specializing in cytology, may be designated Cytotechnician.

Supervised by: PATHOLOGIST or MEDICAL TECHNOLOGIST, CHIEF.

Promotion from: No formal line of promotion.

Promotion to: No formal line of promotion.

PROFESSIONAL AFFILIATIONS

American Society of Medical Technologists
Suite 25, Hermann Professional Building
Houston, Tex. 77025

Clinical Laboratories Department   Hematologist   078.231 T

HEMATOLOGIST

JOB DUTIES

Directs and supervises analysis and testing of blood specimens; interprets test results to provide a basis for treatment of disease; and directs the operations of the hospital blood bank:

Trains and supervises HEMATOLOGY TECHNOLOGISTS and hematology technicians in performance of blood tests and microscopic analysis of blood smears or makes tests and prepares materials for microscopic study. Instructs workers by practical demonstration to correct faulty techniques or to introduce new procedures and equipment. Assists workers with more difficult tests and analysis of unusual test results and performs specialized or highly complex tests. May rerun tests to determine accuracy of results. Reviews and interprets test results, examines blood film slides and cultures under microscope, and writes diagnostic reports for approval by PATHOLOGIST.

Supervises BLOOD BANK TECHNOLOGISTS and blood bank technicians in collection, processing, and dispensing of blood and blood plasma. Participates in educational conferences to exchange information pertinent to latest trends in the field of hematology. May lecture to students of medicine, medical technology, or nursing arts or to interns. May engage in research related to hematological methods and diagnosis.

In some hospital laboratories this job may be performed by a doctor of medicine or osteopathy, particularly a pathologist, who has specialized in hematology. This job may include the duties of HEMATOLOGY TECHNOLOGIST and BLOOD BANK TECHNOLOGIST.

MACHINES, TOOLS, EQUIPMENT, AND WORK AIDS

Laboratory equipment, microscope, work schedules.

EDUCATION, TRAINING, AND EXPERIENCE

Master's degree or doctorate in hematology is usually required. Three years' experience in hematology in a medical laboratory is required.

WORKER TRAITS

Aptitudes: Verbal ability required to instruct workers, conduct lectures, participate in conferences, and consult with PATHOLOGIST.

Form perception required to observe cellular structure of specimens under microscope.

Color discrimination required to perceive color variations and characteristic changes of treated solutions.

Interests: A preference for scientific and technical activities to perform tests and to conduct research in the field of hematology.

A preference for activities carried on in relation to processes and techniques to complete the necessary steps in conducting tests, and in the diagnosis of the nature and extent of diseased conditions.

Temperaments: Capability to direct, control, and plan the activities of workers in the hematology section of the clinical laboratory.

Capable of diagnosis of the nature and extent of disease conditions which requires worker to evaluate information against both measurable and judgmental criteria.

Must attain exacting medical standards when conducting all laboratory tests.

Physical Demands and Working Conditions: Work is light. Lifts and carries relatively light articles short distances.

Reaches for, handles, and fingers a great variety of laboratory equipment and supplies.

Talking and hearing essential to discuss problem cases with a pathologist, participate in conferences, and give instructions to workers.

Near-visual acuity required to examine specimens.

Color vision required to detect characteristic color changes in treated specimens.

Works inside.

Subject to infection from careless handling of diseased specimens; exposure to odorous chemicals and specimens.

JOB RELATIONSHIPS

Workers supervised: BLOOD BANK TECHNOLOGIST; HEMATOLOGY TECHNOLOGIST.

Supervised by: PATHOLOGIST.

Promotion from: No formal line of promotion.

Promotion to: No formal line of promotion. May be promoted to PATHOLOGIST in charge of clinical laboratory, if holding an M.D. degree.

PROFESSIONAL AFFILIATIONS

American Medical Association
535 Dearborn Street
Chicago, Ill. 60610

American Osteopathic Association
212 East Ohio Street
Chicago, Ill. 60611

American Society of Clinical
  Pathologists
445 North Lake Shore Drive
Chicago, Ill. 60611

American Osteopathic College of
  Pathologists
3921 Beecher Road
Flint, Mich. 48504

American Society of Medical
  Technologists
Suite 25, Hermann Professional
  Building
Houston, Tex. 77025

Clinical Laboratories Department   Hematology Technologist   078.281

HEMATOLOGY TECHNOLOGIST

medical technologist, hematology

JOB DUTIES

Performs blood tests and studies morphology of constituents of blood to obtain data for use in diagnosis and treatment of disease:

Receives blood specimens sent to laboratory or draws blood from patient's finger or earlobe, or by venipuncture, observing strict principles of asepsis and antisepsis to prevent infection of patient and contamination of specimens. Centrifuges blood specimens in test tubes and capillary tubes to separate cells and sediment from blood serum. Measures blood quantitatively by pipettes, making necessary dilutions in accordance with standard procedures.

Performs such tests as red and white blood cell counts, platelet counts, differential white blood cell counts, reticulocyte counts, sickle cell counts, hemoglobin estimations, fragility tests, and determinations of color index, sedimentation rate, coagulation time, bleeding time, clot reaction time, volume index, and mean corpuscular, using specialized laboratory equipment, such as photometer, sedimentation rate stand, and fibrometer. Records direct scale readings or converts readings to percent and grams, using converting tables. Consults with HEMATOLOGIST or PATHOLOGIST regarding difficult analyses or abnormal findings.

Transfers blood from pipettes to counting chambers in making cell counts, and counts number of cells within ruled squares of chamber as reviewed through a microscope. Calculates number of cells per cubic millimeter of blood sample. Stains blood sample cells for clearer definition and to distinguish between various types of cells.

Adds prescribed reagents to blood sample and compares resultant color with standard color scales, such as those representing blood containing various amounts of hemoglobin, or makes color comparisons in a colorimeter or photometer, and converts scale readings into percent and grams.

Groups or types blood by mixing red cells of person to be typed with typing serums, and noting if clumping of cells occurs. Cross-matches donors and patients blood to determine compatibility.

Studies morphology of red blood cells in terms of proportion of cells in various stages of development and other characteristics of red corpuscles which may be related to disease processes. Studies slides made from bone marrow specimens.

May calculate prothrombin time by drawing blood samples into anticoagulant solution of specific strength and measuring, with a stopwatch, appearance of a coagulum upon addition of thromboplastin. May prepare and examine thick and thin blood film slides for malaria or other parasites such as filaria and trypanosomes.

May prepare solutions and reagents used in conducting blood tests. Records all results of tests conducted in laboratory log or record.

This job is frequently included in with that of HEMATOLOGIST or BLOOD BANK TECHNOLOGIST.

MACHINES, TOOLS, EQUIPMENT, AND WORK AIDS

Centrifuge, counter, laboratory equipment, logbook, microscope, pipettes, stains, timers.

EDUCATION, TRAINING, AND EXPERIENCE

Three years of college with courses in biology, chemistry, and mathematics, plus 1 year of training in a school of medical technology approved by the American Society of Clinical Pathologists.

Must be registered as a Medical Technologist by the Registry Board of the American Society of Clinical Pathologists.

Some states require a license issued by the state board of health in order to practice.

WORKER TRAITS

Aptitudes: Verbal ability required to use and understand medical terminology and to prepare reports in technical language.

Numerical ability required to count blood cells in slide samples and to calculate solution reaction and physical test time.

Form perception required to perceive pertinent details of cellular structure under microscope and to count platelets and red and white cells in specimen samples.

Color discrimination required to perceive colors, shadings, and hues within constituents of blood during morphological examinations and in preparing stains.

Interests: A preference for scientific and technical activities in order to master hematological duties and keep abreast of the latest innovations in the field of hematology.

A preference for activities carried out in relation to processes and techniques to perform tests.

Temperaments: Accuracy to perform tests involving the evaluation of information against measurable criteria.

Laboratory testing requires precise and accurate job performance carried out according to established laboratory procedures.

Physical Demands and Working Conditions: Work is light. Lifts and carries laboratory equipment about the laboratory.

Occasionally walks throughout the institution to obtain blood specimens from hospital patients.

Reaches for, handles, and fingers laboratory equipment.

Near-visual acuity required to read test results and to study specimens.

Color vision required to detect shadings in blood samples in solutions for various types of identification.

Works inside. Exposed to infection from contaminated blood and to odorous chemicals.

JOB RELATIONSHIPS

Workers supervised: MEDICAL LABORATORY ASSISTANT specializing in hematology, who may be designated as Hematology Technician.

Supervised by: HEMATOLOGIST or MEDICAL TECHNOLOGIST, CHIEF.

Promotion from: No formal line of promotion.

Promotion to: No formal line of promotion.

PROFESSIONAL AFFILIATIONS

American Society of Medical
Technologists
Suite 25, Hermann Professional
Building
Houston, Tex. 77025

American Society of Clinical
Pathologists
445 North Lake Shore Drive
Chicago, Ill. 60611

Clinical Laboratories Department   Histopathologist   041.181

HISTOPATHOLOGIST

JOB DUTIES

Directs and supervises preparation of tissue specimens and examines specimens to provide data on body functions or cause and progress of disease:

Trains and supervises laboratory personnel in fixing, embedding, cutting, staining, and mounting tissue sections or prepares tissue materials from surgical and diagnostic cases or from autopsies. Examines tissue section under microscope to detect changes indicative of disease in tissues and all structures. Assists personnel with more difficult tissue sections and directs use of special stains and methods for isolation, identification, study of functions, morphology, and pathology of obscure cells, tissues, and connecting fibers. Writes diagnostic reports of microscopic examinations for approval by PATHOLOGIST. May lecture to students of medicine, medical technology, or nursing, or to interns. May conduct autopsies to select tissue specimens for study. May engage in research to develop new histopathological methods and new stains to bring out special tissue structure of chemical components. May study formation of organs and related problems to obtain data on body functions.

This job is frequently combined with that of PATHOLOGIST.

MACHINES, TOOLS, EQUIPMENT, AND WORK AIDS

Laboratory supplies, microscope, microtome, reports.

EDUCATION, TRAINING, AND EXPERIENCE

Master's degree or doctorate in histopathology is usually required.

Three years of experience in histopathology in a medical laboratory is required.

WORKER TRAITS

Aptitudes: Verbal ability required to supervise laboratory personnel engaged in histopathology, to prepare reports, and to lecture.

Form perception required to observe details of tissue under microscopic study.

Finger dexterity required to manipulate testing equipment.

Color discrimination required to perceive color variations of specimens being analyzed.

Interests: A preference for scientific activities is required in analyzing tissue to detect diseases.

A preference for activities carried on in relation to established processes and techniques is required to complete the various steps in preparation of slides and diagnosis of the nature and extent of disease conditions.

Temperaments: Administrative ability to direct, control, and plan the activities of personnel in the histology section of the clinical laboratories.

Stability to perform adequately under stress when rapid preparation and examination of slides on surgical specimens are required.

Must attain exacting medical standards in conducting all laboratory tests.

Physical Demands and Working Conditions: Work is light. Lifts and carries relatively light articles short distances.

Reaches for and handles a great variety of laboratory equipment.

Near-visual acuity required to observe specimens and prepared slides.

Color vision required to examine suitability of stains on specimens.

Works inside. Handles tissue which may be capable of transmitting disease. Exposed to odorous chemicals and specimens.

JOB RELATIONSHIPS

Workers supervised: HISTOLOGICAL TECHNOLOGIST and HISTOLOGICAL TECHNICIAN.

Supervised by: PATHOLOGIST.

Promotion from: No formal line of promotion.

Promotion to: No formal line of promotion. May be promoted to PATHOLOGIST in charge of clinical laboratory, if histology training includes M.D. degree and experience in other branches of pathology.

PROFESSIONAL AFFILIATIONS

American Medical Association
535 Dearborn Street
Chicago, Ill. 60610

American Society of Clinical
  Pathologists
445 North Lake Shore Drive
Chicago, Ill. 60611

American Society of Medical
  Technologists
Suite 25, Hermann Professional
  Building
Houston, Tex. 77025

Clinical Laboratories Department   Cleaner, Laboratory Equipment 381.887

LABORATORY AIDE

clean up man
equipment washer
laboratory attendant
laboratory helper
tester helper
utility man, laboratory

JOB DUTIES

Cleans laboratory equipment, such as glassware, metal instruments, sinks, tables, and test panels, using solvents, brushes, and rags; assists MEDICAL TECHNOLOGIST by performing routine duties in the clinical laboratories:

Mixes water and detergents or acids in container to prepare cleaning solutions according to specifications. Washes used glassware and instruments in container by rinsing them in water and drying, using cloth, hot air drier, or acetone bath. Examines cleaned equipment to detect breakage and discards damaged or broken equipment. Carries cleaned items to the appropriate section of clinical laboratories for storage. May sterilize glassware and instruments, using autoclave.

Pours, measures, and mixes liquid, powder, and crystalline chemicals to prepare simple stains, solutions, and culture media, following established formulas and using uninvolved chemical and bacteriological procedures. May label tubes and bottles and fill them with specified solutions.

As assigned, and under close supervision, may perform such simple laboratory tests as qualitative determinations of sugar and albumin in urine. Adds specific reagents to urine sample and notes change in color or appearance of precipitate.

Collects patients' specimens from wards and returns them to laboratory for analysis. Assembles equipment used in collecting communicable disease specimens. Distributes supplies and laboratory specimens to designated area, using hand truck. Keeps records of specimens held in the laboratory. Maintains inventory of supplies. Repairs laboratory apparatus, using hand tools. Scrubs walls, floors, shelves, tables, and sinks, using cleaning solutions and brush. May tend still that provides the laboratory with distilled water.

In smaller hospitals the duties of ANIMAL CARETAKER may be combined with this job.

MACHINES, TOOLS, EQUIPMENT, AND WORK AIDS

Autoclave, chemicals, cleaning supplies, hot air drier, glassware, instruments, records, scales.

EDUCATION, TRAINING, AND EXPERIENCE

High school education is required, preferably including chemistry and bacteriology.

Experience is not essential, although worker usually requires approximately 2 months' training in a clinical laboratory to be capable of normal productivity.

WORKER TRAITS

Aptitudes: Finger dexterity required to manipulate small objects, such as test tubes and microscope slides during cleaning and sterilization duties.

Manual dexterity required to place and arrange articles in sterilizer and cabinets and on shelves. Worker must also handle laboratory glassware carefully to avoid breakage.

Interests: A preference for activities dealing with things and objects to wash and repair laboratory equipment.

A preference for routine, organized activities, to assist MEDICAL TECHNOLOGIST.

Temperaments: Work situation involves doing things only under close supervision, allowing very little room for independent action in working out job problems.

Worker must attain precise tolerances and standards when conducting simple laboratory tests.

Physical Demands and Working Conditions: Work is light. Walking and standing most of day.

Reaches for, lifts, and carries laboratory equipment and materials weighing up to 20 pounds.

Near-visual acuity to examine laboratory glassware for breakage.

Works inside. Worker is subject to unpleasant laboratory odors and to danger of burns and cuts from laboratory apparatus and equipment.

JOB RELATIONSHIPS

Workers supervised: None.

Supervised by: MEDICAL TECHNOLOGIST, or may be supervised by MEDICAL TECHNOLOGIST, CHIEF.

Promotion from: No formal line of promotion. This is an entry job.
Promotion to: No formal line of promotion.

PROFESSIONAL AFFILIATIONS

None.

Clinical Laboratories Department   Medical Laboratory Assistant   078.381

MEDICAL LABORATORY ASSISTANT

assistant laboratory technician
biochemistry technician
blood bank technician
cytotechnician
hematology technician
laboratory assistant
microbiology technician
serology technician

JOB DUTIES

MEDICAL LABORATORY ASSISTANTS in the larger hospitals, and those who are engaged in research may work in only one of several fields of clinical pathology. Thus they would be classified according to field of specialization such as HISTOLOGICAL TECHNICIAN, BIOCHEMISTRY TECHNICIAN, CYTOTECHNICIAN, HEMATOLOGY TECHNICIAN, MICROBIOLOGY TECHNICIAN, SEROLOGY TECHNICIAN, or BLOOD BANK TECHNICIAN. In smaller hospitals, assistant may work in one or a combination of areas depending upon the size and scope of the laboratory activity. Thus they would be classified in the broader, general category of MEDICAL LABORATORY ASSISTANT.

Conducts routine tests in clinical laboratories for use in treatment and diagnosis of disease and performs related duties:

Performs routine tests in various areas such as serology, hematology, chemistry, microbiology, histology, and cytology using standard techniques and equipment. May make qualitative determination of sugar in urine, by adding prescribed reagents to specimens and noting change of color or appearance of precipitate; make blood cell counts by adding reagents to sample and comparing with standard color scales or color comparisons in a colorimeter; or separate plasma from whole blood, using a centrifuge. Stores and labels plasma. May tend automatic equipment, such as diluting-titrating machine, blood cell counter, and spectrophotometer to prepare specimens and perform analytical tests.

Prepares sterile media such as agar in plates, jars, or test tubes, for use in growing bacterial cultures. Incubates cultures for specific times at prescribed temperatures. May make preliminary identification of common types of bacterial cultures for confirmation by supervisor. Cleans and sterilizes laboratory equipment, glassware, and instruments. Prepares solutions, reagents, and stains, following standard laboratory formulas and procedures. Maintains laboratory stock of chemicals and glassware. May collect specimens from patients. Keeps detailed records of all tests performed and reports laboratory findings to all persons authorized to receive such information.

MACHINES, TOOLS, EQUIPMENT, AND WORK AIDS

Glassware, laboratory equipment, reagents, and records.

EDUCATION, TRAINING, AND EXPERIENCE

High school graduation with courses in chemistry and biology plus 1 year of training in a school approved by the Board of Certified Laboratory Assistants, from which worker must also be certified.

WORKER TRAITS

Aptitudes: Form perception required to perceive details in test samples when conducting laboratory tests.

Finger and manual dexterity required to handle specimens and small pieces of laboratory equipment.

Color discrimination required to denote different colors and shadings when observing test samples.

Interests: A preference for working with things and objects for handling test devices and laboratory equipment.

A preference for technical activities to perform the various laboratory tests.

A preference for activities carried on in relation to processes and techniques, used in conducting laboratory tests.

Temperaments: Accuracy, since worker evaluates test samples against known criteria to determine the exact nature of the sample being tested.

Worker must adjust to following standard procedures and techniques when conducting laboratory tests.

Physical Demands and Working Conditions: Work is light. Lifts and carries laboratory equipment about the laboratory.

Reaches for, handles, and fingers specimens and laboratory equipment.

Near-visual acuity to read and prepare formulas of solutions and reagents, examine test results with or without the use of a microscope, and record test results.

Color vision necessary to make color comparisons of tested fluids and materials against established standards.

Works inside. Exposed to infection from disease-bearing specimens and to odorous chemicals and specimens.

JOB RELATIONSHIPS

Workers supervised: None.
Supervised by: MEDICAL TECHNOLOGIST.
Promotion from: No formal line of promotion.
Promotion to: No formal line of promotion.

PROFESSIONAL AFFILIATIONS

Board of Certified Laboratory Assistants
9500 South California Avenue
Evergreen Park, Ill. 60642

Clinical Laboratories Department   Medical Technologist   078.281

MEDICAL TECHNOLOGIST

JOB DUTIES

In large hospitals, and those engaged in research, MEDICAL TECHNOLOGISTS may be responsible for tests and examinations in only one of several fields of clinical pathology. Thus, they would be classified according to field of specialization such as HISTOLOGICAL TECHNOLOGIST, BIOCHEMISTRY TECHNOLOGIST, HEMATOLOGY TECHNOLOGIST, MICROBIOLOGY TECHNOLOGIST, SEROLOGY TECHNOLOGIST, CYTOTECHNOLOGIST or BLOOD BANK TECHNOLOGIST. In smaller hospitals, technologists may perform clinical tests in any one or a combination of areas of specialization depending on the size and scope of the laboratory activity. Thus they would be classified in the broader, general category of MEDICAL TECHNOLOGIST.

Performs various chemical, microscopic, and bacteriological tests to obtain data for use in diagnosis and treatment of disease:

Receives written requisitions from physician for routine or special laboratory tests. Sets up and adjusts laboratory equipment and apparatus, such as chemical glassware, balance, microscope, slides, and reagents.

Obtains laboratory specimens, such as urine, blood, and sputum, from wards or directly from patient, using established laboratory techniques. Adds reagents or indicator solutions, and subjects specimens for processing to operations such as heating, agitating, filtering, or titrating according to established procedures. Prepares slides for microscopic analysis as necessary. Observes reactions, changes of color, or formation of precipitates; studies slides using microscope; or subjects treated specimens to automatic analyzing equipment to make qualitative and quantitative analyses. Posts all test findings to laboratory slips for study by PATHOLOGIST or other laboratory supervisor. Also posts results of laboratory analyses to record cards and files reports. Indicates amount to be charged to patient's account. Identifies and labels all specimens to be retained and files them for further reference or research.

MACHINES, TOOLS, EQUIPMENT, AND WORK AIDS

Autoanalyzer, balance, Bunsen burner, centrifuge, colorimeter, cryostat, laboratory equipment, logbook, laboratory slips, slides, and reports.

EDUCATION, TRAINING, AND EXPERIENCE

Three years of college with courses in biology, chemistry, and mathematics, plus 1 year of training in a school of medical technology approved by the American Society of Clinical Pathologists.

Must be registered as a Medical Technologist by the Registry Board of the American Society of Clinical Pathologists.

Some states require a license issued by the state board of health in order to practice.

WORKER TRAITS

Aptitudes: Numerical ability required to calculate test results, using standard formulas, and to measure prescribed quantities of samples during tests.

Form perception required to notice pertinent details of specimens under microscopic study.

Color discrimination required to stain slides and to distinguish various shades and colors of specimens.

Interests: A preference for scientific and technical activities required to perform a great variety of laboratory tests and to keep abreast of the latest innovations in methods of testing.

A preference for activities carried out according to established processes and techniques in performing laboratory tests.

Temperaments: Keen judgment to evaluate information against measurable criteria in the performance of tests.

Laboratory testing requires precise and accurate job performance carried out according to established laboratory procedures.

Physical Demands and Working Conditions: Work is light. Lifts and carries relatively light laboratory equipment, containers of reagents, and specimens.

Reaches for, handles, and fingers specimens, glassware, controls on equipment, and laboratory slips.

Near-visual acuity required to read detailed instructions and to examine specimens.

Color vision required to detect color changes of specimens and stains used on specimens.

Works inside. Exposed to infection from disease-bearing specimens and to odorous chemicals and specimens.

JOB RELATIONSHIPS

Workers supervised: MEDICAL LABORATORY ASSISTANT; may supervise LABORATORY AIDE.

Supervised by: MEDICAL TECHNOLOGIST, CHIEF or PATHOLOGIST.

Promotion from: No formal line of promotion.

Promotion to: MEDICAL TECHNOLOGIST, CHIEF.

PROFESSIONAL AFFILIATIONS

American Society of Medical Technologists
Suite 25, Hermann Professional Building
Houston, Tex. 77025

MEDICAL TECHNOLOGIST, CHIEF
laboratory supervisor

JOB DUTIES

In large hospitals, and those engaged in research, the MEDICAL TECHNOLOGIST, CHIEF would be responsible for supervision and performance of tests in only one of several fields of clinical pathology. Thus, he would be classified according to field of specialization, such as HISTOLOGICAL TECHNOLOGIST, CHIEF; BIOCHEMISTRY TECHNOLOGIST, CHIEF; MICROBIOLOGY TECHNOLOGIST, CHIEF; HEMATOLOGY TECHNOLOGIST, CHIEF; SEROLOGY TECHNOLOGIST, CHIEF; CYTOTECHNOLOGIST, CHIEF; or BLOOD BANK TECHNOLOGIST, CHIEF. In smaller hospitals the MEDICAL TECHNOLO-GIST, CHIEF would be responsible for supervision and the performance of tests in any one or a combination of areas of specialization depending upon the size and scope of the laboratory activity. Thus they would be classified in the broader, general category of MEDICAL TECH-NOLOGIST, CHIEF.

Supervises, coordinates, and participates in activities of workers performing various chemical, microscopic, and bacteriological tests of body fluids, exudates, skin scrapings, or autopsy and surgical specimens to obtain data for diagnosis and treatment of disease.

Consults with PATHOLOGIST to plan priorities of work to be completed each day. Prepares work schedules and assigns duties to workers in the laboratory. Supervises workers in assigned section or area of specialization in clinical laboratory. Checks validity and accuracy of test results obtained by laboratory personnel on a sample basis by performing the same test and comparing results. Keeps records pertaining to tests performed and charts test results to insure that variation in test results and standards are within acceptable quality control ranges. May keep time records and make ratings and recommendations for promotions. Gives instructions to new workers in procedures and techniques of performing tests. May direct training and instruction of students of medical technology. May interview and hire new laboratory workers.

Performs experimental testing procedures and submits reports to PATHOLOGIST suggesting changes to increase validity and reliability of tests. Demonstrates to personnel newly approved methods to implement standard procedures. Studies current medical laboratory literature to obtain information on new test methods and procedures.

May assist PATHOLOGIST during autopsies. May schedule appointments. Orders replacements to maintain stock of equipment and supplies.

Performs all duties of MEDICAL TECHNOLOGIST.

MACHINES, TOOLS, EQUIPMENT, AND WORK AIDS

Autoanalyzer, balance, Bunsen burner, centrifuge, colorimeter, cryostat, laboratory equipment, logbook, laboratory slips, slides, reports, and work schedules.

EDUCATION, TRAINING, AND EXPERIENCE

Three years of college with courses in biology, chemistry, and mathematics, plus 1 year of training in a school of medical technology approved by the American Society of Clinical Pathologists.

Must be registered as a Medical Technologist by the Registry Board of the American Society of Clinical Pathologists.

Some states require a license issued by the state board of health in order to practice.

Usually requires from 2 to 5 years' experience in a clinical laboratory.

WORKER TRAITS

Aptitudes: Verbal ability required to supervise laboratory personnel and to discuss experimental test procedures and other matters with PATHOLOGIST.

Numerical ability required to calculate test results, use formulas, and measure prescribed quantities of samples during tests.

Form perception required to see details of specimens under microscopic study.

Clerical ability required to accurately record, transcribe, and compare test results.

Color discrimination required to stain slide and to distinguish various shades and colors of specimens.

Interests: A preference for scientific and technical activities to perform a great variety of laboratory tests, to keep abreast of the latest innovations in methods of testing, and to develop new and improved methods for conducting laboratory tests.

A preference for activities carried out according to established processes and techniques to perform laboratory tests.

Temperaments: Sufficient administrative ability for the direction, control, and planning of activities of clinical laboratories' personnel.

Ability to evaluate information against measurable criteria in the performance of tests.

Laboratory testing requires precise and accurate job performance carried out according to established laboratory procedures.

Physical Demands and Working Conditions: Work is light. Lifts and carries relatively light laboratory equipment, containers of reagents, and specimens.

Reaches for, handles, and fingers specimens, glassware, controls on equipment, work schedules, and laboratory slips.

Talking and hearing essential to direct laboratory personnel and to discuss problems with PATHOLOGIST.

Near-visual acuity required to detect color changes of specimens and stains used on specimens.

Works inside. Exposed to infection from disease-bearing specimens and to odorous chemicals and specimens.

JOB RELATIONSHIPS

Workers supervised: MEDICAL TECHNOLOGISTS, MEDICAL LABORATORY ASSISTANTS, and LABORATORY AIDES.

Supervised by: PATHOLOGIST.

Promotion from: MEDICAL TECHNOLOGIST.

Promotion to: No formal line of promotion.

PROFESSIONAL AFFILIATIONS

American Society of Medical Technologists
Suite 25, Hermann Professional Building
Houston, Tex. 77025

Clinical Laboratories Department   Microbiologist   041.081

MICROBIOLOGIST

medical bacteriologist

JOB DUTIES

Directs and supervises cultivation, classification, and identification of microorganisms found in patient body fluids, exudates, skin scrapings, or autopsy and surgical specimens, to provide data on cause, cure, and prevention of disease:

Trains and supervises MICROBIOLOGY TECHNOLOGISTS and microbiology technicians in collecting swabs and smears from patients and preparing bacterial growth under microscope. Assists technologists with more difficult cultures and analyses and studies and identifies less common bacteria, rickettsiae, fungi, protozoa, and viruses. Posts all test findings and writes diagnostic reports for approval by PATHOLOGIST. Performs research to develop new or improved bacteriological methods for discovering and identifying pathogenic organisms. Correlates laboratory findings with clinical data supplied by hospitals and medical practitioners regarding human illnesses. May supervise inoculation of small animals as a means of determining infectious nature, virulence, and course of diseases. May lecture to students of medicine, medical technology, or nursing or to interns. May investigate biology, distribution, and mode of transmission of bacteria and nature and efficiency of chemotherapeutic treatment. Maintains production records including data pertinent to total number of cultures and interpretation of specific cultures.

This job is frequently combined with that of SEROLOGIST and may also include the duties of MICROBIOLOGY TECHNOLOGIST.

MACHINES, TOOLS, EQUIPMENT, AND WORK AIDS

Autoclave, Bunsen burner, incubator, laboratory equipment, microscope, pipettes, and stains.

EDUCATION, TRAINING, AND EXPERIENCE

Bachelor's degree in bacteriology or microbiology is essential; master's or doctor's degree is desirable and frequently required.

Some employers may require certification by the American Board of Microbiology of the American Academy of Microbiology (doctorate degree level) or the National Registry of Microbiologists of the American Board of Microbiology (bachelor's degree level).

At least 3 years' experience in microbiology in a medical laboratory is usually required.

Aptitudes: Verbal ability required to instruct laboratory personnel, understand technical terminology, and write diagnostic reports.

Form perception required to see pertinent details of specimens under microscope.

Color discrimination required to aid in identification of various types of bacteria.

Interests: A preference for scientific and technical activities to prepare cultures and identify microorganisms.

A preference for activities in relation to processes and techniques, to prepare bacteria cultures, and to study and identify bacterial growth under microscope.

Temperaments: Ability to plan, control, and direct the activities of all personnel in the microbiology section of the clinical laboratories.

Good judgment to evaluate information against measurable criteria, when performing research to develop new or improved bacteriological methods for discovering and identifying pathogenic organisms.

Accuracy in identifying pathogens is critical to prevent incorrect diagnosis and treatment of patients.

Physical Demands and Working Conditions: Work is light. Lifts and carries laboratory equipment and supplies about the laboratory.

Reaches for, handles, and fingers specimens, equipment, and materials.

Talking and hearing essential to discuss cases with PATHOLOGIST and to issue instructions to assistant.

Near-visual acuity required for minute detail of specimens under microscope.

Color discrimination required to identify types of stains and characteristics in the growth of microorganisms.

Works inside. Works with specimens capable of transmitting diseases. Exposed to odorous chemicals and specimens.

JOB RELATIONSHIPS

Workers supervised: MICROBIOLOGY TECHNOLOGISTS.

Supervised by: PATHOLOGIST.

Promotion from: No formal line of promotion.

Promotion to: No formal line of promotion. Promotion is through additional administrative and supervisory duties.

PROFESSIONAL AFFILIATIONS

American Academy of Microbiology
P.O. Box 897
Vero Beach, Fla. 32960

American Society for Microbiology
115 Huron View Boulevard
Ann Arbor, Mich. 48103

MICROBIOLOGY TECHNOLOGIST

bacteriology technologist
medical technologist, microbiology

JOB DUTIES

Cultivates, isolates, and assists in identifying bacterial and other microorganisms present in body fluids, exudates, skin scrapings, or autopsy and surgical specimens and performs various bacteriological, mycological, virological and parasitological tests to provide data on cause and progress of disease:

Cultivates and identifies microorganisms found in body materials. Receives specimens of human or animal body materials, such as feces, sputum, pus, urine, and serous fluids from autopsies, diagnostic cases, or directly from patients. Injects and incubates cultures for prescribed length of time under aseptic conditions in suitable media such as meat extracts, sugars, and body products and discharges. Makes periodic observations of material derived from cultures, and identifies type of bacterial colonies found by determination of cultural requirements and biochemical reactions in chemically defined media.

Places specimen from culture on microscopic slides with platinum wire sterilized over gas burner. Collects swabs from nose, ear, throat, rectum, and similar areas of patient under the supervision of physician, and makes direct smears on slides of materials collected. Stains specimens under examination to define essential features more clearly, using one or a combination of standard stains, and dries with blotting paper. Mounts slides on microscope; studies, identifies, and counts bacteria or other microorganisms present and writes reports of findings. Discusses findings and consults with MICROBIOLOGIST or PATHOLOGIST when results are conflicting or do not fall into recognized patterns. May examine growth to identify pathogens. Performs macroscopic and microscopic agglutination and precipitation tests to detect presence of pathological bacteria in human hosts through identification of specific antibodies that are found. May cultivate and identify fungi, rickettsiae, protozoa, and viruses.

Prepares culture media according to established formulas, titrating them to determine degree of acidity. Sterilizes media under standard conditions. Stores all media in refrigerators. Prepares bacteriophage (agents which destroy microorganisms) by filtering feces or pus through special filters. Tests potency of phage by adding various dilutions to test tubes containing growth of organisms and noting reactions. Sterilizes equipment and apparatus.

May inoculate animals: Injects material derived from patients either directly or after cultivation into mice, rats, guinea pigs, or rabbits. Observes disease produced in these animals and determines nature, pathogenicity, and virulence of bacteria or other agents.

The job duties of Microbiology Technician may be combined with this job; it is also frequently combined with that of MICROBIOLOGIST.

MACHINES, TOOLS, EQUIPMENT, AND WORK AIDS

Autoclave, Bunsen burner, incubator, platinum loop, laboratory equipment, microscope, pipettes, and stains.

EDUCATION, TRAINING, AND EXPERIENCE

Three years of college with courses in biology, chemistry, and mathematics, plus 1 year of training in a school of medical technology approved by the American Society of Clinical Pathologists.

Must be registered as Medical Technologist by the Registry Board of the American Society of Clinical Pathologists.

Some states require a license issued by the state board of health in order to practice.

WORKER TRAITS

Aptitudes: Verbal ability required to understand and use medical terminology for preparing written reports in technical language and for periodic review of test instructions and literature.

Numerical ability required to examine and count the number of bacteria in specimens.

Form perception required to observe minute detail of secimens under microscopic study.

Color discimination required to distinguish colors, shades, and hues in identifying microorganisms and in preparing stains.

Interests: A preference for scientific and technical activities in order to master microbiological duties and to keep abreast of the latest innovations in microbiology.

A preference for activities carried on in relation to processes and techniques, required to conduct microbiological tests.

Temperaments: Performance of tests requires the evaluation of information against measurable criteria.

Laboratory testing requires precise and acurate job performance carried out according to established laboratory procedures.

Physical Demands and Working Conditions: Work is light. Lifts and carries relatively light equipment about the laboratory.

Walks through the institution to obtain specimens from hospital patients.

Reaches for, handles, and fingers laboratory equipment and materials.

Near-visual acuity required to study specimens under microscope.

Color vision required to distinguish colors of stains used in microscopic study.

Works inside. Exposed to odorous chemicals and specimens and to infection from contaminated specimens.

JOB RELATIONSHIPS

Workers supervised: MEDICAL LABORATORY ASSISTANT, specializing in microbiology, may be designated Microbiology Technician.

Supervised by: MICROBIOLOGIST or MEDICAL TECHNOLOGIST, CHIEF.

Promotion from: No formal line of promotion.

Promotion to: No formal line of promotion.

PROFESSIONAL AFFILIATIONS

American Society of Medical Technologists
Suite 25, Hermann Professional Building
Houston, Tex. 77025

Clinical Laboratories Department   Morgue Man   355.887

MORGUE ATTENDANT

diener

JOB DUTIES

Assists PATHOLOGIST in performing autopsies in hospital morgue and maintains morgue room and equipment in clean and orderly condition:

Transfers body from compartment tray of morgue refrigerator to the autopsy table, using a wheeled stretcher. Lifts body manually or using portable hoist from stretcher to the autopsy table. Lays out cutting and surgical instruments, glass specimen jars, and test tubes to prepare for autopsy. Writes information such as date and name of deceased on specimen labels and in autopsy logbook for identification and record purposes. Hands PATHOLOGIST surgical instruments, such as knives, saws, scalpels, forceps, and linens, as needed or directed in order that PATHOLOGIST need not divert his attention from field of study. Flushes blood and body fluids from body, using water and suction evacuation hoses. Occasionally performs minor prosecting duties, such as opening the skull, using electric band saw. Weighs organs removed from body and posts weights for use of PATHOLOGIST in making diagnostic reports. Places organs and specimens in prelabeled specimen containers. May photograph specimens. Locates and ties off major arteries and stumps of organs and closes incision in body cavities to prepare body for the undertaker. May fill cranium with plaster. Preserves body in refrigerated storage area until removal by the undertaker.

Cleans the surgical instruments, equipment, and morgue area, using water, sterilizing equipment and solutions, and cleaning equipment. Selects powders and liquids and mixes in prescribed proportions to replenish supply of preserving solutions. Gathers soiled linens for laundering and replaces with fresh supply. Requisitions supplies from the storeroom to maintain stock in the morgue.

Receives bodies of deceased patients in morgue and assists porters in placing bodies in compartment trays, taking care to verify identification of body by armband, compartment label, and record-of-death form accompanying the body. Releases body to authorized person.

MACHINES, TOOLS, EQUIPMENT, AND WORK AIDS

Cleaning solutions, electric band saw, laboratory equipment, preservative solutions, scales, stretcher, suction-evacuator, surgical tools.

EDUCATION, TRAINING, AND EXPERIENCE

High school graduation is usually required.

Usually requires no previous experience. Some employers may require some morgue room experience.

Three months' on-the-job training is required.

WORKER TRAITS

Aptitudes: Numerical ability required to weigh and measure organs and specimens removed from body.

Form perception required to perceive structural details of organs and tissues during autopsy.

Finger dexterity required to manipulate small instruments to tie off arteries and organs and to close body cavity after autopsy.

Interests: A preference for things and objects to perform cleaning tasks in hospital morgue room and to assist PATHOLOGIST in the autopsy.

A preference for routine, organized activities to perform everyday tasks in the hospital morgue room.

Temperaments: Aptitude for work involving repetitive activities carried out according to set procedures, such as assisting in the autopsy, preserving specimens, and preparing solutions.

Work is performed under specific instructions of the PATHOLOGIST, allowing little room for independent action by the worker.

Physical Demands and Working Conditions: Work is heavy. Moves bodies to and from the morgue compartments, stretchers, and autopsy tables.

Reaches for and handles instruments used in performing autopsies.

Fingering and feeling are essential to locate and tie major arteries and stumps of organs removed from the body.

Talks to and listens to PATHOLOGIST to follow instructions.

Near-visual acuity required to read label and post data in logbook.

Works inside. Worker is exposed to hazards from handling of diseased organs and tissues. Subject to noxious odors from deceased bodies and penetrating odors of preservative chemicals.

JOB RELATIONSHIPS

Workers supervised: None.
Supervised by: PATHOLOGIST.
Promotion from: No formal line of promotion. This may be an entry job.
Promotion to: No formal line of promotion.

PROFESSIONAL AFFILIATIONS

None.

SEROLOGIST

JOB DUTIES

Directs and supervises preparation of serums used in treatment and diagnosis of infectious diseases and immunization against these diseases; performs or directs laboratory tests to identify diseases, based on characteristic reactions of various serums:

Trains and supervises SEROLOGY TECHNOLOGISTS and serology technicians in collecting specimens from hospital patients, making serums by inoculating laboratory animals, and conducting serological tests to identify bacteria causing infectious diseases. Observes workers during performance of tasks to determine that established procedures are utilized. Conducts or assists with more difficult tests and devises improved methods for preparing serums and diagnostic antigens and antibodies. Writes diagnostic reports for approval by PATHOLOGIST. Investigates safety of new commercial antibiotic products and accuracy of therapeutic claims. Directs immunology tests and injections, investigates problems of allergy, and conducts tests to determine therapeutic and toxic dosages and most effective methods of administering serums, vaccines, antibiotics, antitoxins, antigens, and related drugs, using laboratory animals as controls. May lecture interns or students of medicine, medical technology, or nursing. Participates in educational conferences to exchange information pertinent to trends in bacteriology, serology, and immunology.

This job is frequently combined with that of MICROBIOLOGIST. The job duties of SEROLOGY TECHNOLOGIST may be included with SEROLOGIST.

MACHINES, TOOLS, EQUIPMENT, AND WORK AIDS

Centrifuge, balance, incubator, laboratory equipment, microscope, work schedules.

EDUCATION, TRAINING, AND EXPERIENCE

Bachelor's degree in bacteriology or serology is essential; master's degree or doctor's degree desirable and frequently required.

At least 3 years of experience in serology in a medical laboratory is usually required.

WORKER TRAITS

Aptitudes: Verbal ability required to instruct and lecture, to participate in conferences, and to consult with PATHOLOGIST.

Numerical ability required to calculate serum formulas.

Form perception required to observe pertinent details of specimens under microscope.

Color discrimination required to aid in identificaton of various types of bacteria.

Interests: A preference for scientific and technical activities to devise new methods for preparing serums and diagnostic antigens and antibodies.

A preference for activities carried on according to processes and techniques, used in performing laboratory tests and in preparing serum.

Temperaments: Capability to plan, control, and direct the activities of the serology section of the clinical laboratory.

Accuracy to evaluate information against measurable criteria when determining the effectiveness of serums used in the diagnosis and treatment of disease.

Must attain exacting medical standards when conducting laboratory tests and in preparing serums.

Physical Demands and Working Conditions: Work is light. Lifts and carries relatively light equipment about the laboratory.

Reaches for, handles, and fingers equipment, materials, and specimens.

Talking and hearing essential to communicate with subordinates and to discuss cases with PATHOLOGIST.

Near-visual acuity required to read and prepare reports and to study reactions of treated specimens.

Color vision used to detect color changes of specimens.

Works inside. Exposed to infection from disease-bearing specimens and to odorous chemicals and specimens.

JOB RELATIONSHIPS

Workers supervised: SEROLOGY TECHNOLOGISTS.
Supervised by: PATHOLOGIST.
Promotion from: No formal line of promotion.
Promotion to: No formal line of promotion. Promotion may be through increased administrative and supervisory duties.

PROFESSIONAL AFFILIATIONS

American Society for Microbiology
115 Huron View Boulevard
Ann Arbor, Mich. 48103

DIETETIC DEPARTMENT

PURPOSE: To provide complete dietetic treatment to all patients, including patient therapy and education, and to plan, prepare, and serve nutritious and appetizing food for patients, personnel, and visitors. To train dietetic and other hospital personnel and to maintain close working relationships with other hospital activities and community agencies.

RESPONSIBILITY: To plan, organize, and direct all phases of the dietetic operation which includes menu planning; food preparation and service; budget estimates; cost control and administrative record-keeping; patient therapy and education; analysis and appraisal of personnel requirements; and safety and sanitation programs. The department is responsible for keeping informed of advancements and changes in equipment and food for possible application.

It is a responsibility of the Dietetic Department to specify quantity and quality of food through use of commodity specifications. Meals must supply basic physiological needs and also have aesthetic appeal to the patient. For efficiency in operations, all diets can be built around general diets by additions and modifications.

Files of recipes for quantity cooking are maintained to facilitate preparation and cost control. The recipes should contain formulas to be followed and indicate yields in terms of number and size of servings, and costs of both total recipe and single servings. A diet manual, prepared or recommended by the department and approved by the medical staff, must be available for use by physicians and nurses.

Food preparation and service constitute a large part of the work of the Dietetic Department. All foods should be prepared under strictly sanitary conditions in accordance with local and State public health regulations. Foods should be prepared preserving full color, flavor, and nutritional value; meals should be attractively served. Trays must be inspected so that patients on modified diets will receive proper meals. Dishwashing and housekeeping in main kitchen, floor kitchen, and other dietetic areas usually are also functions of this department.

Another function is that of formal and informal education. Dietetic interns are trained in many hospitals. Nurses, medical and dental students, and interns and residents are instructed in principles of nutrition and diet therapy. The department is also responsible for teaching patients and their families nutrition and modified diet requirements.

Infant formulas may be prepared by the Dietetic Department or preprepared formulas purchased from vendors.

Other dietetic services include visiting patients in nursing units to determine their food preferences both as to type of food and manner in which it is prepared; advising patients with special dietetic problems prior to their discharge from the hospital, or as referred from the outpatient clinic; cooperating with medical staff in planning, preparing, and serving metabolic research diets.

Dietetics is an important aspect of hospital medical care. To be effective, the Dietetic Department must develop a planned program, efficient organization and administration, and close coordination with other hospital activities. The program must be flexible enough to take advantage of current developments in medicine, dietetics, and the food-service industry.

AUTHORITY: The Dietetic Department is under the direction of a DIRECTOR, FOOD SERVICE, who reports directly to the ADMINISTRATOR or to an ASSOCIATE ADMINISTRATOR. Administrative policies, budgetary controls, and procedures for carrying out the dietetic program are determined by the ADMINISTRATOR in cooperation with the DIRECTOR, FOOD SERVICE and heads of other departments involved such as Nursing, Housekeeping, or Laundry. The DIRECTOR, FOOD SERVICE is then delegated full authority for implementing the dietetic program.

INTERRELATIONSHIPS AND INTRARELATIONSHIPS: The Dietetic Department maintains operating relationships with most of the medical care and administrative activities of the hospital. Close relationships are maintained with the medical staff on special dietetic needs of patients, with nursing services on provisions of regular and modified diets and between-meal nourishment, and with the ADMINISTRATOR on management matters. The department usually takes an active part in formal and informal educational programs of the hospital and works closely with physicians, interns, residents, nurses, student nurses, dietetic interns, and other employees. The department may have an opportunity to conduct instructive courses in dietetics for the general public.

STANDARDS: The Joint Commission on Accreditation of Hospitals has developed minimum standards for Dietetic Departments in hospitals, which include standards on organization, facilities, personnel, foodhandling practices, records, and policies.

The American Dietetic Association has developed standards for the education of dietetic interns and has established specified educational requirements for qualified dietitians.

In most States, it is required by law that those involved with food service shall be subject to physical examinations to determine that they are free of communicable diseases. Local or State Health Departments require that the premises and personnel conform to ordinances and regulations. All employees must wear hair nets and/or caps when handling and preparing food.

PHYSICAL FACILITIES AND STAFFING: Modern food service in a hospital requires not only the necessary space for main and area kitchens, storage, refrigeration, modified diet preparation, infant for-

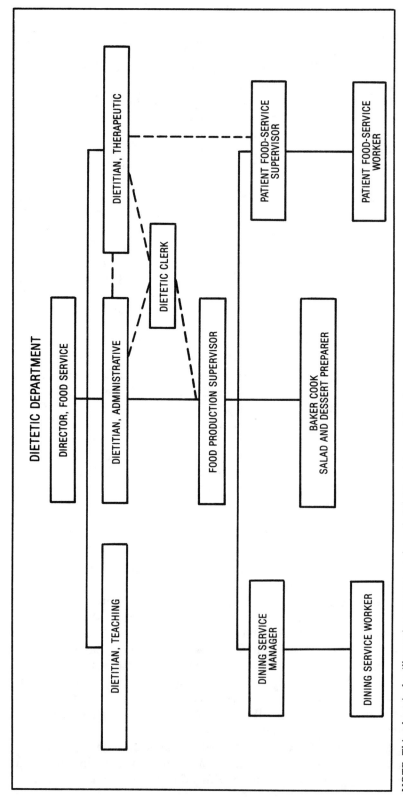

DIETETIC DEPARTMENT

DIRECTOR, FOOD SERVICE

DIETITIAN, TEACHING

DIETITIAN, ADMINISTRATIVE

DIETITIAN, THERAPEUTIC

DIETETIC CLERK

FOOD PRODUCTION SUPERVISOR

PATIENT FOOD-SERVICE SUPERVISOR

PATIENT FOOD-SERVICE WORKER

BAKER COOK SALAD AND DESSERT PREPARER

DINING SERVICE MANAGER

DINING SERVICE WORKER

NOTE: This chart is for illustrative purposes only and should not be considered a recommended pattern of organization.

mula room, dining room for employees and visitors but also should take into consideration such factors as location, utilities, transportation of food, garbage disposal, dishwashing, and general cleaning. Employee locker rooms and restroom facilities are also necessary. Careful consideration should be given to laborsaving devices and to location and arrangement of equipment.

A DIRECTOR, FOOD SERVICE heads the department and must possess requisite qualifications. The number of staff is determined by such factors as average number of hospital patients, number of modified diets, type of service, number of personnel served, extent of educational programs, and physical capacities of the department.

GENERAL WORKING CONDITIONS: Workers may be subject to cuts, burns, muscle sprains, and falls. Handtrucks are available for moving heavy food supplies, garbage, and trash cans. Much of the work in the department is interchangeable, and personnel work according to an assigned schedule.

Dietetic Department   Dietitian, Chief 077.118

DIRECTOR, FOOD SERVICE
chief dietitian
director, dietetics

JOB DUTIES

Plans, directs, and coordinates activities of Dietetic Department to provide dietetic services for patients and hospital employees:

Establishes departmental regulations and procedures, in conformance with administrative policies, and develops standards for organization and supervision of dietetic service. Determines quality and quantity of food required, plans menus, and controls food costs. Reviews regular diet menus as to cost and suitability to type of hospital, and standardized recipes for menu requirements. Makes frequent inspections of all work, storage, and serving areas to determine that regulations and directions governing dietetic activities are followed. Recommends or institutes changes in techniques or procedures for more efficient operation. Develops and prepares policies and procedures governing handling and storage of supplies and equipment, sanitation, and for records and compiling reports. Prepares job descriptions, organization charts, manuals, and guidebooks covering all phases of departmental operations for use by employees. Makes final determination of kinds and amounts of supplies and equipment needed.

Interviews and makes final selection of applicants for employment. Reviews work schedules for personnel and job performance ratings.

Selects, upon recommendation, personnel for transfer, promotion, and special training to insure most effective utilization of individual skills and employee development.

Reviews records and reports covering number and kinds of regular and therapeutic diets prepared, nutritional and caloric analyses of meals, costs of raw food and labor, computation of daily ration cost, inventory of equipment and supplies. Develops and directs cost control system. Prepares and submits department budget.

Confers with other department heads regarding technical and administrative aspects of dietetic service. Establishes effective relationships with medical staff, nursing, and other patient care services. Attends hospital staff conferences and transmits information to department staff regarding new developments and trends.

Delegates authority to supervisory staff for task details to facilitate smooth flow of materials and services.

Attends professional meetings and conferences to keep informed of current practices and trends in fields of dietetics and nutrition. May prepare articles for publication in professional journals and lecture on various aspects of dietetic operations. May discuss dietetic problems with patients or their families and explain diet therapy for specific case.

In smaller hospitals the duties of DIETITIAN, ADMINISTRATIVE and/or DIETITIAN, THERAPEUTIC may be combined with this job.

MACHINES, TOOLS, EQUIPMENT, AND WORK AIDS

Dietetic personnel records, inventory records, purchase requisitions, recipes, other records and reports, and work schedules.

EDUCATION, TRAINING, AND EXPERIENCE

Bachelor's or advanced degree from an accredited institution, with major in foods, nutrition, or food-service administration.

May have completed an internship in hospital offering dietetic internship approved by The American Dietetic Association or have met necessary experience requirements.

Varied experience in dietetics and administration is required.

WORKER TRAITS

Aptitudes: Verbal ability required to understand medical and scientific terminology in order to communicate with professional staff regarding technical aspects of the department; ability to understand policies, principles, and procedures of dietetics and hospital administration; ability to communicate with personnel of all levels; and ability to solve problems.

Numerical ability required to evaluate and prepare statistical material for budget, cost control, and other purposes.

Interests: A preference for contacts with people to confer with administrative personnel regarding department activities and to direct work of department personnel.

Temperaments: Suitability to direct, control, and plan all activities in the department.

Able to deal with people, for conferring with other department heads, supervisors, and patients.

Physical Demands and Working Conditions: Work is light.

Talking and hearing essential to consult with departmental personnel and applicants, to confer with other hospital department heads, and to represent department in hospital staff meetings.

Works inside.

JOB RELATIONSHIPS

Workers supervised: All employees assigned to the department.

Supervised by: ADMINISTRATOR or an ASSOCIATE ADMINISTRATOR.

Promotion from: DIETITIAN, ADMINISTRATIVE; DIETITIAN, TEACHING, or DIETITIAN, THERAPEUTIC.

Promotion to: No formal line of promotion. May be promoted to an ASSOCIATE ADMINISTRATOR.

PROFESSIONAL AFFILIATIONS

American Society for Hospital Food
  Service Administrators
840 North Lake Shore Drive
Chicago, Ill. 60611

The American Dietetic Association
620 North Michigan Avenue
Chicago, Ill. 60611

DIETITIAN, ADMINISTRATIVE

assistant director, food service
food production manager

JOB DUTIES

Directs and supervises hospital personnel concerned with planning, preparing, and serving food to patients, staff, and visitors:

Plans basic menus considering such factors as variety, season of the year, availability of foods, known food preferences of the group, nutritional and caloric content, and food costs. Estimates number of people to be served and computes quantity of food to be prepared to insure that individual portions will be in conformance with dietetic standards. Prepares daily menus and portion specification orders for guidance of the staff and inspects prepared food to insure adherence to specifications, observing appearance, quantity, and temperature, and sampling the food to estimate its palatability.

Develops and implements work standards, sanitation procedures, and personal hygiene requirements consistent with institutional rules; local, State and Federal regulations; and foodhandling principles. Inspects food preparation and serving areas, equipment, and storage facilities, observes the appearance and personal habits of the staff to detect deviations and violations of current health regulations, and orders corrective measures as necessary.

Prepares daily work schedules and assigns duties and responsibilities, through supervisors, to dietetic staff. Employs dietetic personnel, directs orientation and training, and initiates, recommends, and approves personnel actions, such as transfers, promotions, and separations, according to procedures established by hospital administration.

Responsible for records and reports concerning technical and administrative operations, such as number of meals served, menus, analyses of diets, food costs, supplies issued, repairs to dietetic equipment, maintenance service and costs, personnel data, and continuous inventory of supplies on hand. Suggests revisions or adaptations of procedures for more efficient performance of department and for training of employees.

Reviews technical publications, studies journals, and confers with food industry representatives regarding new developments in food packing and processing, new and modified equipment, and new nutritional concepts. Selects those with merit for possible incorporation into the hospital programs.

Depending on the size and organization of the Dietetic Department, may directly supervise the food preparation personnel, overseeing the cooking, serving, and cleaning tasks. May also supervise all dietetic personnel not specifically assigned to patient food service or modified diet preparation. May direct the employee food-service activity.

In smaller hospitals, the duties of DIRECTOR, FOOD SERVICE or DIETITIAN, THERAPEUTIC may be combined with this job.

MACHINES, TOOLS, EQUIPMENT, AND WORK AIDS

Food preparation reports, inventory records, menus, personnel records, recipes, work schedules, and all institutional kitchen equipment.

EDUCATION, TRAINING, AND EXPERIENCE

Bachelor's or advanced degree from an accredited college or university with major in foods, nutrition, or food-service administration.

May have completed a dietetic internship approved by The American Dietetic Association or have met necessary experience requirements.

Varied experience in dietetics and administration is required.

WORKER TRAITS

Aptitudes: Verbal ability required to direct work activities and to utilize hospital and dietetic terminologies.

Numerical ability required to calculate nutritional values of foods, plan work schedules, develop requisitions, and estimate food purchasing requirements.

Form perception required to judge adherence to portion-size specifications.

Interests: A preference for contacts with people, to direct departmental personnel and their activities and to resolve problems related to departmental activities.

Temperaments: Capable of the direction, control, and planning of the food production activities of the department.

Able to deal with people, for supervising staff, conducting on-the-job training, and conferring with associates.

Physical Demands and Working Conditions: Work is light. Stands and walks much of working day.

Talking and hearing essential to give assignments and work instructions to subordinates and to resolve dietary matters with associates. Works inside.

JOB RELATIONSHIPS

Workers supervised: All employees of food production unit.

Supervised by: DIRECTOR, FOOD SERVICE.

Promotion from: No formal line of promotion. May be promoted from staff level position.

Promotion to: DIRECTOR, FOOD SERVICE.

PROFESSIONAL AFFILIATIONS

American Society for Hospital Food
    Service Administrators
840 North Lake Shore Drive
Chicago, Ill. 60611

The American Dietetic Association
620 North Michigan Avenue
Chicago, Ill. 60611

Dietetic Department   **Dietitian, Teaching 077.128**

DIETITIAN, TEACHING

assistant director, dietetic education

JOB DUTIES

Plans, organizes, and conducts dietetic educational programs for nurses, medical and dental interns, medical residents, dietetic interns, and other personnel:

Plans schedule of instruction and on-the-job training. May conduct classes in subjects such as nutrition, diet therapy, sanitation, infant nutrition, marketing, menu planning, food procurement, food cost control, and supervisory techniques. Arranges for additional lectures by medical staff, teachers of dietetic subjects in colleges and universities, and members of professional associations. Supervises dietitians in any teaching or training functions they may perform in connection with the program for teaching in the area of dietetics.

May recommend and supervise procedures in orientation and on-the-job training of food-preparation and food-service workers: Institutes orientation program to acquaint employees with work assignments, schedules, and required performance standards.

Selects textbooks and reference materials for subjects to be presented in classroom and prepares course outlines. Prepares manuals and guidebooks for use in on-the-job training. Prepares and presents visual aids to supplement textbook information and to portray on-the-job methods.

Requests, from accredited colleges, universities, and professional associations, literature on trends and practices in fields of dietetics and nutrition.

Participates in meetings of professional associations.

In smaller hospitals the duties of this job may be combined with those of DIETITIAN, ADMINISTRATIVE; DIETITIAN, THERAPEUTIC; or DIRECTOR, FOOD SERVICE.

MACHINES, TOOLS, EQUIPMENT, AND WORK AIDS

Course outlines, dietetic literature, files, manuals, visual aids, textbooks, and written examinations.

EDUCATION, TRAINING, AND EXPERIENCE

Bachelor's and master's degrees from accredited institution with major in foods, nutrition, or food service management. Completion of courses in methods and principles of teaching required.

May have completed an internship in hospital offering dietetic internship approved by The American Dietetic Association or equivalent approved experience. At least 1 year's experience as instructor in one or more phases of dietetics in a college or institution is preferred.

WORKER TRAITS

Aptitudes: Verbal ability required to read and comprehend complex principles of dietetics and to be able to develop and prepare course outlines, conduct class lectures, prepare examinations, and rate student performance.

Interests: A preference for working with people and the communication of ideas to conduct educational program.

A preference for scientific and technical activities to present such subject matter as nutrition, sanitation, and diet therapy.

Temperaments: Leadership required to plan, control, and direct all phases of the educational program relating to dietetics.

Capable of guiding students in their opinions, attitudes, and judgments in teaching dietetics.

Physical Demands and Working Conditions: Work is light. Intermittent standing, walking, and sitting to conduct classes and observe activities of students.

Talking and hearing essential in lecturing to students and answering questions. Works inside.

JOB RELATIONSHIPS

Workers supervised: All trainees and dietetic personnel who take part in training activities.

Supervised by: DIRECTOR, FOOD SERVICE.

Promotion from: No formal line of promotion. May be promoted from staff level position.

Promotion to: No formal line of promotion. May be promoted to DIRECTOR, FOOD SERVICE.

PROFESSIONAL AFFILIATIONS

The American Dietetic Association
620 North Michigan Avenue
Chicago, Ill. 60611

DIETITIAN, THERAPEUTIC
assistant director, therapeutic dietetics

JOB DUTIES

Plans and directs preparation of modified diets prescribed by medical staff for patients with therapeutic diet needs:

Reviews medical orders for modified diets required for patients. May interview patients to obtain information regarding food habits and preferences for guidance in planning diets. Advises on types and quantities of foods and methods of preparation for therapeutic diets. May instruct personnel regarding type and quantity of food to be prepared and any special techniques to be employed. May inspect meal assembly so that trays conform to prescribed diet and meet standards and directions as to quality, quantity, temperature, and appearance. May instruct patients and/or their relatives, regarding diet therapy to be applied during and subsequent to hospitalization. Initiates referral of specific patients to community agencies for follow-up, with physician's approval.

Is responsible for records and reports concerning technical and administrative operations, such as number of meals served, menus, analyses of modified diets, and food costs.

In smaller hospitals, the duties of this job may be combined with those of DIETITIAN, ADMINISTRATIVE or DIRECTOR, FOOD SERVICE.

MACHINES, TOOLS, EQUIPMENT, AND WORK AIDS

Diet manuals, diet lists, diet orders, menus, and related reference and research publications.

EDUCATION, TRAINING, AND EXPERIENCE

Bachelor's or advanced degree from accredited institution with a major in foods and nutrition.

May have completed an internship in hospital offering dietetic internship approved by The American Dietetic Association or have had equivalent approved experience.

WORKER TRAITS

Aptitudes: Verbal ability required to comprehend dietetic course work, practices, principles, and theories; to communicate effectively with medical personnel and staff; and to explain dietetic restrictions to patients.

Numerical ability required to compute dietetic values of food and to work with dietetic chemical formulas.

Interests: A preference for dealing with people and the communication of ideas, to instruct patients and/or their relatives regarding diet therapy to be followed after hospitalization.

A preference for scientific and technical activities to perform duties requiring a knowledge of chemistry, caloric values, and physical properties of foodstuffs, as well as understanding the medical basis for dietetic restrictions.

Temperaments: Capable of the direction, control, and planning of duties of personnel concerned with meals served in the modified diet unit.

Ability to deal with people to explain dietetic restrictions to patients and the necessity for following such restrictions.

Physical Demands and Working Conditions: Work is light.

Talking and hearing essential to discuss food preparation with cooking personnel and section staff, to explain dietetic restrictions to patients, and to discuss diet plans with supervisor or attending medical personnel.

Works inside.

JOB RELATIONSHIPS

Workers supervised: All employees of therapeutic or modified diet unit.

Supervised by: DIRECTOR, FOOD SERVICE.

Promotion from: No formal line of promotion. May be promoted from a staff level position.

Promotion to: No formal line of promotion. May be promoted to DIRECTOR, FOOD SERVICE.

PROFESSIONAL AFFILIATIONS

The American Dietetic Association
620 North Michigan Avenue
Chicago, Ill. 60611

Dietetic Department
Executive Chef 313.168
Kitchen Supervisor 310.138

FOOD PRODUCTION SUPERVISOR

chef
chief cook
first cook
head cook

JOB DUTIES

Supervises and coordinates activities of kitchen workers preparing and cooking foods for hospital patients, staff, and visitors:

Plans or participates in planning menus and utilization of foodstuffs and leftovers, taking into consideration number and types of meals to be served, marketing conditions, and recency of menus. Estimates food consumption and requirements to determine type and quantity of meats, vegetables, and other foods to be prepared. Supervises cooking personnel and coordinates their assignments to insure economical and timely food preparation. Reviews menus and determines food quantities, labor, and overhead costs in cooperation with the DIETITIAN, ADMINISTRATIVE. Observes methods of food preparation, cooking, and sizes of portions to insure food is prepared in prescribed manner. Tests cooked foods by tasting and smelling. May develop and standardize recipes.

May inspect trays for attractiveness, palatability, and temperature of food.

Inspects purchased foods for standards of quality.

May train new food service employees. Keeps records of work assignments and hours worked of personnel under his supervision.

MACHINES, TOOLS, EQUIPMENT, AND WORK AIDS

Various types of food preparation equipment, menus, work schedules, and records and reports.

EDUCATION, TRAINING, AND EXPERIENCE

High school education. In addition, may have completed a special 1-year course which includes such subjects as sanitation, hygiene, quantity food preparation, supervisory techniques, estimating requirements, purchasing food, and managing kitchen and storeroom.

WORKER TRAITS

Aptitudes: Verbal ability is required to read and comprehend menus and to issue clear and concise instructions when supervising kitchen employees.

Numerical ability is required in estimating daily food requirements and in calculating amount of foodstuffs to be purchased to augment existing stocks or for replenishment.

Manual dexterity is required to demonstrate easily and skillfully food preparation and cooking techniques.

Color discrimination is required to recognize freshness from appearance of meats and other foods; also to determine the accepted degree of palatability from color shadings of cooked foodstuffs.

Interests: A preference for managerial activities for the direction and supervision of personnel involved with cooking.

A preference for multiple operations in order to produce satisfactorily finished, palatable meals.

Temperaments: Versatility to adapt to frequent changes in job duties covering a broad range of kitchen occupations, including supervisory responsibility as well as actual preparation and cooking of foods.

A sense of responsibility for the planning and control of an extensive program for feeding a large number of hospital patients, in an expeditious manner, and according to set procedures and stringent sanitation conditions.

Physical Demands and Working Conditions: This work is light.

Stands and walks short distances most of working day.

Stoops, reaches for, and lifts kitchen equipment.

Handles and uses kitchen utensils.

Tastes and smells food to determine its quality and palatability.

Talking and hearing for supervising staff.

Near-visual acuity and color discrimination for examining cooked and stored foods to determine quality.

Works inside. Work area may be warm and humid.

JOB RELATIONSHIPS

Workers supervised: Employees concerned with preparation of food.

Supervised by: DIETITIAN, ADMINISTRATIVE or DIETITIAN, THERAPEUTIC.

Promotion from: COOK or BAKER.

Promotion to: No formal line of promotion.

PROFESSIONAL AFFILIATIONS

None.

Dietetic Department   Food Service Supervisor 319.138

DINING SERVICE MANAGER

cafeteria food-service supervisor
counter service manager
manager, cafeteria

JOB DUTIES

Supervises and coordinates activities of dietetic personnel who serve meals in a cafeteria, dining room, or coffee shop:

Assigns tasks to employees and arranges work schedules. Sees that service is prompt and courteous, and makes adjustments following complaints.

Directs the setup of tables in the dining room and the preparation and serving of food for regular and special luncheons and dinners. Inspects cafeteria, dining room, coffee shop, and equipment for cleanliness.

Interviews and recommends employment of new workers, assigns them to various duties, and instructs them in work procedures. Maintains record of meals served. Keeps cost records and makes periodic reports of operating expenses. Orders food, supplies, and equipment; assists in menu planning.

MACHINES, TOOLS, EQUIPMENT, AND WORK AIDS
Menus, order books, time records, work schedules.

EDUCATION, TRAINING, AND EXPERIENCE
High school graduation preferred. Some college education is desirable but not essential. Courses in foods and nutrition and personnel management or supervisory training are desirable.

Six months to 1 year of supervisory experience in a hospital department of dietetics, as manager of a cafeteria or dining room of a hotel or restaurant.

One to 3 months' on-the-job training provided to learn policies and procedures of the establishment.

WORKER TRAITS
Aptitudes: Verbal ability is required in supervising and explaining job duties to workers.

Numerical ability at level of simple arithmetic in order to work out time schedules and prepare inventory control.

Clerical perception for the maintenance of records and reports.

Interests: A preference for contact with people.

Temperaments: Capability to direct, control, and coordinate the activities of dietetic personnel engaged in serving food.

Cooperative, to work with staff, associates, and supervisors in resolving food-service problems.

Physical Demands and Working Conditions: Work is light. Constant walking and standing.

Reaches for and handles dishes, utensils, and other equipment to inspect for cleanliness and to demonstrate work methods.

Talking and hearing to communicate with employees and supervisors.

Visual acuity and color discrimination for judging appearance, condition, and attractiveness of foods and displays.

Works inside.

JOB RELATIONSHIPS
Workers supervised: All workers engaged in serving meals in the cafeteria, dining room, or coffee shop.

Supervised by: FOOD PRODUCTION SUPERVISOR or DIETITIAN, ADMINISTRATIVE.

Promotion from: Qualified worker in the department.

Promotion to: No formal line of promotion.

PROFESSIONAL AFFILIATIONS
None.

PATIENT FOOD-SERVICE SUPERVISOR
kitchen steward
patient tray-line supervisor
sanitation supervisor

JOB DUTIES

Trains and supervises personnel who serve trays to patients and maintain cleanliness of food service areas and equipment, and otherwise assists DIETITIAN, THERAPEUTIC, as directed:

Instructs workers in methods of performing duties and assigns and coordinates work of employees to promote efficiency of operations.

Observes filled trays to assure that foods are properly apportioned and attractively garnished and arranged on trays. Directs workers in loading trays on carts or in automatic conveyor units, in dispatching to nursing stations, and in serving food trays to patients.

Interviews and recommends employment of new workers. Visits patients to learn of food preferences. Calculates routine modified diets.

MACHINES, TOOLS, EQUIPMENT, AND WORK AIDS
Menus, time records, work schedules.

EDUCATION, TRAINING, AND EXPERIENCE

High school graduation preferred. Some college education is desirable but not essential. Courses in foods, nutrition, and personnel management, or supervisory training are desirable.

Six months to 1 year of supervisory experience in a hospital food preparation unit.

One to 3 months' on-the-job training is provided to learn policies and procedures of the establishment.

WORKER TRAITS

Aptitudes: Verbal ability is required in supervising and explaining job duties to workers.

Numerical ability at the level of simple arithmetic is required in order to work out time schedules and prepare inventory control.

Clerical perception for the maintenance of records and reports.

Interests: A preference for contact with workers, in preparing and serving meals to patients.

Temperaments: Capability to direct, control, and coordinate the activities of dietetic personnel engaged in preparing and serving food.

Deals with staff, associates, and supervisors in resolving food-service problems.

Physical Demands and Working Conditions: The work is light. Constant walking and standing.

Reaches for and handles dishes, utensils, and other equipment to inspect for cleanliness and to demonstrate work methods.

Talking and hearing to communicate with subordinates and supervisors.

Near-visual acuity and color discrimination for judging appearance, condition, and attractiveness of foods and displays.

Works inside.

JOB RELATIONSHIPS

Workers supervised: PATIENT FOOD-SERVICE WORKERS.

Supervised by: FOOD PRODUCTION SUPERVISOR or DIETITIAN, THERAPEUTIC.

Promotion from: PATIENT FOOD-SERVICE WORKER.
Promotion to: No formal line of promotion.

PROFESSIONAL AFFILIATIONS

None.

HOUSEKEEPING DEPARTMENT

PURPOSE: To maintain the hospital facilities in a clean, sanitary, orderly, and attractive condition, to provide a suitable environment for the care of patients and for the work of the hospital staff and employees.

RESPONSIBILITY: Clean, sanitary, pleasant environment and facilities are essential to medical and nursing care of patients, and to hospital staff. The responsibility for providing such surroundings in as economic a manner as possible falls in a large measure upon the housekeeping staff of the hospital. Housekeeping is a complex activity requiring constant attention to many different details and to an over-all plan which provides for the utilization of personnel, procedures, and material in an efficient and effective manner.

More specifically, responsibilities of the Housekeeping Department include:

1. Establish and maintain a regularly scheduled cleaning program throughout the hospital complex. Patient-care areas, intensive-care units, surgical suites, and other specialized areas require that a high level of sanitation and sterilization be maintained.

2. Recruit, select, and train personnel for this purpose.

3. Study new techniques for improving housekeeping services; evaluate, select, and provide proper equipment and supplies for efficient and economical operation of the housekeeping services.

4. Provide qualified supervision and direction to scheduled work activities in the most effective utilization of manpower.

5. Establish and maintain procedures which will insure acceptable standards of quality. This includes routine cleaning of windows, walls, floors, fixtures, and furnishings as well as responsibility for disposal of ordinary and contaminated refuse; disinfection of contaminated areas; pest and rodent control; taking bacteriological surface samplings; and carrying out pertinent infection-control procedures.

6. Utilize good interior design principles with regard to decorating and choice of furniture and furnishings, and attend to furniture repairs, refinishing, and upholstering or replacement of equipment and supplies. May move and relocate furniture.

7. Maintain linen selection, distribution, control, and repair.

8. Be aware of common safety precautions and correct or report safety hazards to the correct authority.

9. Coordinate department activities with those of all other departments.

10. Report building repair needs to the Engineering and Maintenance Department.

The Housekeeping Department may also be responsible for the following services: Hospital security; elevator operation; operation

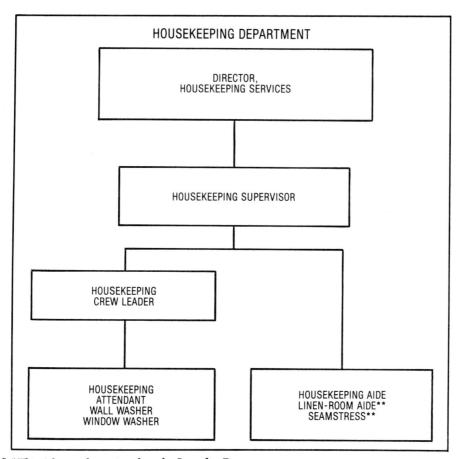

HOUSEKEEPING DEPARTMENT

DIRECTOR,
HOUSEKEEPING SERVICES

HOUSEKEEPING SUPERVISOR

HOUSEKEEPING
CREW LEADER

HOUSEKEEPING
ATTENDANT
WALL WASHER
WINDOW WASHER

HOUSEKEEPING AIDE
LINEN-ROOM AIDE**
SEAMSTRESS**

* *This job may be assigned to the Laundry Department.

NOTE: This chart is for illustrative purposes only and should not be considered a recommended pattern of organization.

of the laundry; and control of service contracts for services provided by nonhospital personnel.

AUTHORITY: While the housekeeping function is performed within every department of the hospital, it should be the sole responsibility of the DIRECTOR, HOUSEKEEPING SERVICES who reports to an ASSOCIATE ADMINISTRATOR.

INTERRELATIONSHIPS AND INTRARELATIONSHIPS: Cleanliness, sanitation, and pleasant appearance of facilities are vital to the well-being and safety of patients. Housekeeping services must be coordinated with activities of other departments so that minimal disturbance is caused to patients, staff, and employees.

Functions of the Housekeeping Department must be clearly identified and understood by other departments to avoid duplication of services or misunderstanding resulting in loss of services to patients and staff.

PHYSICAL FACILITIES AND STAFFING: The Housekeeping Department requires adequate space and facilities according to the functions under its jurisdiction. An office should be provided for the head of the department, clerical and supporting staff, and housekeeping supervisors. A central storeroom for supplies and equipment is required as well as supply rooms and closets with sinks, shelving, and storage space on every floor and near strategic areas. There should be locker rooms for all personnel, sewing repair rooms, and workrooms of various kinds.

The department is headed by a DIRECTOR, HOUSEKEEPING SERVICES who may have a number of assistants and supervisors as well as a clerical staff. Work must be planned and carefully allocated to prevent overlapping and unbalanced distribution. The DIRECTOR is responsible for training and supervision of all departmental personnel and advises personnel in other departments who may necessarily perform housekeeping duties.

Housekeeping Department   Executive Housekeeper 187.168

DIRECTOR, HOUSEKEEPING SERVICES

administrative housekeeper

director, environmental services

executive housekeeper

JOB DUTIES

Directs and administers the housekeeping program to maintain the hospital environment in a sanitary, attractive, and orderly condition:

Establishes standards and work procedures for the housekeeping staff in accordance with the establishd policies of the hospital. Plans work schedules and assigns hours and areas of work to insure adequate service for all areas of the hospital. Interviews, selects, hires, evaluates, and terminates personnel and is responsible for their training and supervision.

Inspects and evaluates the physical condition of the hospital; recommends painting, repairs, furnishings and refurnishing, relocation of equipment, and reallocation of space to improve sanitation, appearance, and efficiency. Reports any unsafe conditions. Conducts research to improve housekeeping technology. Investigates and evaluates new housekeeping supplies and equipment. Takes, processes, and analyzes microbiological samples of air and surfaces to evaluate housekeeping methods and materials.

Conducts staff meetings and meets with members of other departments to coordinate housekeeping activities with those of other departments. Serves on the Infection Control Committee and other committees as requested.

Prepares budgets, work reports, and other administrative guides. Inventories housekeeping supplies and equipment, and selects and requisitions new or replacement supplies and equipment. Is responsible for maintaining the records of the Housekeeping Department.

MACHINES, TOOLS, EQUIPMENT, AND WORK AIDS

Records and reports.

EDUCATION, TRAINING, AND EXPERIENCE

A high school education is the minimum formal education required; a college degree is desirable. In addition, special courses in housekeeping or institutional management are desirable.

Experience as a Housekeeping Supervisor or as an Assistant Director of Housekeeping is required.

WORKER TRAITS

Aptitudes: Verbal ability is needed to comprehend and communicate with housekeeping personnel and to prepare reports in concise, understandable language.

Numerical ability is required to perform arithmetic operations in keeping work records, preparing budgets, in requisitioning supplies, and in preparing and balancing workloads.

Color discrimination is needed in the preparation of decorative recommendations.

Interests: A preference for working with people in order to supervise them and to coordinate housekeeping activities with those of other departments.

A preference for activities resulting in the satisfaction of maintaining the hospital in a clean, orderly, attractive, and safe condition.

Temperaments: Ability to direct, control, and plan the total activity of the entire housekeeping department.

Able to communicate with people beyond giving instructions, as in coordinating activities with other department heads and staff.

Physical Demands and Working Conditions: Work is light. There is extensive walking and standing.

Frequent talking and hearing when giving instructions and explanations and in receiving oral information.

Color vision is necessary for determining harmonious color schemes.

Works inside.

JOB RELATIONSHIPS

Workers supervised: All personnel assigned to the Housekeeping Department either directly or through supervisors.

Supervised by: ASSOCIATE ADMINISTRATOR or ADMINISTRATOR.

Promotion from: HOUSEKEEPING SUPERVISOR.

Promotion to: ASSOCIATE ADMINISTRATOR.

PROFESSIONAL AFFILIATIONS

Institute of Sanitation Management
1710 Drew Street
Clearwater, Fla. 33515

National Executive Housekeepers
   Association
204 Business and Professional
   Building
Second Avenue
Gallipolis, Ohio 45631

Housekeeping Department   Housekeeper 321.138

HOUSEKEEPING SUPERVISOR

assistant housekeeper

housekeeper

JOB DUTIES

Supervises work activities of cleaning personnel to ensure clean, orderly, and attractive conditions in the hospital:

Prepares daily assignment schedules to include established routine duties, as well as special areas to be cleaned to maintain adequate service at all times to all areas. Tours hospital periodically, covering each assigned area to observe cleaning crews at work and to determine that instructions are followed and safety rules are observed. Inspects hospital premises to determine next assignments such as preparation of vacated rooms for next patient, and to insure that trash and garbage disposal meet safety, health, and sanitation regulations. Occasionally, takes cultures from bed linens, floors, beds, or other equipment and submits them for laboratory analysis.

Introduces and instructs personnel in use of new equipment and cleaning methods to provide most efficient and economical methods of maintaining hospital. Trains new employees, assigns them to tasks, and closely supervises them until fully trained. Recommends personnel actions, such as employing, transfering. or termination.

Maintains an inventory of cleaning materials, supplies, and equipment, and prepares requisitions for replacement of items "used up" or in need of repair. Inspects hospital equipment and furnishings such as beds, cabinets, chairs, screens, and fans, and prepares requisition for maintenance.

Determines that collection and distribution of linen meet needs of the hospital.

Keeps records of rooms and other areas of the hospital that have been cleaned.

May be responsible for keeping a lost-and-found department for the convenience of patients, visitors, and employees. Also may keep personnel records on workers such as hour and wage data.

MACHINES, TOOLS, EQUIPMENT, AND WORK AIDS

Linens and household cleaning supplies, wheeled equipment, tools, mops, and similar items.

EDUCATION, TRAINING, AND EXPERIENCE

High school graduation is required. Courses in hospital housekeeping or institutional management are helpful.

Experience in functions to be supervised is essential, whether gained from employment or practical training. Must have demonstrated leadership potential.

WORKER TRAITS

Aptitudes: Verbal ability is needed to supervise workers.

Clerical ability is needed to keep departmental records in good order.

Interests: A preference for working with people to supervise, instruct, and maintain harmony among workers .

A preference for activities resulting in tangible, productive satisfaction, such as maintaining hospital areas in clean, orderly, and pleasant condition.

Temperaments: Ability to direct and control housekeeping activities, and evaluate cleanliness and neatness of work against established procedures.

Physical Demands and Working Conditions: Work is light. Extensive walking and standing while supervising workers or inspecting for cleanliness of area.

Bending and stooping for inspecting work areas.

Talking and hearing are required in giving and receiving instructions and explanations.

Near-visual acuity needed to inspect hospital areas for cleanliness.

Works inside.

JOB RELATIONSHIPS

Workers supervised: Supervises housekeeping personnel.
Supervised by: DIRECTOR, HOUSEKEEPING SERVICES.
Promotion from: HOUSEKEEPING AIDE.
Promotion to: DIRECTOR, HOUSEKEEPING SERVICES.

PROFESSIONAL AFFILIATIONS

Institute of Sanitation Management
1710 Drew Street
Clearwater, Fla. 33515

National Executive Housekeepers
  Association
204 Business and Professional
  Building
Second Avenue
Gallipolis, Ohio 45631

Housekeeping Department   Porter, Head 381.137

HOUSEKEEPING CREW LEADER

group leader

head porter

lead houseman

JOB DUTIES

Supervises, coordinates activities of, and works with cleaning crews engaged in housekeeping activities:

Receives special work assignments for crew or individuals under his supervision from the DIRECTOR, HOUSEKEEPING SERVICES or the HOUSEKEEPING SUPERVISOR. Establishes daily work schedule for special and routine assignments, assigns duties, issues supplies and equipment, and inspects completed work. Leads and works with cleaning crew in housekeeping services in patient rooms, locker rooms, cast rooms, utility storage, treatment rooms, offices, storage rooms, and specialty areas such as, operating rooms, delivery rooms, and clinics. May work on ladders or scaffolding when washing walls and ceilings.

Inspects equipment used, to determine needs for new parts, repairs, overhaul, replacement, and for cleanliness before and after use. Recommends needs for equipment additions, changes, or dispositions. Inspects and takes corrective action in supply needs. Prepares cleaning and disinfectant solutions as prescribed. Enters in record book supplies, material, and equipment dispersed to workers.

Trains new employees by demonstrating use of cleaning materials and equipment; explains methods of cleaning and insures most efficient and economical use of materials and manpower. Recommends personnel actions such as promotions, demotions, transfers, or discharges.

Reviews, continuously, procedures to assure standardized work methods. Records work accomplished, schedules work for semiannual completion reports or machine-record unit cards. Completes requisitions for supplies to be issued from stock.

MACHINES, TOOLS, EQUIPMENT, AND WORK AIDS

Floor scrubbing and polishing machines; pressurized wall-washing equipment, vacuum cleaners, ladders and scaffolds; cleaning supplies such as mops, pails, and solvents.

EDUCATION, TRAINING, AND EXPERIENCE

Employers' requirements range from grammar school to high school graduation.

Up to 2 years' experience as a HOUSEKEEPING ATTENDANT in a hospital.

From 1 to 4 months' on-the-job training to become familiar with all housekeeping duties, to acquire working knowledge of cleaning procedures, record-keeping, adjustment and maintenance of power equipment.

WORKER TRAITS

Aptitudes: Verbal ability is necessary to discuss assignments with workers and supervisors, to train new workers and to demonstrate new techniques and equipment.

Numerical ability is necessary to measure ingredients and to learn dilution ratios; ability to measure square area and to count out supply items.

Motor coordination is necessary to be able to operate floor scrubbing and polishing machines and to move equipment safely within the confines of patients' rooms and heavily traveled hallways.

Manual and finger dexterity is necessary to reach for, handle, lift, and carry housecleaning supplies and equipment and to finger equipment controls.

Interests: An interest in working with people to supervise, instruct, and maintain harmony among workers.

A preference for activities resulting in the satisfaction of maintaining hospital areas in clean, orderly, pleasant conditions.

Temperaments: Ability to direct and control housekeeping personnel activities, evaluating quality and quantity of work against established criteria.

Physical Demands and Working Conditions: Work is heavy, involving lifting and carrying supplies, equipment, and materials weighing up to 100 pounds.

Extensive standing and walking.

Pushing and pulling on handles of floor polishers to steer along hallways, floors, and corridors.

Stoops, kneels, and crouches to sweep floors, pick up waste and litter, and to polish fixtures and fittings.

Talking and hearing necessary to train new workers, supervise cleaning crews, and discuss work schedules with supervisor.

Visual acuity is required for inspection of surfaces and observation of procedures. Works inside.

Subject to injury from moving parts of housecleaning equipment and falls from scaffolds or ladders.

JOB RELATIONSHIPS

Workers supervised: Members of cleaning crew.

Supervised by: HOUSEKEEPING SUPERVISOR or DIRECTOR, HOUSEKEEPING SERVICES.

Promotion from: A member of the cleaning crew.

Promotion to: HOUSEKEEPING SUPERVISOR.

PROFESSIONAL AFFILIATIONS

None.

LAUNDRY DEPARTMENT

PURPOSE: To collect and launder hospital linens, garments, and all washables in order to provide adequate supplies of clean, sanitary linens to all departments.

RESPONSIBILITY: Collecting and processing linens according to the particular system in use, checking condition of linens for worn spots or tears, and weighing for production records. Linens are then sorted on the basis of type of washing to be used and processed through washer-extractor-dryer equipment after load limits have been determined. The laundry is finished by one of two methods — dried in dry tumblers or ironed by a flatwork ironer, hothead presses, or hand iron. During these finishing processes each item of laundry will be checked for stains and damage and, where necessary, returned for rewashing or mending.

In some hospitals, the Laundry Department is assigned responsibility for storing, issuing, and inventorying all linens to maintain centralized control. In other hospitals, laundered articles are returned to the Housekeeping Department for distribution. SEAMSTRESS and LINEN-ROOM AIDE may be found in either department.

AUTHORITY: The Laundry Department is usually an independent department under the supervision of a LAUNDRY MANAGER who has full authority over laundry functions and reports to either the ADMINISTRATOR or an ASSOCIATE ADMINISTRATOR.

INTERRELATIONSHIPS AND INTRARELATIONSHIPS: Every effort should be made to emphasize the importance of clean linens in care and treatment of patients and of the coordinated effort required in providing adequate supplies. Linens are furnished to many departments and units of the hospital, necessitating close coordination between the laundry and various users of linens. Work schedules should be set up in cooperation with department heads, and consideration given to over-all requirements and daily distribution of finished laundry. The LAUNDRY MANAGER should recommend and advise on purchase of hospital linens and laundry equipment.

STANDARDS: The National Association of Institutional Laundry Managers, the American Institute of Laundering, and the Laundry Manual of the American Hospital Association recommend washing formulas and supplies. Periodic bacteriological counts are taken to test for presence of bacteria and germs in washing and pressing areas of the laundry. In some hospitals a Sanitarian periodically reviews the laundering and distribution process.

PHYSICAL FACILITIES AND STAFFING: Adequate space, equipment, and staff necessary to meet the established objectives of the laundry must be provided.

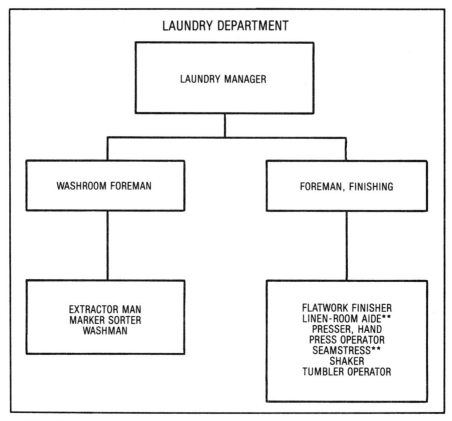

* *See Housekeeping Department.

NOTE: This chart is for illustrative purposes only and should not be considered a recommended pattern of organization.

Laundry Department   Laundry Foreman 361.138

LAUNDRY MANAGER

director, laundry and linen

JOB DUTIES

Supervises and coordinates activities of laundry personnel:

Determines the amount of laundry to be processed and plans daily work schedule accordingly. Schedules work loads and assigns workers to maintain even flow of work. Inspects the area periodically and observes laundry equipment in use. Ascertains that standards are being met. When repairs are needed, notifies Maintenance Department. Adjusts workflow as required.

Establishes procedures for examination of finished laundry in the interest of quality control. Arranges for distribution and storage of finished laundry to insure adequate supplies of clean laundry for all departments.

Tests samples of water periodically to determine hardness of water and effectiveness of cleaning agents and stain removers.

Changes formulas as needed. Charts and logs quantities of laundry collected and processed on daily and monthly basis for departmental charges, and to aid in scheduling work. Prepares charts indicating quantities of detergents, soaps, bleaches, and other materials used on a daily basis to aid in maintenance of inventory. Prepares written formulas indicating quantity of washing and rinsing compounds required and posts them for use by washing section personnel. Posts temperatures and pressures required for effective operation of equipment.

Inspects and inventories supplies to estimate consumption and orders accordingly. Prepares requisitions and checks quantities delivered. May order replacements for worn linens.

Records hours worked by each laundry worker and submits report to payroll office. Maintains production records and computes operating costs. Interviews new employees to determine amount and type of experience, and assigns workers to tasks accordingly. Trains new workers to operate equipment in order to secure a maximum of transferability among workers in case of absenteeism and during peakloads. Inspects laundered articles and evaluates worker efficiency. Corrects faulty techniques by demonstration.

Investigates new equipment and procedures in laundry operations and recommends changes and additions.

May supervise workers directly or through forelady or foreman, in washing, extracting, and finishing sections. May perform any laundry operation where needed. May remove stains or handle isolation wash requiring special treatment.

MACHINES, TOOLS, EQUIPMENT, AND WORK AIDS

Washers, extractors, tumblers, ironers, laundry washing agents, and compounds.

EDUCATION, TRAINING, AND EXPERIENCE

Preference will be given to a graduate of a laundry school or to one who holds a certificate of professional laundry manager.

A minimum of 1 year's laundry supervision, or 5 years' general laundry work with ability to supervise workers is required.

A new LAUNDRY MANAGER should be given on-the-job training in procedures and practices of specific institution.

WORKER TRAITS

Aptitudes: Verbal ability is necessary to understand hospital reports and directives, prepare reports and schedules, issue oral instructions, and demonstrate processing techniques and methods and use of equipment.

Numerical ability is necessary to calculate anticipated laundry needs in personnel and supplies, keep records, and prepare administrative reports.

Manual dexterity is necessary to use hands rapidly to handle laundry and operate switches and controls of machines.

Color discrimination is necessary to determine cleanliness of laundry.

Interests: A preference for activities that follow a definite routine through the entire laundry process.

A preference for working with people, in a supervisory capacity.

Temperaments: Ability to plan and coordinate all laundry activities, using judgmental and verifiable criteria to evaluate performances of workers and equipment and various aspects of the laundry program.

Physical Demands and Working Conditions: Work is light. Considerable walking about the building, observing the performance of workers and equipment.

Reaching, handling, fingering, feeling, and stooping are required in inspecting operations.

Near-visual acuity and color vision are important for setting dials, testing water samples, and detecting stains or discolorations.

Works inside where area is noisy, hot, and humid. Exposed to hot equipment and wet floors.

JOB RELATIONSHIPS

Workers supervised: All laundry department workers.
Supervised by: ADMINISTRATOR or an ASSOCIATE ADMINISTRATOR.
Promotion from: WASHROOM FOREMAN.
Promotion to: No formal line of promotion.

PROFESSIONAL AFFILIATIONS

National Association of Institutional
   Laundry Managers
P.O. Box 11486
Philadelphia, Pa. 19111

American Institute of Laundering
Doris and Chicago Avenues
Joliet, Ill. 60434

Laundry Department   Flatwork Foreman 361.138

FOREMAN, FINISHING

forelady, finishing

JOB DUTIES

Supervises and coordinates activities of workers engaged in shaking out, tumbling, flatwork feeding and catching, pressing, folding, packing, and distributing garments and articles for use by hospital staff and patients:

Plans work schedule based on production requirements and availability of workers. Assigns workers to routine tasks, allowing for interchanging of jobs, to relieve monotony and maintain workflow.

Orients and instructs new workers, emphasizing the importance of adhering to prescribed methods, techniques, and procedures to avoid spread of infection. Observes workers in performance of duties and demonstrates techniques to improve production and maintain workflow.

Inspects articles for cleanliness, routes those not meeting standards for rewashing and notifies supervisor of repeated washing discrepancies.

Performs any of the operations supervised, to maintain production schedule.

May perform any of the following tasks: Hire, transfer, and discharge worker; maintain linen stock, inventories, and payroll records; prepare requisitions for linen supplies for various departments.

MACHINES, TOOLS, EQUIPMENT, AND WORK AIDS

Handiron, flatwork ironer, presser machine, folding machine.

EDUCATION, TRAINING, AND EXPERIENCE

Grammar school education, with ability to understand laundry procedures.
Minimum of 1 year's experience in a laundry is preferred.
One to 3 months on the job to become proficient in supervisory methods.

WORKER TRAITS

Aptitudes: Verbal ability is necessary for discussing laundry finishing procedures and problems with supervisor and subordinates; for issuing instructions for successful performance of duties in coordination with activities of other departments.

Form perception is necessary to detect stains, tears, and other imperfections in articles.

Motor coordination and manual dexterity are necessary to coordinate eyes and hands, and move fingers and hands to manipulate articles rapidly and easily to maintain steady workflow.

Interests: A preference for activities in supervising workers in the routine process of finishing laundered articles.

Temperaments: Ability to be alert to a variety of activities, such as hand or machine ironing, shaking of articles, folding and packing.

Ability to plan and direct various activities of finishing section.

Physical Demands and Working Conditions: Work is light. Standing and walking between work stations.

Talking and hearing for supervisory duties.

Reaching for, handling, fingering, feeling, stooping, and turning are all necessary for the variety of duties either performed or supervised.

Works inside. Area is hot, humid, and noisy. Subject to burns from hot equipment.

JOB RELATIONSHIPS

Workers supervised: Members of flatwork ironing crew, folders of tumbled work, and handironers and pressers.

Supervised by: LAUNDRY MANAGER.

Promotion from: Any member of the finishing section.

Promotion to: LAUNDRY MANAGER.

PROFESSIONAL AFFILIATIONS

National Association of Institutional Laundry Managers
P.O. Box 11486
Philadelphia, Pa. 19111

Laundry Department   Washroom Foreman 361.138

WASHROOM FOREMAN

chief washman

JOB DUTIES

Supervises and coordinates activities of workers engaged in sorting and washing soiled linens, garments, drapes, and other hospital articles in electrically powered machines and extracting excess water to prepare them for the finishing operations:

Plans, in cooperation with LAUNDRY MANAGER, wash schedule and priorities, and assigns workers to duties, such as collecting soiled laundry from laundry chute areas, weighing and sorting laundry, and washing and extracting. Trains new workers in use of supplies and equipment by demonstrating use, explaining operating techiques, and assisting in actual operations.

Sorts, or directs workers to segregate, laundry according to volume, degree of stain or soil, and types of articles. Places heavily stained articles in cart for pre-washing. Manually loads articles into washer or washwheel until machine is loaded to designated capacity. Sets water-level control and turns valve to admit water heated to a degree intended to reduce soil and infectious bacteria. Closes washer doors and starts machine. Adds soaps, detergents, bleach, and/or bluing through trough, according to treatment required for wash. Drains sudsy water, admits clean water after each washing cycle, and rerinses as required, adding specified washing chemicals to each step, as necessary.

Assists workers in loading and unloading washers and extractors. Observes and listens to operation of machines and makes minor adjustments, or reports malfunctioning to LAUNDRY MANAGER. Keeps records of total weight of wash processed each day for each hospital department, for budgetary charge purpose.

Inspects wash at various stages of processing for cleanliness, advises workers or recommends changes in washing and rinsing procedures to effect a clean and sanitary wash.

Is responsible for isolation wash.

May shut down all equipment at end of daily operation.

Rotates workers within washroom or arranges for rotation with finishing section to relieve monotony and to maintain workflow.

MACHINES, TOOLS, EQUIPMENT, AND WORK AIDS

Semiautomatic and automatic washers and extractors; laundry solutions, such as soaps, detergents, bleaches; logbook.

EDUCATION, TRAINING, AND EXPERIENCE

Grammar school education, with ability to understand laundry procedures.
Minimum of 1 year's experience as WASHMAN is required.
One to 3 months' on-the-job training to become proficient in supervisory methods.

WORKER TRAITS

Aptitudes: Verbal ability is necessary for discussing washing procedures and problems with supervisor and subordinates; for issuing instructions for successful performance of washroom workers in coordination with activities of other departments and laundry sections.

Some numerical ability is necessary for proper measuring of such laundry agents and chemicals as soaps, detergents, bleaches.

Form perception is necessary to discern stains, tears, and other discrepancies in laundry articles when sorting or determining type of washing treatment necessary.

Motor coordination and manual dexterity are necessary to coordinate eyes and hands rapidly; sort, load, unload, and tend machines; and add detergents and other chemical solutions to wash. Must move rapidly to maintain flow of work to finishing section.

Interests: A preference for activities of supervisory workers in the routine process of loading, tending, and unloading washers and extractors.

Temperaments: Ability to plan and direct activities of washing sections.

Ability to determine type of wash necessary for different stains, materials, and colors for clean and sanitary wash.

Physical Demands and Working Conditions: Work can be heavy. Standing and walking from washer to washer, checking machine operation, and observing performance of workers.

Stooping, crouching, turning, reaching for, and lifting, in the process of handling laundry and tending machines.

Talking and hearing for supervisory duties.

Near-visual acuity and color vision are required to detect stains, and sort by color.

Works inside. Area is hot, humid, and noisy. Subject to burns from hot equipment and water, and falls due to wet floors.

JOB RELATIONSHIPS

Workers supervised: All workers assigned to washroom.
Supervised by: LAUNDRY MANAGER.
Promotion from: WASHMAN or EXTRACTOR MAN.
Promotion to: LAUNDRY MANAGER.

PROFESSIONAL AFFILIATIONS

National Association of Institutional Laundry Managers
P.O. Box 11486
Philadelphia, Pa. 19111

RADIOLOGY — NUCLEAR MEDICINE DEPARTMENT

PURPOSE: To provide an adjunct diagnostic and therapeutic radiology service as required in examination, care, and treatment of hospital patients.

RESPONSIBILITY: Taking, processing, examining, and interpreting radiographs and fluorographs. Radiographs may be taken for diagnostic purposes or to study physiological processes. Fluoroscoping may be done to study action of internal physiological processes, localize foreign bodies, or for related medical purposes. Radioisotopes are used to indicate the course of compounds introduced into the human body. Radiographs and fluorographs must be examined, and the extent and significance of their pathology or deviation from the normal interpreted. Roentgenotherapy and therapy by radium and radioactive substances are also a responsibility of this department. In large research or teaching hospitals there may be a separate Department of Nuclear Medicine concerned with medical diagnosis and therapy through the use of radioisotopes, as well as research in radiochemical analysis, radiation biology research, instrumentation and monitoring techniques, radioactive waste disposal, control and reduction of occupational and environmental exposures, and special health problems of nuclear propulsion.

In addition to these functions, the department is responsible for planning and carrying out policies and procedures to insure protection to all hospital personnel in contact with radiation modalities; providing consultation and advice to clinicians in interpreting diagnostic roentgenological findings; planning diagnostic X-ray procedures and other pertinent matters; administering therapeutic treatment; participating in research programs; presenting films at autopsies and making additional post mortem examinations as required to complete records; participating in hospital's educational program; and maintaining accurate and complete records.

AUTHORITY: The authority for the radiological services of the hospital rests with a DIRECTOR OF RADIOLOGY or RADIOLOGIST (depending upon the size of the department) who reports to the administration on administrative matters and to the Chief of the Medical Staff on professional practices. The DIRECTOR is delegated authority for organization, operation, and training of personnel so that an effective organization is established and maintained. While standardizing agencies recommend medical supervision, the administrative functions may be assigned to the RADIOLOGIC TECHNOLOGIST, CHIEF.

In those hospitals where nuclear medicine has evolved as a separate department, the CHIEF OF NUCLEAR MEDICINE is delegated authority for those workers concerned with theory, research, techniques, and procedures of nuclear medicine. However, few hospitals have developed this separate department with its own staff. The reasons given for this lack of evolution in more hospitals are: (1) Complexity of new techniques, procedures, and equipment; (2) cost of the equipment; (3) necessity for a highly trained staff skilled in the use of these procedures, techniques, and equipment; (4) a relatively small number of cases that require such radiologic services. This is a fast-changing and rapidly advancing segment of medical science. What is written today may well be outmoded tomorrow.

In this study, because of similarity of purpose, responsibility, equipment, and techniques, and since both processes utilize the properties of radioactive substances, nuclear medicine has been combined with radiology.

INTERRELATIONSHIPS AND INTRARELATIONSHIPS: An effective diagnostic and therapeutic radiological program is accomplished through sound planning of the program and its supporting policies and procedures, efficient internal administration and organization, and cooperation and liaison with other hospital activities. The department serves inpatients, and outpatients, and hospital personnel. There must be close coordination between activities of this department and all clinical activities of the hospital. Contact and cooperation with Outpatient Department, nursing service, and medical staff are essential. The DIRECTOR or RADIOLOGIST serves as a member of the medical staff as well as an administrative department head. This department participates in the total hospital program of patient care, research, education, and community health programs.

STANDARDS: The American College of Surgeons and American College of Radiology have cooperated in establishing minimum standards for hospital roentgenological service. To meet the minimum standards, the radiology program should have adequate space and equipment, qualified personnel, proper records and reports, and sufficient authority and personnel to carry out an acceptable program.

The American Registry of Radiologic Technologists and Council of Medical Education and Hospitals of the American Medical Association have formulated standards for technologists and it is recommended that hospitals adopt these standards, which also constitute qualifications for registry by the accrediting agency. Many hospitals conduct their own schools for training RADIOLOGIC TECHNOLOGISTS and other technical workers in the department. These schools are under the direction of a RADIOLOGIST and must meet standards formulated by the Council on Medical Education of the American Medical Association, in conjunction with the American Registry of Radiologic Technologists and American College of Radiology. The Committee on Hospitals of the Bureau of Professional Education of the American Osteopathic Association has established minimum standards of similar scope for hospital roentgenological services.

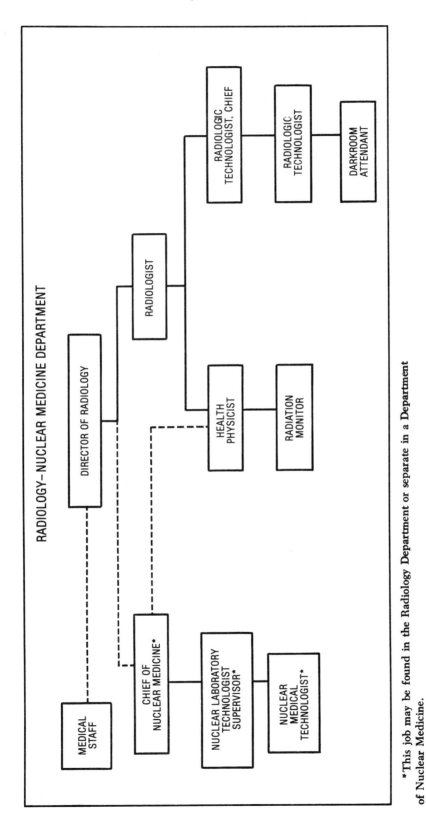

RADIOLOGY–NUCLEAR MEDICINE DEPARTMENT

MEDICAL STAFF

DIRECTOR OF RADIOLOGY

RADIOLOGIST

RADIOLOGIC TECHNOLOGIST, CHIEF

RADIOLOGIC TECHNOLOGIST

DARKROOM ATTENDANT

HEALTH PHYSICIST

RADIATION MONITOR

CHIEF OF NUCLEAR MEDICINE*

NUCLEAR LABORATORY TECHNOLOGIST SUPERVISOR*

NUCLEAR MEDICAL TECHNOLOGIST*

*This job may be found in the Radiology Department or separate in a Department of Nuclear Medicine.

NOTE: This chart is for illustrative purposes only and should not be considered a recommended pattern of organization.

PHYSICAL FACILITIES AND STAFFING: The Radiology Department usually consists of therapeutic radiology, physics, and diagnostic radiology sections. All three provide specialized services to the clinical activities of the hospital.

With the growth of the department's functions, in most instances, it is necessary to provide offices for the DIRECTOR OF RADIOLOGY, RADIOLOGIST, CHIEF OF NUCLEAR MEDICINE, and possibly one for the HEALTH PHYSICIST, who is responsible for protecting the workers in the department by monitoring programs and controlling radiation hazards. Space should be provided for a viewing room; a waiting room; dressing rooms; a dark room; a file room; roentgenography, roentgenoscopy, and roentgenotherapy (one or more rooms); and storage and usage of radioactive materials. In the smaller hospital these rooms may be variously combined. Equipment may be located in a single convenient area or may be dispersed in operating rooms and near outpatient clinics. Portable units can be brought to bedside. Technical equipment should be modern and paced to technological advances but will vary with type and activity of the hospital.

The problems of contamination and exposure to radiation are, of course, present but safety regulations are enforced. All radiology employees wear badges to measure the exact amount of radiation to which they are exposed. Fluoroscopy treatment offers the greatest radiation hazard, and lead aprons and gloves are worn to protect the worker. The badges are checked monthly by the RADIATION MONITOR and resulting information recorded in the Radiology Department records. Radiation hazards can be reduced to a minimum as a result of safety precautions. The Atomic Energy Commission has specific regulations for those workers in nuclear medicine who handle radioisotopes and other radioactive substances.

Responsibility for all radiological examinations, diagnosis, and treatment rests with the department head who may be DIRECTOR OF RADIOLOGY assisted by RADIOLOGIST and CHIEF OF NUCLEAR MEDICINE. All three should hold a degree of Doctor of Medicine or Osteopathy from an accredited medical school or school of osteopathy and have qualifications in radiology acceptable to the Council on Medical Education and Hospitals of the American Medical Association or the Committee on Hospitals of the Bureau of Professional Education of the American Osteopathic Association. A part-time RADIOLOGIST who periodically visits the hospital and makes necessary interpretations of X-ray films is the usual practice followed in the small hospital, although this does not preclude the study and interpretation of films by a qualified attending staff physician. If a member of the medical staff with fundamental training in radiology is assigned to supervise the service, a RADIOLOGIST should be engaged and called upon to interpret obscure findings. RADIOLOGIC

TECHNOLOGISTS and NUCLEAR MEDICAL TECHNOLOGISTS operate radiologic equipment for diagnosis and therapy. The films are processed by the DARKROOM ATTENDANT.

Radiology—Nuclear Medicine Department   Director of Radiology
                                                                070.118 T

DIRECTOR OF RADIOLOGY

chief of radiology

JOB DUTIES

Administers radiology programs and directs and coordinates department activities in accordance with accepted national standards and administrative policies:

Plans scope, emphasis, and objectives of the radiology programs, conferring with administrators, directors of other departments, and medical staff to ascertain hospital needs. Participates with personnel of other departments in planning joint administrative and technical programs and recommends methods and procedures for coordinating radiological services with other patient care services. Investigates and studies trends and developments in radiologic practices and techniques and develops operation manuals, outlining methods, procedures, and techniques reflecting applicable advances in the field to guide professional and technical staff. Establishes and enforces, through subordinate supervisors, safety regulations for the department to insure that both patients and hospital personnel receive maximum protection from the hazardous effects of roentgen rays and radioactive materials used in diagnosis and therapy.

Prepares budget estimates of personnel, supplies, and equipment and prepares narrative and statistical reports of activities and expenditures. Recommends and approves personnel actions, such as hirings, transfers, and promotions, usually interviewing and hiring the professional applicants. Resolves problems requiring administrative authority or professional knowledge, and outlines policies, procedures, and methods for resolving lesser problems by subordinate personnel.

Instructs students and interns in theory and practice of radiology, lecturing, conducting diagnostic seminars, or providing individual instruction and on-the-job training.

The director's actual involvement in providing diagnostc and therapeutic radiology service for patients depends on the size of the radiology staff and hospital organization. He may, in small hospitals, be a director in name only, having responsibility for the department's activities, aspects of which are required by law, and advising the staff on technical matters but delegating actual administrative duties to the RADIOLOGIC TECHNOLOGIST, CHIEF, so that he may devote his time to performing the duties of a RADIOLOGIST. He may, in large hospitals, confine his clinical activities to a single specialty, such as radiation therapy, nuclear medicine, or diagnosis. He may limit his activities to those furthering a specific research project or act solely as a consultant to assist staff radiologists and the medical staff with unusual or complex cases. His services as consultant, adviser, and coordinator may, in some communities, extend to other hospitals, especially if the other hospitals have limited radiological services. His research activities are also determined by the size and kind of hospital as well as by his own interests and abilities. He may, in a large hospital, determine the nature of research to be performed and assign specific projects to staff members.

MACHINES, TOOLS, EQUIPMENT, AND WORK AIDS

The administrative duties of this occupation do not require any machines, tools, equipment, or work aids. However, if he is performing any diagnostic or therapeutic radiology, he will use what the specific procedure requires, such as X-rays and an X-ray viewer for diagnostic work.

EDUCATION, TRAINING, AND EXPERIENCE

Graduation from a medical school recognized by the Council on Medical Education and Hospitals of the American Medical Association or Committee on Hospitals of the Bureau of Professional Education of the American Osteopathic Association. License to practice medicine or osteopathy in State where located.

For certification by the American Board of Radiology, applicant must have 3 years' special training in radiology in clinics, hospitals, or dispensaries recognized and approved by the Board and by the Council on Medical Education and Hospitals of the American Medical Association.

Four to 6 years' radiology specialization, 1 or more of which was in supervisory or administrative capacity.

WORKER TRAITS

Aptitudes: Verbal ability is required to read and understand professional and technical radiologic and medical material; to communicate with administrative and medical personnel; to write administrative reports and technical manuals; and to lecture to students.

Numerical ability is required to prepare budget estimates and statistical reports of department activities.

Interests: A preference for business contacts with people, in coordinating department services with other departments for the best patient care services.

A preference for communicating ideas, in planning emphasis and objectives of radiology programs, preparing manuals, and lecturing to students.

Temperaments: Ability to plan and control activities and personnel of the radiology department.

Ability to deal with people in planning and coordinating work programs and in making diagnostic recommendations based on measurable and verifiable criteria.

Physical Demands and Working Conditions: Work is sedentary.

Reaching for and handling X-rays and reports.

Talking and hearing when lecturing, interviewing applicants, and attending patients.

Near-visual acuity, depth perception, and accommodation in reading radiographs and conducting examinations and therapy treatments.

Works inside. Radiation hazards are fewer for this worker than for others in the department, since exposure is less frequent.

JOB RELATIONSHIPS

Workers supervised: All persons assigned to Radiology Department (professional, technical, clerical, and paramedical).

Supervised by: ASSOCIATE ADMINISTRATOR for administrative purposes, and Chief of Medical Staff for professional practice.

Promotion from: RADIOLOGIST.

Promotion to: No formal line of promotion.

PROFESSIONAL AFFILIATIONS

American Medical Association
535 North Dearborn Street
Chicago, Ill. 60610
American Osteopathic Association
212 East Ohio Street
Chicago, Ill. 60611

American College of Radiology
20 North Wacker Drive
Chicago, Ill. 60606

Radiology—Nuclear Medicine Department   Radiologic Technologist, Chief
078.168

RADIOLOGIC TECHNOLOGIST, CHIEF

chief X-ray technologist

JOB DUTIES

Plans, directs, and supervises all technical aspects of the department in regard to services, programs, and evaluations of such programs:

Maintains radiologic services in accordance with standards established by the hospital and with State, local, and Federal standards which may apply. Is responsible for the technical aspect of radiologic safety in the hospital, recommending programing, monitoring, and location of warning or identifying devices in carrying out recommendations of the radiation safety officer.

Recommends equipment modification, new equipment, and essential construction within the department. Is responsible for existing equipment and such contractual services as may be required. Coordinates departmental purchasing and is responsible for stock level, storage, and utilization.

Administers preparation of reports, documents, payroll records, statistical surveys, and other data required. Provides for recruitment, selection, training, supervision, and other personnel matters in the department. Makes work assignments and coordinates requests for radiologic service with hospital routine. Evaluates accuracy and technical quality of X-rays; demonstrates and explains difficult or new techniques and procedures to the technical staff. Delegates responsibilities to designated staff.

Assists RADIOLOGIST with difficult radiologic procedures and performs general technical duties when workload is heavy.

MACHINES, TOOLS, EQUIPMENT, AND WORK AIDS

Diagnostic and therapeutic radiographic units, reports and records, and protective garments.

EDUCATION, TRAINING, AND EXPERIENCE

High school graduation or equivalent. Satisfactory completion of formal radiologic technology training in an AMA-approved school and able to meet the requirements for registry by the American Registry of Radiologic Technologists (ARRT).

At least 5 years' experience with appropriate broad experience within the department to be familiar with all aspects of departmental policy and administrative procedures.

WORKER TRAITS

Aptitudes: Verbal ability is necessary to read and understand medical and technical materials and instructions; to communicate with medical, technical, and clerical personnel as well as hospital administrators and patients; and to lecture to students.

Numerical ability is necessary to compile statistical data and prepare reports relating to operating costs, purchases, and services rendered.

Clerical perception is necessary to detect errors in written material and statistical data and when writing and proofreading records and reports.

Spatial perception is necessary to visualize relationships of internal organs in relation to X-ray tube and film in order to obtain radiographs of diagnostic value.

Form perception is necessary to perceive detail in X-rays to determine acceptability of exposure.

Manual dexterity is necessary to adjust machine controls and arrange, attach, and adjust supportive devices.

Interests: A preference for scientific and technical activities to master principles, techniques, and procedures of radiology.

A preference for processes, machines, and techniques to direct RADIOLOGIC TECHNOLOGIST in obtaining radiographs, developing X-ray film, and performing diagnostic tests using radioisotopes.

A preference for people and for communicating ideas in supervising department personnel and assisting them in solving technical problems.

Temperaments: Ability to direct, control, and plan an entire activity and activities of others in the Radiology Department.

Able to evaluate processed X-rays against measurable and verifiable criteria.

Physical Demands and Working Conditions: Work is of medium demand. Stands when supervising technologists and sits when preparing reports.

Reaching for and handling machine controls and setting up equipment.

Talking and hearing to converse with patients and staff and to conduct training classes.

Near-visual acuity, accommodation, and depth perception for setting up X-ray equipment, and preparing and maintaining radiologic records and reports.

Works inside. Electrical and radiant energy hazards are present. Wears protective gloves and apron during certain procedures. May wear film badge and have periodic blood counts to detect effects of radiation.

JOB RELATIONSHIPS

Workers supervised: DARKROOM ATTENDANT, RADIOLOGIC TECHNOLOGIST, NUCLEAR MEDICAL TECHNOLOGIST, clerical assistants, and student technologists.

Supervised by: RADIOLOGIST.

Promotion from: RADIOLOGIC TECHNOLOGIST, NUCLEAR MEDICAL TECHNOLOGIST.

Promotion to: No formal line of promotion.

PROFESSIONAL AFFILIATIONS

American Society of Radiologic
  Technologists
645 North Michigan Avenue
Chicago, Ill. 60611

American Registry of Radiologic
  Technologists
2600 Wayzata Boulevard
Minneapolis, Minn. 55404

Radiology—Nuclear Medicine Department   Chief of Nuclear Medicine
                                                                           070.118T

CHIEF OF NUCLEAR MEDICINE
director of radioisotope laboratory

JOB DUTIES

Coordinates and directs activities of radioisotope laboratory; instructs students and interns in theory and techniques of nuclear medicine; serves as specialist in diagnosis, internal, and nuclear medicine; and performs nuclear medical research:

Interviews, selects, and hires staff for radioisotope laboratory. Participates in hospital staff meetings to maintain liaison between department and medical staff and to recommend methods and procedures for coordinating functions of the Nuclear Medical Department with other patient care services. Prepares budgets indicating estimated cost of new equipment, maintenance, and personnel costs. Formulates and directs policies and procedures to be followed by staff personnel to provide best possible patient care. Establishes and enforces, through subordinate supervisors, safety regulations for the department to insure that patients and hospital personnel receive maximum protection from the hazardous effects of roentgen rays and radioactive materials used in diagnosis and therapy.

Formulates and conducts teaching program, conferences, and seminars on nuclear medicine for students and interns. Studies technical and trade journals; attends local and national nuclear medicine seminars and medical conferences to acquire and contribute knowledge of procedures and methods.

Examines new patients and discusses diagnoses with attending physicians to determine courses of treatment. Reads medical charts and reports of examinations and tests (made in own department and in other departments) and makes recommendations for treatment plan according to organs or tissues involved and type of radioisotope applicable. Writes instructions on patients' charts to be followed by technologist or technician. Studies scans (X-ray type pictures of a malfunctioning organ or area reproduced in small squares on film plate by the Magna-Scanner and utilizing gamma rays emanating from radioisotopes injected into the patient's body) and X-rays, interprets findings, and records data for hospital records and information of referring physician. Is available to other physicians for discussions, conferences, and advice to benefit patients and to further knowledge of nuclear medicine.

Conducts research in nuclear medicine to discover ways and means of utilizing radioisotopes in diagnosis and treatment of disease. Studies current unsolved medical problems or observes patients' needs and notes area of medicine needing research to select a project in which use of radioisotopes could be applied. Studies similar research projects and reviews known information to become familiar with related aspects of the proposed research. Studies properties of all available isotopes, considering source, half-life (a measure of the rate of decay), and expense to select the one which is specifically adaptable to proposed research. Considers function of organ or tissue involved to select a carrier (an agent — chemical or natural — selected according to its affinity for the involved organ and to, or with, which the isotope is bound or combined to introduce it to the area to be scanned), if one is needed. Assembles all information and writes a protocol to present to the research reviewing board for approval. Delegates authority to technologist or technician to carry out technical aspects of the project according to plan. Writes final report at completion of research and publishes results in medical journals, prepares paper for presentation at seminars, and adapts data obtained to practical use for benefit of patients.

MACHINES, TOOLS, EQUIPMENT, AND WORK AIDS
Radioactive compounds and research laboratory equipment and apparatus.

EDUCATION, TRAINING, AND EXPERIENCE
Graduation from a medical school recognized by the Council on Medical Education and Hospitals of the American Medical Association or Committee on Hospitals of the Bureau of Professional Education of the American Osteopathic Association. License to practice medicine or osteopathy from State where located.

For certification by the American Board of Radiology, applicant must have 3 years' special training in radiology in clinics, hospitals, or dispensaries recognized and approved by the Board and by the Council on Medical Education and Hospitals of the American Medical Association.

Four to 6 years' specialization in nuclear medicine or radiology, of which 1 or more years was in supervisory or administrative capacity.

WORKER TRAITS
Aptitudes: Verbal ability is required to read and understand professional and technical radiologic and nuclear medical materials; to communicate with administrative and medical personnel; to write administrative reports and technical research papers; and to lecture to students.

Numerical ability is required to prepare budget estimates and to apply mathematical formulas in computing radioactive materials.

Manual and finger dexterity is needed to use laboratory instruments and apparatus for research.

Interests: A preference for contacts with people, in coordinating department services with other departments for the best patient care services.

A preference for scientific and technical activities to conduct research to discover ways and means of combating disease with radioactive materials.

Temperaments: Ability to plan, direct, and control activities of the nuclear medical laboratory and its personnel.

Ability to deal with people in planning and coordinating work programs and in making diagnostic recommendations based on measurable and verifiable criteria.

Capable of working to exact tolerances and standards when performing nuclear medical research.

Physical Demands and Working Conditions: Work is light. Standing and walking when lecturing to students and supervising activities of the department.

Reaching for and handling equipment when performing research.

Talking and hearing when lecturing, interviewing applicants, and attending patients.

Near-visual acuity, depth perception, and accommodation in conducting examinations and in performing research.

Works inside. Rigid adherence to established laboratory techniques and standards prescribed by the Atomic Energy Commission is vital to minimize hazards to the worker. Must wear protective clothing.

JOB RELATIONSHIPS

Workers supervised: All persons assigned to Nuclear Medical Laboratory (professional, technical, clerical, and paramedical).

Supervised by: DIRECTOR OF RADIOLOGY and Chief of Medical Staff.

Promotion from: No formal line of promotion.

Promotion to: No formal line of promotion.

PROFESSIONAL AFFILIATIONS

American College of Radiology
20 North Wacker Drive
Chicago, Ill. 60606
American Medical Association
535 North Dearborn Street
Chicago, Ill. 60610

American Osteopathic Association
212 East Ohio Street
Chicago, Ill. 60611

Radiology—Nuclear Medicine Department   Nuclear Laboratory
Technologist Supervisor 078.221T

NUCLEAR LABORATORY TECHNOLOGIST SUPERVISOR
radioisotope laboratory supervisor

JOB DUTIES

Supervises and directs activities of personnel engaged in diagnostic laboratory testing, instructs medical students in nuclear medical technology, and performs the technical aspects of nuclear medical research:

Assigns work schedules, explains duties, and interprets policies and regulations. Reviews appointment schedules, suggesting or effecting changes necessary to provide for maximum use of facilities and staff and most efficient service to patients and physicians. Demonstrates and explains procedures and techniques involved in using radioisotopes in diagnostic studies, such as how to compute doses, operate equipment, and minimize the possibility of excessive radiation exposure, for the purpose of training new technologists and improving work performance of regular staff.

Evaluates work performance of staff and makes recommendations for promotions, transfers, or other personnel actions.

Instructs medical students in procedures and techniques in nuclear medical technology, demonstrating laboratory machines and equipment and following a course designed to supplement theoretical instruction.

Performs assigned phases of nuclear research, under direction of CHIEF OF NUCLEAR MEDICINE, concerned with isotopes, carriers, and organs to be studied in terms of research objectives. Injects test doses into the test subject (usually a rabbit); counts and traces the radioactivity, using spectrometer and Magna-Scanner; and records all pertinent data in specified report form.

Insures a sufficient stock of radioisotopes at all times by weekly review of appointment schedules, listing isotope requirements for each test and using knowledge of nuclear medicine. Computes remaining radioactivity of stock on hand and, considering known rate of decay, determines supplementary isotopes needed and prepares requisition.

MACHINES, TOOLS, EQUIPMENT, AND WORK AIDS

Magna-Scanner, X-ray machine; spectrometer and laboratory equipment; and glassware, protective clothing.

EDUCATION, TRAINING, AND EXPERIENCE

High school graduation or equivalent. Satisfactory completion of formal radiologic technology training in an AMA-approved school and ability to meet requirements for registry by the American Registry of Radiologic Technologists (ARRT).

WORKER TRAITS

Aptitudes: Verbal ability is needed to give training and work instructions to subordinate personnel, lecture to medical students, and discuss nuclear medical technology with professional medical personnel.

Numerical ability is needed to apply mathematical formulas in computing radioactivity of radioisotopes and dosages.

Spatial ability is needed to visualize spatial relationships of internal organs for proper focus of X-ray machine and to adjust detector head of scanner.

Manual and finger dexterity is needed to adjust machine controls and to use small laboratory instruments for research.

Interests: A preference for scientific and technical activities to master principles of radiology and elements of radiologic procedures, and to perform research in nuclear medicine.

A preference for processes, machines, and techniques of handling radioisotopes in performing diagnostic tests and research.

Temperaments: Ability to direct and control activities of technologists.

Able to evaluate work performance of staff against measurable and verifiable criteria.

Qualified to work to exact tolerances and standards when performing nuclear medical research.

Physical Demands and Working Conditions: Work is light. Standing and walking when demonstrating equipment, lecturing to students, and supervising department activities.

Reaching for, handling, and fingering laboratory glassware and machine dials.

Talking and hearing to instruct students and subordinates, to supervise, and to converse with medical staff.

Visual acuity and depth perception to read machine dials and to distinguish markings on scans.

Works inside.

Exposed to radioactivity while preparing doses to be administered to patients and while handling body products containing isotopes. Protective lead shielding and constant monitoring of laboratory by Geiger counter to safeguard work surroundings. Sensitized film badges are worn by all isotope personnel to measure cumulative radiological exposures. Worker wears disposable gloves and uses metal tongs when preparing isotope doses. Rigid adherence to established laboratory techniques and standards prescribed by the Atomic Energy Commission to minimize hazards to the worker.

JOB RELATIONSHIPS

Workers supervised: NUCLEAR MEDICAL TECHNOLOGISTS.
Supervised by: CHIEF OF NUCLEAR MEDICINE.
Promotion from: NUCLEAR MEDICAL TECHNOLOGIST.
Promotion to: No formal line of promotion.

PROFESSIONAL AFFILIATIONS

Registry of Medical Technologists
P.O. Box 2544
Muncie, Ind. 47304
American Society of Radiologic
    Technologists
645 North Michigan Avenue
Chicago, Ill. 60611

American Registry of Radiologic
    Technologists
2600 Wayzata Boulevard
Minneapolis, Minn. 55405

INDEX